Quality Management in the Assisted Reproduction Laboratory

Da Li • Yingzhuo Gao

Quality Management in the Assisted Reproduction Laboratory

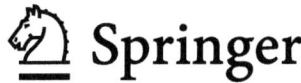 Springer

Da Li
Reproductive Medicine
Shengjing Hospital
Shenyang, China

Yingzhuo Gao
Reproductive Medicine
Shengjing Hospital
Shenyang, China

ISBN 978-981-99-6661-5   ISBN 978-981-99-6659-2   (eBook)
https://doi.org/10.1007/978-981-99-6659-2

Preface

Looking back on the past 40 years, reproductive medicine practitioners have been forging ahead with their founding principles. As we look around the world, reproductive medicine and assisted reproductive technology have made remarkable advances in all aspects. Reproductive medicine, as a special discipline, stands out for its dependence on and synergy with assisted reproduction laboratory techniques. The assisted reproduction laboratory is a place for new lives to begin. Its stable operation is critical to achieving the goal of assisted reproduction treatment, which is singleton, full-term, healthy live births. Comprehensive and effective quality control and management of assisted reproduction laboratories and laboratory techniques are critical.

The concept of quality control was first widely used in industrial production and has been gradually introduced into reproductive medicine over the last two decades. The purpose of implementing quality control in assisted reproduction laboratories is to establish practice specifications for all operational steps aiming toward consistency and stability. Managing assisted reproduction laboratories requires mastery of the "big picture" and an emphasis on details. Given the many factors affecting assisted reproduction laboratories and technologies and the complexity of the operational process, how to ensure comprehensive and detailed control has been an issue of constant concern in reproductive medicine. Nevertheless, when reading the assisted reproductive technology books released by the leading global publishing groups in recent years, those that provide a holistic overview of the quality management in assisted reproduction laboratories are lacking. Although only a few studies have covered these topics, they have focused more on personnel management and have only briefly described the core technologies of assisted reproduction laboratories. The publication of this book will thus not only fill this market gap but also present important theoretical and practical values.

This book is grounded on literature and clinical practice. It is closely integrated with work experience, international consensus, and the latest research. Various aspects affecting assisted reproduction laboratories and corresponding management approaches are elaborated, and key points of laboratory operations and quality control measures are presented in detail. The authors aim to address practical problems encountered in real-world clinical work and provide a scientific, advanced, helpful, and reader-friendly professional resource to help reproductive medicine practitioners establish a disciplined quality management system for assisted reproduction laboratories and techniques. Furthermore, this book is intended to be a well-rounded guide to the scientific operation and management of assisted reproduction laboratories for scientific teams involved in reproductive medicine.

As we look at the evolution of assisted reproduction laboratories, conventional in vitro fertilization-embryo transfer, intracytoplasmic sperm injection, preimplantation genetic testing, and embryo cryopreservation and thawing have accomplished the technical transformation from initial exploration to today's routine clinical application. Meanwhile, assisted reproduction laboratories have largely transitioned from experimental and technical investigation to serving clinical medical needs. From the perspective of evolving with the times, the term "Clinical Embryology Center" seems more accurate than "Assisted Reproduction Laboratory." In this fast-paced era, constantly evolving theoretical knowledge instructs and optimizes in vitro embryo culture techniques. In parallel, new technologies are emerging and being swiftly transferred for application in assisted reproduction laboratories. Furthermore, the inevitable greater challenges for the medical staff and embryologists in "Clinical Embryology Centers" necessitate us always acquiring new knowledge and introducing new technologies that will improve the safety and efficiency of assisted reproductive treatments. The future is in sight as we keep stepping forward!

All editors have made every effort to be accurate during the preparation of this book. However, with limited time and knowledge, we would appreciate corrections from colleagues and readers for any omissions.

Shenyang, China   Da Li
                                                                   Yingzhuo Gao

Contents

Introduction of Quality Control and Risk Management in IVF Laboratory

Assisted reproductive technology (ART) refers to medical interventions for infertile couples to have a baby. The assisted reproduction laboratory, also known as in vitro fertilization (IVF) laboratory, is an integral part of the assisted reproduction process and critically affects the IVF clinical outcomes. Its workflow is shown in Fig. 1.1. In the process of an in vivo gestation, the formation and development of an embryo always occur in a light-proof, constant temperature, and low-oxygen environment and are protected by the mother. However, in the case of an in vitro process, the protection provided by the mother is not available, and the development potential of an embryo may be affected by any external factors, from volatile organic compounds (VOCs) to changes in humidity, the pH value, or the osmotic pressure, etc. Therefore, a reliable and high-quality IVF laboratory would provide an essential safeguard for the viability and development of gametes and embryos.

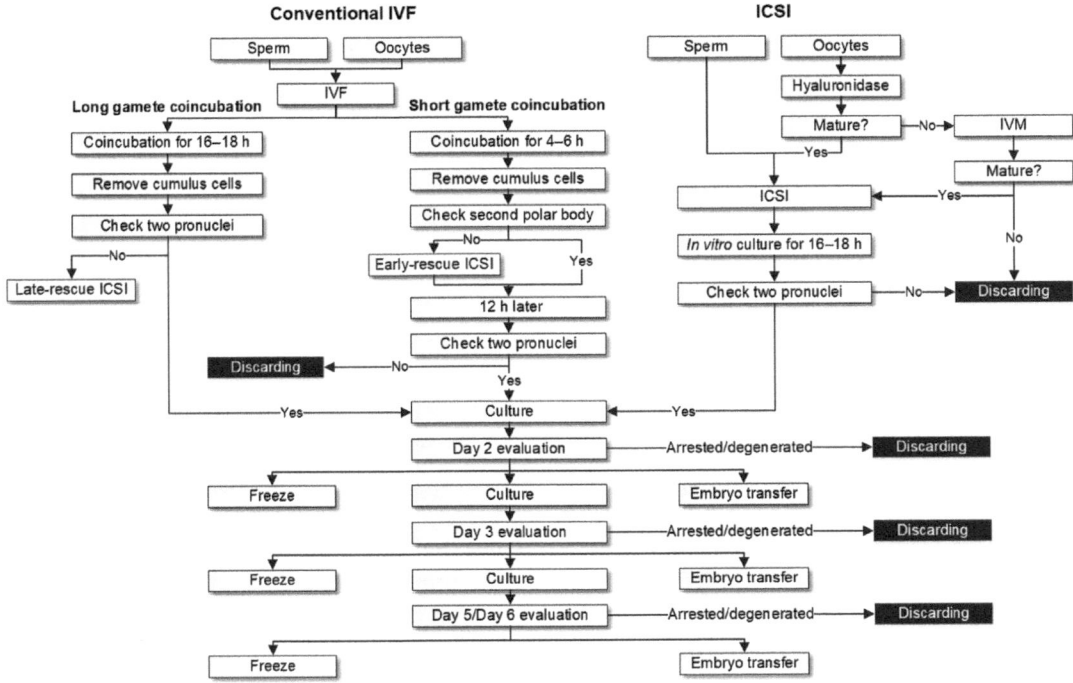

Fig. 1.1 IVF laboratory workflow. Abbreviations: *ICSI* intracytoplasmic sperm injection, *IVM* in vitro mature

1.1 ISO9001 Accreditation and the Reproductive Medicine

Reproductive medicine is a particular medical specialty with a highly complex treatment process involving clinical reproductive medicine department, an embryo laboratory, an andrology laboratory, reproductive nursing, and many other aspects. The treatment targets include the patients and their gametes and embryos, while the outcomes involve the safety of infertile patients and their biological offspring. There are numerous risks throughout the treatment process.

The concept of quality management was initially widely applied to manufacturing industries and, during the last two decades, has been gradually introduced to the management system of reproductive medicine centers. For IVF laboratories, quality management is a series of practical rules developed for every procedure component to achieve consistency and stability in every practical step. Given this concept, it is vital for IVF laboratories to have an integrated quality management system that operates robustly and effectively. A sound quality management system should consider not only the clinical outcomes, for example, clinical pregnancies and the live birth rate, but also regular evaluations of personnel, equipment, and consumables in the entire reproductive medicine center. The critical elements of a quality management system include workflow diagrams, standard operating procedures (SOPs), organizational charts, employee job descriptions, key performance indicators (KPIs), etc. A reproductive medicine center's medical standard and service quality may only be ensured when the IVF laboratory operates within the framework of a stringent quality management.

At IVF laboratories, the quality management system should clearly outline the work specifications of embryologists, including but not limited to the following: the embryologists must turn on the clean bench, the heating plate, the heating stage, and air decontamination equipment 30 min in advance of starting the work. It should closely monitor and record the CO_2 concentration and temperature in the incubator and the temperature and humidity in the culture room, as well as record abnormal conditions inside and outside the laboratory and their causes. The staff should check the incubator operating status and gas supply each morning and evening. All manipulations on gametes or embryos should be double-checked. When performing intracytoplasmic sperm injection (ICSI), frequent personnel movement and door opening and closing shall be prohibited. The operation must be stopped immediately if a patient's identity is found questionable or the specimens are in disorder. Using embryotoxic chemicals and radioactive sources shall be prohibited within IVF laboratories. Using gametes or embryos for scientific research without the patient's informed consent and sex selection without medical indications shall also be prohibited.

Out of the quality management systems, ISO9001 is an international standard developed by the International Organization for Standardization's Technical Committee on Quality Management and Quality Assurance, which was transformed from the world's first quality management system standard, BS5750. Currently, it is a standardized quality system that is the most internationally recognized and proven. The ISO9001 quality management system may be considered a complete revolution and upgrade over the traditional hospital management model. For example, the conventional hospital management model implements a local quality control approach, where each medical department serves as a primary quality management entity and designated quality managers are responsible for quality control, while only a limited number of personnel is involved in quality management and is trained in quality control matters. In contrast, ISO9001: 2008 has the fol-

lowing characteristics: the standard emphasizes total quality control with top administrators being at the core of quality management, effecting full participation in quality management and conducting quality training for all employees. Implementing the ISO9001 quality management system provides a powerful tool for standardizing and systematizing the laboratory's quality management system.

Years ago, some countries, such as Australia and Spain, provided that the ISO9001: 2008 certification shall be a mandatory requirement for the assisted reproductive centers to apply for admission. In China, only some hospitals in Hong Kong were accredited with ISO9001 in the early days. In 2010, CITIC-Xiangya Reproductive and Genetic Hospital introduced and implemented the ISO9001 quality management system, promoting the standardization of the internal management functions of the reproductive center. It was successfully accredited by the authorities in March 2014, making itself the first ISO9001: 2008-certified fertility center in China. During 2017–2018, several reproductive medicine centers, including CITIC-Xiangya Reproductive and Genetic Hospital and Peking University Third Hospital, were upgraded or accredited with the ISO9001: 2015 quality management system. Compared to the 2008 version of ISO9001 quality accreditation, the 2015 version introduces the concept of a risk-based mentality and focuses more on controlling risks and challenges while adopting a process management approach that combines the plan-do-check-act (PDCA) cycle (Fig. 1.2) with the risk-based thinking and provides sufficient resources to ensure continuous improvement.

It is worth noting that the purpose of the ISO9001 accreditation for reproductive medicine centers is not just to gain international recognition but to establish a trustworthy standardized and refined platform for holistic quality management, to improve quality management, and to improve the workflow and to attain sustainable development.

Fig. 1.2 Schematic diagram of the PDCA cycle

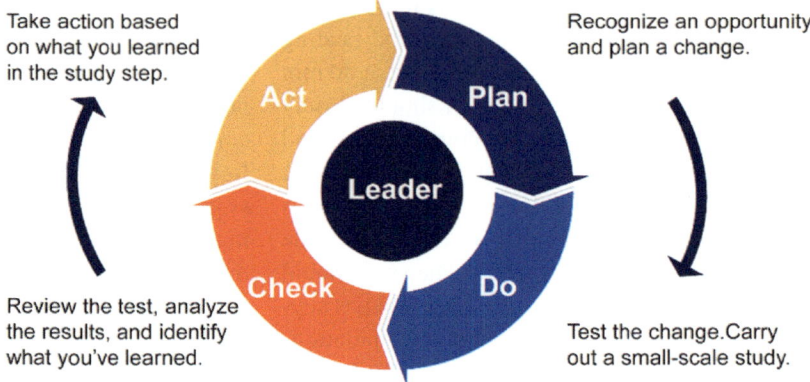

1.2 Organizational Structure and Personnel Characteristics

An IVF laboratory has a linear organizational structure with three major sections: the embryology laboratory, the andrology laboratory, and the genetics laboratory led by IVF Laboratory Director. This results in a relatively straightforward structure with well-defined responsibilities and a clear delegation of authority and accountability (Fig. 1.3).

How do we choose or train a good embryologist? For many years, national and international experts have agreed that it is often the personality traits rather than the training or experience that make the embryologists the most suitable candidates. A fundamental medical and reproductive biology background and formal training are certainly required, but this is only an entry-level selection criterion. Essentially, an excellent clinical embryologist needs to have most, if not all, of the following characteristics: (a) they are a natural leader; (b) they have a good sense of responsibility; (c) they can work independently; (d) they are self-motivated; (e) they are a good team player; (f) they love challenges; (g) they are a perfectionist; (h) they have a strong empathic ability; (i) they are energetic; (j) they are honest; (k) they are intelligent and creative; (l) they know what they are doing and why they are doing it [1–3].

At IVF laboratories, laboratory employees' professional profiles may be used to determine their roles and responsibilities as well as define their duties and the scope of work. The IVF laboratory verification system, the assessment system, the assessment protocol, and the delineation of responsibility should be set up to provide guidance and constraints, encouragement and incentives, rules and procedures. Basic posts (the clerical post, assistant post, the morning quality control post), more or less fixed operation posts (semen processing, oocyte retrieval, solution preparation), operation posts (embryo-related manipulations: fertilization, oocyte denudation, observation, freezing, and thawing), various working groups (the risk control group, the reagents, and consumables quality control group, the equipment management group), etc. can be set up, and daily laboratory scheduling shall be carried out according to the work posts.

It is important to note that, for an IVF laboratory to function well, it is not only necessary to have a top-notch team of embryologists, but it is also necessary to foster a willingness to cooperate and work together with a view to achieving the set goals and ensuring the technical compatibility of all team members. It is also worth noting that this "teamwork" spirit is a core value of a modern business and commercial operations. Beyond a solid intra-team collaboration, it is also essential to keep an eye on the career planning and future professional development of laboratory team members. Only by adequately implementing these points can an IVF laboratory operate reliably and efficiently.

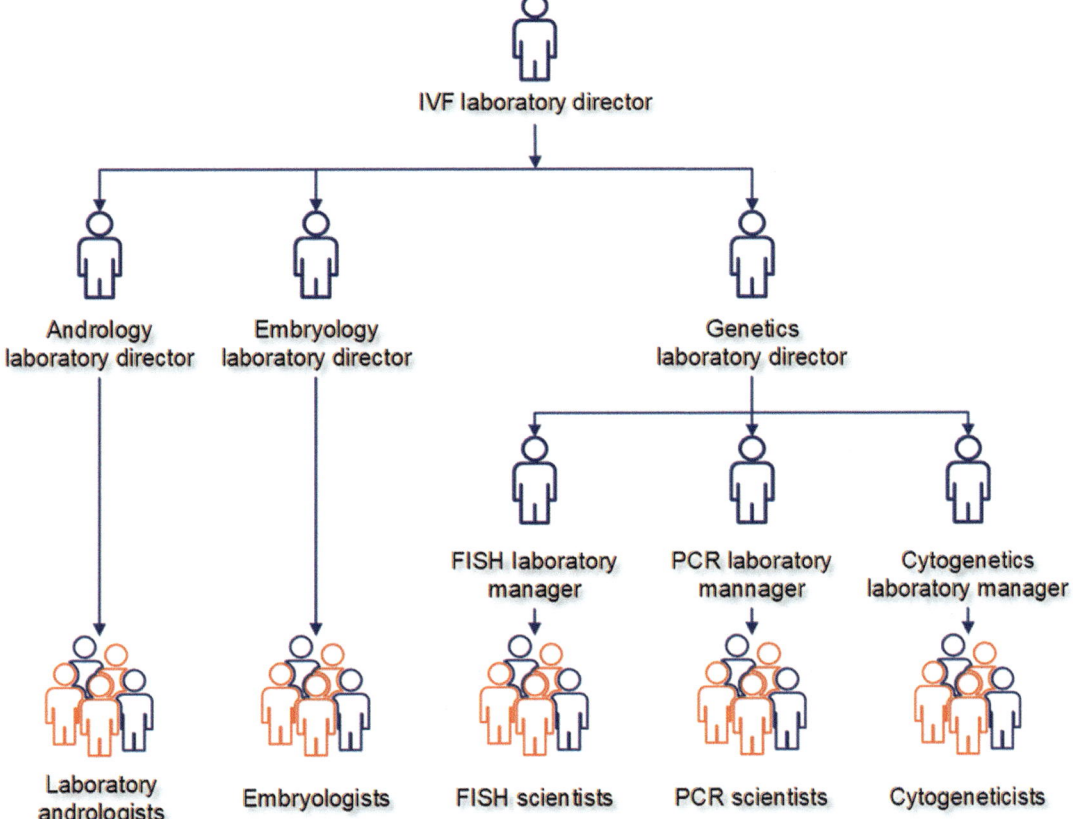

Fig. 1.3 Organizational structure of the IVF laboratory

1.3   Space Area and Environment

The space area and the environment of the IVF laboratory shall be controlled to provide a safe culture setting for the development of gametes/embryos.

1.3.1   Air Quality

The critical equipment in a clean room is the recirculating heating, ventilation, and air conditioning (HVAC) system. The system uses a series of air filters that have increasing filtering effectiveness to minimize the amount of suspended particulate matter and microorganisms in the environment air. It also purifies the room using the air circulation control system. It is an effec-

tive, safe, and easy-to-operate device to remove bacteria.

1.3.2   Room Temperature and Humidity

In addition to purifying the air, the HVAC system is also tasked with regulating the room temperature and humidity. It is recommended to maintain the laboratory room temperature at $23 \pm 2\,°C$ and humidity at 40–60% because too high a temperature would affect the regular operation of the equipment and cause discomfort to laboratory personnel. In contrast, the overly high humidity would cause mold formation and reduce the service life of metal-containing equipment. In this case, the low humidity may easily cause an increase in the osmolality of the culture medium, which will adversely affect the development of gametes and embryos.

1.3.3 Materials that Are in Direct Contact with Gametes and Embryos

1. Culture medium: Bicarbonate-buffered systems are commonly used as a medium for fertilization, embryo cleavage, and blastocyst. Therefore, CO_2 is required to maintain a physiological pH, which needs to be equilibrated overnight before use. In contrast, the medium used for in vitro handling of gametes and embryos is generally buffered with 4-(2-hydroxyethyl)-1-piperazineethanesulfonic acid (HEPES) or 3-(N-morpholino)-propanesulfonic acid (MOPS), which can be exposed to the air and keep a stable physiological pH. A culture medium may typically be used for 4 weeks under normal storage conditions. The batch number and opening time of the medium should be recorded in detail. The medium should be used within the specified valid time after opening the vial, as per the manufacturer's recommendations. Aside from that, the culture medium should not be used for more than 48 h after the overnight equilibration.
2. Density gradient centrifugation medium: After being taken out from a 4 °C refrigerator, it needs to be equilibrated to room temperature before use.
3. Tissue culture oil: The tissue culture oil is often used to cover culture medium microdroplets to prevent changes in the osmolality of the culture medium due to evaporation. Before use, it needs to be subjected to equilibration by temperature and CO_2.
4. ICSI-related reagents and consumables: The hyaluronidase used in the process of removing cumulus granulosa cells from oocytes and polyvinyl pyrrolidine (PVP) for sperm immobilization and their analogs are often stored at a temperature of 2–8 °C and should be equilibrated at the temperature of 37 °C for at least 1 h before use. The injection pipettes and holding pipettes are stored at room temperature.
5. Culture dishes/tubes: It is recommended to use IVF-specific culture dishes/tubes that have passed the mouse embryo assay test.
6. Handheld instruments: Pasteur pipettes, oocyte retrieval needles, oocyte denudation pipettes, embryo transfer catheters, etc.
7. Sterile water: UPS grade medical water that is free of antimicrobial reagents, endotoxins, polyvinyl chloride, and dioctyl phthalate should be used. It should be preheated to 37 °C before installation into the workstation and incubator to prevent cold stress on the incubation equipment.
8. Laboratory gases.

1.4 Management of Consumables and Equipment

It is crucial to ensure that all the disposable consumables that are used in the IVF laboratory are non-toxic and have the tissue culture grade, including oocyte retrieval needles and follicular fluid collection systems, ICSI pipettes, pipette tips, culture containers (culture dishes and tubes, etc.), and the catheters that are used for insemination or embryo transfer. Other points to take notice of are listed as follows:

1. Consumables should be stored in a spacious storage room that is away from high temperature/direct sunlight, and those consumables that have been sterilized should be left alone for some time to allow the complete release of VOCs.
2. Reagents (e.g., culture media, etc.) should be shipped at a controlled temperature, and cold chain records should be verified for compliance upon receipt.
3. When receiving laboratory supplies, the product names, specifications, and quantities of reagents and consumables should be identified and recorded. The package lot number should be carefully confirmed to ensure that

it matches the item lot number, while the packaging should be checked for integrity. After all the above information is verified, the staff shall sign and record the date of receipt on the delivery note, register the entry and file the record to ensure traceability of all the supplies intended for gamete and embryo manipulation.

4. European Commission (EU) and Food and Drug Administration (FDA)-sourced disposable plastic supplies must pass the endotoxin test before their use and should pass the mouse embryo assay test when conditions permit.

5. It is recommended to use pipette tips that are DNA-RNase-free. However, it should be noted that the EU certification is not quality assurance. It only certifies that the manufacturing process is in compliance with EU standards and is not a guarantee that the product has been tested in cell culture and proven to be non-cytotoxic.

6. Pieces of equipment frequently used in IVF laboratories include IVF workstations, micromanipulation systems, incubators of various types and sizes, and thermostatic equipment (heating plates, thermostatic test tube racks, water baths), dewars, refrigerators, etc. For special items, such as gas cylinders, gas pipelines, dewars, etc., management procedures should be implemented to enable specialized management, and contingency plans should be developed for unexpected emergencies. Critical equipment should have a master control system for continuous monitoring and abnormal warnings. Essential equipment in daily use should be continuously monitored to ensure it is in the best operational condition. Operators should be regularly trained to understand the common failures of the operated equipment and can develop the appropriate emergency plans. According to International Standardization Organization specifications, the manufacturer should provide equipment monitoring and maintenance protocol. The user should accurately document and ensure traceability of the equipment maintenance and calibration process so that it can be fully addressed in clinical outcomes.

Table 1.1 Critical equipment monitoring parameters

Equipment and environment	Parameters to be monitored (5-min intervals)
Incubator	Temperature/CO_2/humidity
Thermostatic equipment	Temperature
Refrigerator	Temperature and opening status
Dewar	Temperature/liquid nitrogen level
Gas supply	Pressure

We need to implement a real-time monitoring system to monitor the following critical parameters (Table 1.1):

1.5 Risk Factors

IVF is a rapidly evolving technical field, making continuous training and competency evaluation processes indispensable. However, even with these strategies, risks and problems cannot be avoided entirely. Based on the experience, we have compiled an exhaustive list of risk factors for IVF laboratories.

1.5.1 Staffing Problems

1. Inadequate staffing: The current lack of IVF laboratory staff worldwide is prevalent.

2. Overwork: To execute all tasks flawlessly and minimize the risk of errors, every embryologist must be on high alert at all times, so overworking (e.g., working more than 48 h per week or more than six consecutive days without a good rest [1]) may increase the chances of occurrence of risk events at work.

3. Lack of training: A comprehensive and consistent training program is of utmost importance, not only for novice and junior staff but also for senior embryologists, so that they can keep up with the new concepts, techniques, and methods owing to their continuous training.

4. Lack of experience and sense of responsibility: Due to the unique nature of IVF work, inexperienced employees unable to recognize

and manage the critical components of the work would cause a risk of serious adverse events. Aside from that, the employees who demonstrate no accountability for the overall IVF process and outcomes should not work at the IVF laboratory.

1.5.2   Resource Issues

1. Inadequate resources: To begin with, if IVF laboratories consider operating with the most limited resources possible (human, material, and financial), the working concept itself has a high risk. This is so because essential culture equipment often needs sufficient volume and space to ensure its safe operation. For example, incubators must not be turned on and off frequently (to avoid temperature/gas concentration fluctuations), and ICSI operations need to be completed within a precisely controlled time frame for the tasks such as oocyte denudation and sperm injection (no delays or waiting time due to human or equipment problems are allowed).
2. Equipment failure: All equipment must be subject to regular preventive maintenance (performance testing, sterilization, etc.). Also, the operational status of all critical equipment, such as dewars, incubators, gas supply, etc., must be monitored continuously. In addition, IVF laboratories must be equipped with an alarm system for non-working hours.
3. Circuit failure: IVF laboratories must have provisions to ensure power continuity for critical equipment. Equipment sensitive to power fluctuations must be protected by line conditioners or uninterruptible power supply (UPS) devices.

1.5.3   Procedural Issues

1. Lack of double-checking: Double-checking is required for any critical operation, especially when transferring gametes or embryos to another culture dish or container.

2. SOP irregularities: Incomplete and irregular SOPs would pose hidden dangers to the operation.
3. Lack of responsibility: IVF laboratories should establish comprehensive and documented notification systems and task lists to ensure that all their staff knows precisely what must be accomplished daily.
4. "Method improvements" that are not fully validated: The so-called method improvements that are not fully validated shall be strictly prohibited. All employees must strictly follow the IVF laboratory SOPs, and any modifications to the SOPs must be authorized by the laboratory director.

1.5.4   Risk Management Issues

Risks usually exist in three forms: a directly perceived risk, a perceived risk through scientific accumulation, and a virtual risk. The directly perceived risk is relatively straightforward. However, the perceived risk through scientific accumulation and the virtual risk are mostly predictions of future risks formulated through processing, analyzing, and organizing the existing theories and knowledge, as well as focusing on the need to know not only "how to do it" but also "why to do it." There is often a consensus as well as a controversy regarding the understanding and management of risks at this level, requiring the ability of the embryologists to analyze, accumulate and reprocess knowledge, which is the only way to conduct the clinical practice better. The following examples provide a better illustration:

1. Understanding "blastocyst transfer" versus "cleavage stage embryo transfer."
   First, it is established that blastocyst culture is more appropriate for cases where a more significant number of oocytes and embryos are obtained during the IVF process or where embryos need to be genetically tested. And second, although some studies suggest that blastocyst transfer can improve the live birth rate compared to cleavage-stage embryos in both fresh [4, 5] and frozen-

thawed [6] implantation cycles (none of the evidence levels are high); some studies have reported that blastocyst transfer can improve the live birth rate in populations with a better prognosis [7], there are several points worth noting: (a) Blastocyst transfer has no significant advantage in non-selective and poor prognosis populations and may increase the risk of having no embryos available [7]; (b) blastocyst transfer has not increased the cumulative pregnancy rate [8, 9]; (c) fresh blastocyst transfer increases the chance of preterm delivery [10–12]; (d) extended in vitro embryo culture still raises concerns about its impact on sex ratio [11], epigenetic alterations during embryo development [11], and even on future fetal safety and congenital disabilities [10, 11, 13]; (e) we cannot ignore that extended culture of an embryo in vitro increases the demand for technical staff competence, generates additional incidence of failing to have embryos available due to other reasons [8], and imposes additional financial and emotional burdens on patients [10].

2. Awareness of "open versus closed carriers."

There are two main categories of carriers used for vitrification: open carriers and closed carriers. There are currently over 30 different carriers available in the carrier field, of which at least 15 are fully commercialized. But most of them involve only minor improvements on the earlier carriers, and many closed carriers are only slightly modified from the earlier open carriers. Meanwhile, it is still not known whether such improvements are practical.

The type of carrier will directly dictate the cooling rate of the oocytes and embryos when frozen. For the best freezing of oocytes and embryos by rapid cooling through direct contact with liquid nitrogen, the first carrier used for vitrification was designed to be open-type. However, in the early 1990s, closed carriers were gradually investigated and applied with the intention of blocking the transmission of pathogens between the frozen objects via liquid nitrogen. In recent years, there have been various "debates" about the advantages and disadvantages of open and closed carriers. But of course, the main focus has been on the cooling rate and pathogen transmission. Nowadays, we hear not only objective evaluations of both technologies but also "biases" from time to time. Such biases may stem from experimental conclusions derived from poor scientific design, interference due to commercial interests, or even overthinking of ethical and legal issues.

Closed carriers have been used primarily for freezing oocytes and embryos. The closure of the carrier will, without a doubt, affect the cooling rate [14, 15]. However, recent studies have almost overwhelmingly suggested that vitrification using closed carriers does not seem to affect various morphological characteristics, developmental potential, or even reproductive outcomes of oocytes [14, 16–21] and embryos [14, 18, 22–25] compared to open carriers. Contrary opinions, on the other hand, are not often reported [26, 27]. But we cannot ignore that most of the previous experimental data are not derived from prospective randomized controlled trials and multicenter studies, for which the level of evidence is not as high.

It is indisputable that pathogens can survive in liquid nitrogen, and some argue that pathogens carried by infertile couples during assisted reproductive treatment may cause cross-infection. Nevertheless, today, the only published incident that can be attributed to pathogenic infections caused by cross-contamination through liquid nitrogen took place in a plastic liquid nitrogen container where large quantities of blood products were stored [28]. Yet, the number of pathogens in such liquid nitrogen containers holding large amounts of blood products is not in the same order of magnitude as the number of pathogens in the liquid nitrogen environment where embryos are stored. And on top of that: (a) It is estimated that at least one million patients per year are taking open carriers for embryo- or oocyte-vitrification, and no cases of pathogen cross-contamination have been reported to date [15]; (b) there is no direct evidence that pathogens can be transmitted between vitrified embryos via liquid nitrogen [14]; (c) there have been no cases of bacterial or fungal contamination in both open and closed carriers [29]; (d) there have been no reports of cross-infection following IVF treatment, in which oocytes are fertilized with sperm and cultured in vitro before being implanted into the female uterine cavity [30, 31]. The most likely explanation is that the level of pathogens in the liquid nitrogen where the gametes or embryos are stored is far from the threshold of infection and that the level of such pathogens is minimal after multiple dilutions and flushes throughout the IVF process. There is data estimating that >500,000 post-vitrification embryo transfer using fully open carriers do not result in a single detectable infection, with an infection probability of less than 0.0002% [15].

In conclusion, we still need a higher level of evidence to fully understand the advantages and disadvantages of open and closed carriers and make a scientific choice of carriers' type after assessing the risks and benefits.

1.6   Embryotoxicity Testing

Validation of physical and chemical parameters (pH and osmolality) must be done for each lot of IVF commercial culture medium upon manufacture. Significant variation in any of these parameters may indicate poor quality control during manufacture and potentially impact clinical outcomes. Also, manufacturers of plastic consumables used in tissue culture may change the chemical composition of their products during the manufacturing process without notice. It should be known that any changes in syringes, filters, and culture dishes may produce embryotoxicity. Therefore, independent in-house testing of commercial reagents and consumables is essential for troubleshooting.

According to guidelines issued by regulatory agencies, culture media and consumables used in IVF laboratories are mandatory to pass adequate biological tests. However, there is still controversy over how to select the appropriate testing system for embryotoxicity testing. And there are several vital points to keep in mind when conducting embryotoxicity testing [1, 2]: (a) testing methods; (b) testing materials; (c) testing fre-

quency; (d) establish standard/routine procedures and schedules for testing; (e) establish acceptable performance ranges; (f) record all test results; (g) review test results periodically; (h) do not use anything that haven't passed the bioassay; and (i) rewrite SOPs for all improvements. Several bioassays for testing embryotoxicity and culture conditions have been applied to human IVF, including:

1.6.1   Mouse Embryo Assay (MEA)

The ambient temperature and humidity of the embryo culture lab, the temperature and performance of the instruments and equipment, and the quality of reagents and consumables must be up to the requirements for in vitro gamete and embryo manipulation and their growth and development. The entire culture system must therefore be tested before proceeding with in vitro manipulation and culture of human embryos. The mouse embryo assay is one of the standard methods to test whether the culture system complies with the requirements for in vitro culture of human embryos. The premise of this assay is the assumption that the requirements of the in vitro culture system are the same for mouse and human embryos. However, mouse embryos develop slightly differently from human embryos (Table 1.2). For example, the endogenous metabolism of the mouse embryo is not very active until the end of the 2-cell stage [32]. As such, there is a correlation between the success of the mouse embryo assay and the mouse strain, the timing of assay initiation (1-cell or 2-cell stage embryos), the culture conditions, and whether the assay is performed following strictly controlled and repeatable procedures. For example, the development of outbred mouse embryos may be arrested at the 2-cell stage in a specific culture medium; mouse zygotes are more sensitive to toxins in the culture environment; and the presence or absence of amino acids and albumins may also affect the sensitivity of the mouse embryo assay. Ideally, the assay should begin with zygotes of inbred mice, which

Table 1.2 Changes in humans and mice during various developmental stages

	Human		Mouse	
Days	Description	Location	Description	Location
1	Zygote	Oviduct	Zygote to cleavage stage (2–4 cells)	Oviduct
2	Cleavage stage (2–4 cells)	Oviduct	Cleavage stage to morula (4–16 cells)	From the oviduct to the uterus
3	Cleavage stage (4–10 cells)	Oviduct	Morula to early blastocyst	Uterus
4	Morula to early blastocyst	From the oviduct to the uterus	Blastocyst	Uterus
5	Blastocyst	Uterus	Egg cylinder	Uterus
6	Hatched blastocyst	Uterus	Advanced egg cylinder stage	Uterus

should be cultured to 2-cell stage embryos in amino acid-free simple culture medium supplemented with albumin, and then continue to the blastocyst stage in a simple culture medium without albumin [1, 2].

The mouse embryo assay should be performed under a strictly controlled reproducible procedure and with a selected strain that is sufficiently sensitive and stable to detect embryotoxicity. The control and embryotoxicity testing groups should be set up; e.g., for embryotoxicity testing of a new culture dish, you may put the same batch of cleavage medium into the old dishes (both the medium and dishes used that have passed MEA) as the control group and put the same batch of cleavage medium into new dishes that will be examined as the embryotoxicity testing group. Depending on the fertilization method, the mouse embryo assay can be divided into in vitro fertilized embryo culture and in vivo fertilized embryo culture. Some experts suggest that although in vitro fertilization is more challenging, it is more sensitive than in vivo fertilization and more suitable for quality management of new centers and new equipment. However, regardless of the type of fertilization, the procedure for superovulation should be the same: The optimal age for superovulation varies among strains, and female mice of the right age should be selected (usually 3–4 weeks old females, but for some strains, such as FVB/BALB/c, 6–8 weeks old females may also be used). These mice should be injected

intraperitoneally with pregnant mare's serum gonadotropin at 10 IU per mouse and 48 h later with human chorionic gonadotropin (hCG) at 10 IU per mouse. For in vivo fertilization, female mice are caged overnight with sexually mature male mice of the same strain in a 1:2 ratio on the day of hCG injection. Mating is checked the next morning, and female mice detected with vaginal plugs are selected for use. 18–22 h after hCG injection, female mice with vaginal plugs will be sacrificed, and zygotes will be collected from the tubal ampulla and transferred to pre-warmed hyaluronidase. Immediately after denudation, these zygotes are rinsed, selected, and further cultured for observation [33]. For in vitro fertilization, female mice are sacrificed 13–16 h after hCG injection, and the oocyte complexes are extruded from the tubal ampulla by incision with a 1 mL syringe needle. Male mice are then sacrificed, and their epididymis and spermatic duct are perforated to allow sperm to swim out. After processing and counting, sperm and oocytes are placed in fertilization dishes so that they can join to form zygotes for further observation. The oocyte cleavage and blastocyst formation are then monitored, and the acceptance criterion is a blastocyst formation rate of ≥80%. If the MEA fails, the item under test cannot be used and needs to proceed MEA again. If it fails again, this information should be promptly fed back to the product distributor, and the unqualified consumables should be returned.

1.6.2 Human Sperm Survival Assay

The human sperm survival assay (HSSA) is used to indirectly determine the potential toxicity of a subject to sperm, oocytes, or embryos by examining the change in sperm viability after co-incubation of human sperm with the subject or its extracts [34]. In contrast to the mouse embryo assay, which is not routinely performed in IVF laboratories, the sperm survival assay is simple and easy to perform. It can be used as a routine quality control test.

The sperm used for HSSA should be collected from healthy males aged 22 to 35. The criteria for semen selection are as follows: homogeneous and off-white appearance; normal morphology sperm $\geq 15\%$; liquefaction within 30 min; pH > 7.2; semen volume >2 mL; sperm concentration $\geq 20 \times 10^6$/mL; sperm motility (percentage of forward-moving sperm) $\geq 50\%$; and round cells concentration $<1 \times 10^6$/mL. The assay should be performed with at least three qualified semen from different donors. There should be a negative control group, a positive control group, and a test group. Sperm samples are prepared by the swim-up method, counted, and assessed for sperm motility (as a percentage of forward-moving sperm divided by the total number of sperm), and the results should be recorded. Semen specimens with sperm motility $\geq 90\%$ are centrifuged and resuspended, and the concentration was adjusted to $(5 \pm 2) \times 10^6$/mL. Aliquots of three portions are added into the tubes of the negative control group, positive control group, and test group, respectively, and then incubated at 37 °C for 24 h. Sperm motility is measured again, and sperm motility index (SMI) is calculated. SMI = sperm motility at the end of the test/ sperm motility at the beginning of the test; relative SMI = SMI of the test sample/ SMI of the negative control group. At the end of the test, sperm SMI ≥ 0.7 in the negative control group and SMI <0.6 in the positive control group is considered valid. Among three valid tests, the effect of the tested subject on human sperm is considered negligible if there are two specimens with SMI ≥ 0.7 and relative SMI ≥ 0.9 in the test group; otherwise, the effect of the tested subject on human sperm is not negligible.

1.6.3 Culture of Mononucleated or Multinucleated Embryo

Oocytes showing abnormal fertilization can be used to test new batches of consumables. Each embryo should be observed and evaluated daily until the sixth day after insemination [1, 2]

In addition to biological assays, since quality differences are often observed between individual wells of tissue culture plastics, rinsing the plastics with a culture medium before use may be an efficient way to reduce potential embryotoxicity. Moreover, some culture supplies often have embryo-safe coatings, making it advisable to carefully inspect all plastic products for packaging damages before use to avoid exposing the embryos to chemical toxins.

1.7 Key Performance Indicators

1.7.1 International Consensus on Key Performance Indicators

Continuous documentation of KPIs is an essential tool for accurate quality control. With this data, we would be able to identify problems in IVF laboratories at an earlier stage and take prompt action to minimize harm. The *Vienna Consensus* developed by the European Society of Human Reproduction and Embryology (ESHRE) and Alpha Expert in 2017 recommends 12 KPIs (Table 1.3) [5].

1.7.2 Quality Control Chart and Result Analysis

In practice, we can draw a Levey-Jennings quality control chart based on KPIs to identify whether changes in KPIs exceed the alert range. The Levey-Jennings quality control chart is a graphical representation of the control sample mean, working range, and other limits, showing the results of control values over time. When plotting a Levey-Jennings quality control chart, the standard deviation is usually used. Quality control limits are set by calculating the mean and

Table 1.3   KPIs for IVF laboratories based on the *Vienna Consensus*

KPI	Calculation method	Competency value	Benchmark value
ICSI damage rate	$\dfrac{\text{No.of damaged or degenerated oocytes} \times 100\%}{\text{All oocytes injected}}$	≤10%	≤5%
ICSI normal fertilization rate	$\dfrac{\text{No.of oocytes with 2PN and 2PB} \times 100\%}{\text{No.of injected MII oocytes}}$	≥65%	≥80%
IVF normal fertilization rate	$\dfrac{\text{No.of oocytes with 2PN and 2PB} \times 100\%}{\text{No.of COC inseminated}}$	≥60%	≥75%
Failed fertilization rate (IVF)	$\dfrac{\text{No.of cycles without fertilization} \times 100\%}{\text{No.of stimulated IVF cycles}}$	<5%	
Cleavage rate	$\dfrac{\text{No.of cleaved embryos on Day 2} \times 100\%}{\text{No.of 2PN / 2PB oocytes on Day 1}}$	≥95%	≥99%
Day 2 embryo development rate	$\dfrac{\text{No.of 4-cell embryos on Day 2} \times 100\%}{\text{No.of normally fertilized oocytes}}$	≥50%	≥80%
Day 3 embryo development rate	$\dfrac{\text{No.of 8-cell embryos on Day 3} \times 100\%}{\text{No.of normally fertilized oocytes}}$	≥45%	≥70%
Blastocyst development rate	$\dfrac{\text{No.of blastocysts on day 5} \times 100\%}{\text{No.of normally fertilized oocytes}}$	≥40%	≥60%
Successful biopsy rate	$\dfrac{\text{No.of biopsies with DNA detected} \times 100\%}{\text{No.of biopsies performed}}$	≥90%	≥95%
Survival rate of frozen-thawed blastocysts	$\dfrac{\text{No.of blastocysts appearing intact} \times 100\%}{\text{No.of blastocysts thawed}}$	≥90%	≥99%
Implantation rate of cleavage stage embryos	$\dfrac{\text{No.of gestational sacs} \times 100\%}{\text{No.of cleavage stage embryos transfered}}$	≥25%	≥35%
Implantation rate of blastocysts	$\dfrac{\text{No.of gestational sacs} \times 100\%}{\text{No.of blastocysts transfered}}$	≥35%	≥60%

PB polar body, *PN* pronucleus, *COC* cumulus-oocyte complexes

standard deviation based on the test results of a certain number of quality-controlled items. These limits are mean ±1 standard deviation, mean ±2 standard deviations, and mean ±3 standard deviations. Large IVF laboratories, with thousands of treatment cycles per year, can therefore calculate their quality control data. Smaller fertility centers may reference national or international standards, but this approach is not recommended given the complexity of IVF treatment.

The interpretation of quality control data is also an issue worth discussing. For example, is exceeding the threshold of ±2 standard deviations from the mean a normal fluctuation or a significant alarming change? The second generation of quality control rules, "Westgard Rules" (http://www.westgard.com/), recom-

mends using a combination of decisions based on five different control rules to solve this dilemma. However, it is still up to each laboratory to reflect and define its own rules and criteria. Meanwhile, IVF laboratories may apply the following "rules" to determine if there is a real problem:

1. The KPI value is below −3 standard deviations from the mean.
2. Two consecutive KPI values are below −2 standard deviations from the mean.
3. Four consecutive KPI values are below −1 standard deviation from the mean.
4. Seven consecutive decreases in KPI values; some values may be within mean ±1 standard deviation.

1.7.3 Establish Early Warning

There is a risk of misinterpreting KPIs if the suggested rules are taken as the sole basis. Also, as treatment outcomes may not be available soon, undetected problems in the laboratory may affect results for a considerable length of time. Therefore, it is prudent to establish laboratory KPIs that can be used as early warnings to enable more rapid detection of problems in the gamete/embryo culture system, such as: (a) Are normally fertilized oocytes completing their first division 26 h after insemination or sperm injection? (b) Is the number of developmental arrests in fertilized oocytes reasonable, and is the percentage of 2-cell embryos that develop into 4-cell embryos normal? It is recommended that the above two parameters be calculated every 20 consecutive IVF and ICSI cycles.

1.8 Troubleshooting and Classic Problem Solving

"Troubleshooting" refers to the logical and systematic search for the origin of a problem so that an effective solution to that problem can be developed. IVF laboratories are integrated with multiple complex systems and problems are often

related to a multitude of factors. We must be continuously aware of all potential influences throughout the culture system that could cause physiological stress to the embryos and reduce their survival potential (Fig. 1.4).

Also of note is that all changes in patient population characteristics, including age, infertility diagnosis, stimulation regimen, drug batch, dose and responsiveness, sperm and oocyte quality, and all changes in culture conditions (incubator/temperature/pH/gas/culture dish/culture medium), can have a significant impact on reproductive outcomes. Accurate and comprehensive documentation is the basis for troubleshooting. To make an accurate assessment of potential problems, continuous and reliable records of manipulations must always be maintained so that parameters can be systematically compared across time. Meanwhile, effective maintenance of the IVF laboratory requires a monitoring system to constantly monitor every aspect of the process and for continuous troubleshooting (Fig. 1.5).

For problems and failures, we can adopt root cause analysis (RCA), a structured problem management approach, to identify the root cause of the problem and solve it step by step instead of focusing on the symptoms of the problem (Fig. 1.6). RCA is a systematic process that

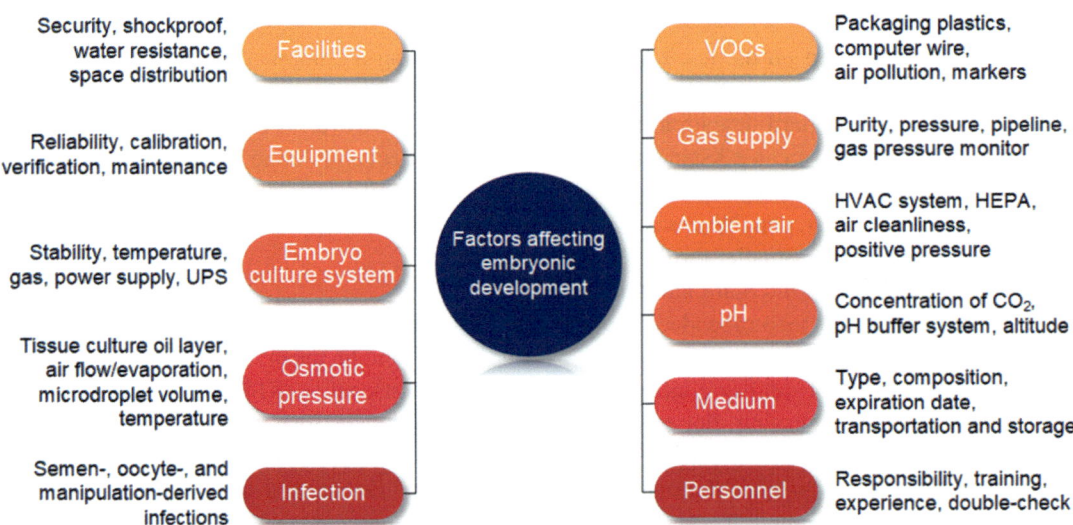

Fig. 1.4 Potential influences on embryo development. *UPS* uninterruptible power supply, *VOCs* volatile organic compounds, *HAVC* heating, ventilation, and air conditioning, *HEPA* high-efficiency particulate air filter

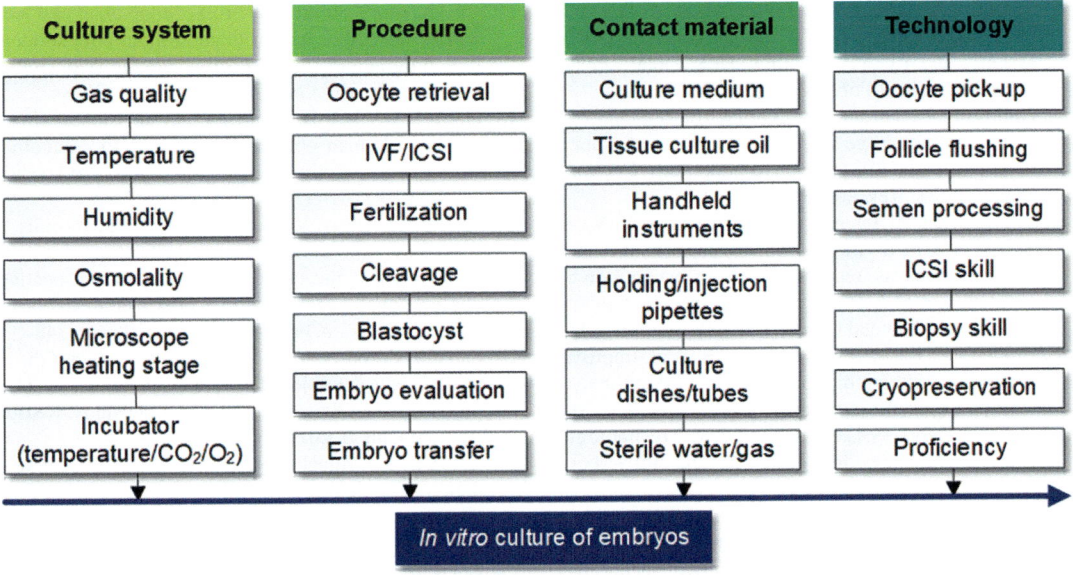

Fig. 1.5 Detailed troubleshooting process

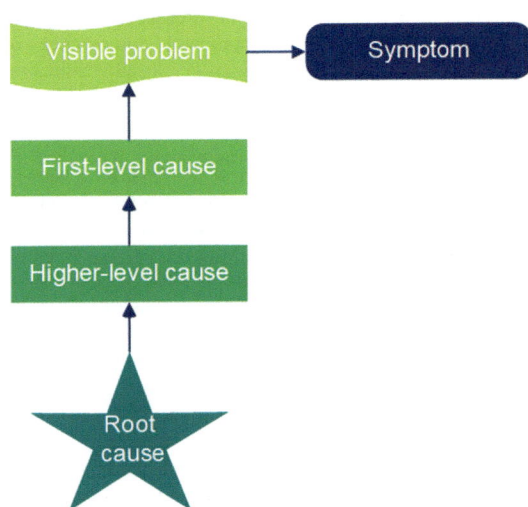

Fig. 1.6 RCA implementation process

involves identifying and analyzing the cause of the problem, finding a solution, and developing preventive measures for that problem.

The goal of RCA is to identify: the problem (what happened); the cause (why it happened); and the measures (what can be done to prevent the problem from happening again). The so-called root cause is the underlying cause that led to the problem of our concern. This is because there are usually many causes of a problem, such as physical conditions, human factors, system behavior, or process factors. Through scientific analysis, we are likely to find more than one root cause of a problem. RCA focuses the analysis on improving the entire system and process rather than being limited to a review of individual performance. By shifting the focus of IVF laboratory quality control from "after-the-fact management" to "before-the-fact management" and "during-the-fact management," the rigor of IVF laboratory work can be continuously improved, defects can be reduced, and new problems can be avoided.

In summary, we have systematically organized and summarized the overall operation, risk factors, quality control measures, and troubleshooting methods and processes in IVF laboratories, which we hope will be helpful to the readers of this book.

References

1. Mortimer ST, Mortimer D. Quality and risk management in the IVF laboratory. 2nd ed. Cambridge: Cambridge University Press; 2015.
2. Elder K, den Bergh MV, Woodward B. Troubleshooting and problem-solving in the IVF laboratory. Cambridge: Cambridge University Press; 2015.

3. Varghese AC, Sjöblom P, Jayaprakasan K. A practical guide to setting up IVF lab and embryo culture systems and running the unit. New Delhi: Jaypee Brothers Medical Publishers; 2013.

4. Glujovsky D, Farquhar C, Quinteiro Retamar AM, et al. Cleavage stage versus blastocyst stage embryo transfer in assisted reproductive technology. Cochrane Database Syst Rev. 2016;6:CD002118.

5. ESHRE Special Interest Group of Embryology and Alpha Scientists in Reproductive Medicine. The Vienna consensus: report of an expert meeting on the development of ART laboratory performance indicators. Reprod Biomed Online. 2017;35(5):494–510.

6. Holden EC, Kashani BN, Morelli SS, et al. Improved outcomes after blastocyst-stage frozen-thawed embryo transfers compared with cleavage stage: a Society for Assisted Reproductive Technologies Clinical Outcomes Reporting System study. Fertil Steril. 2018;110(1):89–94.

7. Practice Committee of the American Society for Reproductive Medicine, Practice Committee of the Society for Assisted Reproductive Technology. Blastocyst culture and transfer in clinically assisted reproduction: a committee opinion. Fertil Steril. 2018;110(7):1246–52.

8. Glujovsky D, Farquhar C. Cleavage-stage or blastocyst transfer: what are the benefits and harms? Fertil Steril. 2016;106(2):244–50.

9. Martins WP, Nastri CO, Rienzi L, et al. Blastocyst vs cleavage-stage embryo transfer: systematic review and meta-analysis of reproductive outcomes. Ultrasound Obstet Gynecol. 2017;49(5):583–91.

10. Martins WP, Nastri CO, Rienzi L, et al. Obstetrical and perinatal outcomes following blastocyst transfer compared to cleavage transfer: a systematic review and meta-analysis. Hum Reprod. 2016;31(11):2561–9.

11. Maheshwari A, Hamilton M, Bhattacharya S. Should we be promoting embryo transfer at blastocyst stage? Reprod Biomed Online. 2016;32(2):142–6.

12. Alviggi C, Conforti A, Carbone IF, et al. Influence of cryopreservation on perinatal outcome after blastocyst- vs cleavage-stage embryo transfer: systematic review and meta-analysis. Ultrasound Obstet Gynecol. 2018;51(1):54–63.

13. Zhu Q, Wang N, Wang B, et al. The risk of birth defects among children born after vitrified blastocyst transfers and those born after fresh and vitrified cleavage-stage embryo transfers. Arch Gynecol Obstet. 2018;298(4):833–40.

14. Castello D, Cobo A, Mestres E, et al. Pre-clinical validation of a closed surface system (Cryotop SC) for the vitrification of oocytes and embryos in the mouse model. Cryobiology. 2018;81:107–16.

15. Vajta G, Rienzi L, Ubaldi FM. Open versus closed systems for vitrification of human oocytes and embryos. Reprod Biomed Online. 2015;30(4):325–33.

16. De Munck N, Belva F, Van de Velde H, et al. Closed oocyte vitrification and storage in an oocyte donation programme: obstetric and neonatal outcome. Hum Reprod. 2016;31(5):1024–33.

17. De Munck N, Santos-Ribeiro S, Stoop D, et al. Open versus closed oocyte vitrification in an oocyte donation programme: a prospective randomized sibling oocyte study. Hum Reprod. 2016;31(2):377–84.

18. Gook DA, Choo B, Bourne H, et al. Closed vitrification of human oocytes and blastocysts: outcomes from a series of clinical cases. J Assist Reprod Genet. 2016;33(9):1247–52.

19. Papatheodorou A, Vanderzwalmen P, Panagiotidis Y, et al. How does closed system vitrification of human oocytes affect the clinical outcome? A prospective, observational, cohort, noninferiority trial in an oocyte donation program. Fertil Steril. 2016;106(6):1348–55.

20. Papatheodorou A, Vanderzwalmen P, Panagiotidis Y, et al. Open versus closed oocyte vitrification system: a prospective randomized sibling-oocyte study. Reprod Biomed Online. 2013;26(6):595–602.

21. Stoop D, De Munck N, Jansen E, et al. Clinical validation of a closed vitrification system in an oocyte-donation programme. Reprod Biomed Online. 2012;24(2):180–5.

22. Chen Y, Zheng X, Yan J, et al. Neonatal outcomes after the transfer of vitrified blastocysts: closed versus open vitrification system. Reprod Biol Endocrinol. 2013;11:107.

23. Hashimoto S, Amo A, Hama S, et al. A closed system supports the developmental competence of human embryos after vitrification: closed vitrification of human embryos. J Assist Reprod Genet. 2013;30(3):371–6.

24. Kuwayama M, Vajta G, Ieda S, et al. Comparison of open and closed methods for vitrification of human embryos and the elimination of potential contamination. Reprod Biomed Online. 2005;11(5):608–14.

25. Panagiotidis Y, Vanderzwalmen P, Prapas Y, et al. Open versus closed vitrification of blastocysts from an oocyte-donation programme: a prospective randomized study. Reprod Biomed Online. 2013;26(5):470–6.

26. Bonetti A, Cervi M, Tomei F, et al. Ultrastructural evaluation of human metaphase II oocytes after vitrification: closed versus open devices. Fertil Steril. 2011;95(3):928–35.

27. Youm HS, Choi JR, Oh D, et al. Closed versus open vitrification for human blastocyst cryopreservation: a meta-analysis. Cryobiology. 2017;77:64–70.

28. Tedder RS, Zuckerman MA, Goldstone AH, et al. Hepatitis B transmission from contaminated cryopreservation tank. Lancet. 1995;346(8968):137–40.

29. Molina I, Mari M, Martinez JV, et al. Bacterial and fungal contamination risks in human oocyte and embryo cryopreservation: open versus closed vitrification systems. Fertil Steril. 2016;106(1):127–32.

30. Savasi V, Oneta M, Parrilla B, et al. Should HCV discordant couples with a seropositive male partner be treated with assisted reproduction techniques (ART)? Eur J Obstet Gynecol Reprod Biol. 2013;167(2):181–4.

31. Vitorino RL, Grinsztejn BG, de Andrade CA, et al. Systematic review of the effectiveness and safety of assisted reproduction techniques in couples serodis-

cordant for human immunodeficiency virus where the man is positive. Fertil Steril. 2011;95(5):1684–90.

32. George MA, Braude PR, Johnson MH, et al. Quality control in the IVF laboratory: in-vitro and in-vivo development of mouse embryos is unaffected by the quality of water used in culture media. Hum Reprod. 1989;4(7):826–31.

33. YY/T 1434-2016. Medical devices for human in vitro assisted reproductive technology—in vitro mouse embryo assay. Former State Administration for Food and Drug Regulation of People's Republic of China, Beijing. 2016.

34. YY/T 1535-2017. Medical devices for human in vitro assisted reproductive technology—biological evaluation—human sperm survival assay. Former State Administration for Food and Drug Regulation of People's Republic of China, Beijing. 2017.

Temperature Control in IVF Culture System

Temperature influences the entire process of in vitro fertilization-embryo transfer. Today, most laboratories keep the embryo culture temperature at 37 °C, which is close to the human basal body temperature and is conducive to the development of gametes and embryos [1–3]. Abnormal temperatures may lead to increased embryonic fragmentation, delayed cell division, and even chromosomal abnormalities and thus compromise pregnancy outcomes. Regardless of whether it is the room temperature, the temperature inside the incubator, the temperature of the instruments, the culture dishes, or all culture media used during embryo development, constant temperature monitoring and control are always vital for maintaining stable ART treatment outcomes by avoiding exposure of gametes and embryos to temperatures either too high or too low.

2.1 Effects of Temperature on Gametes and Embryos

Some studies suggest that the temperature of the human genital tract is lower than the human basal body temperature [4, 5]. Hunter et al. measured preovulatory follicular temperature with a fine thermistor probe in cows. The results indicated that all measured preovulatory follicular fluid temperatures were significantly lower than the rectal temperature [6, 7]. Some studies have shown that during IVF cycles, the highest blasto-

cyst formation rate, embryo implantation rate, and live birth rate are achieved when the follicular fluid temperature before oocyte retrieval is between 36.4 °C and 36.9 °C [8]. Meanwhile, sperm production also requires a temperature slightly below the human body temperature. These studies prompt us to consider whether in vitro culture should be performed slightly below 37.0 °C [9]. However, a lower temperature can profoundly affect metabolism, making 37.0 °C still the preferred embryo culture temperature in most laboratories until more and higher level evidence suggests otherwise.

Temperature affects gametes and embryos from multiple perspectives, particularly by influencing the stability of the spindle during meiosis [10]. During oocyte meiosis and maturation, the spindle controls successive phases of meiosis, maintains the oocyte genome's stability, and ensures proper functions necessary for fertilization and post-fertilization events. The normalcy of the spindle determines the correctness of the cell division process and is crucial for ensuring the accurate distribution of mammalian chromosomes. In case of abnormal chromosome segregation, the fertilized oocyte will develop into an aneuploid embryo, resulting in abnormal embryo development and spontaneous abortion.

Temperature fluctuation affects embryo development. Low temperature can impair the spindle morphology and oocyte metabolism [11, 12]. Some studies have shown that human oocyte

© The Author(s), under exclusive license to Springer Nature Singapore Pte Ltd. 2024
D. Li, Y. Gao, *Quality Management in the Assisted Reproduction Laboratory*,
https://doi.org/10.1007/978-981-99-6659-2_2

spindles will depolymerize or even disappear when exposed to temperatures ranging from 27.1 °C to 31.9 °C [13]. When oocytes are incubated at room temperature or 4 °C for 60 min, respectively, the number of meiotic spindles is significantly reduced in metaphase I (MI) stage and metaphase II (MII) stage oocytes incubated at 4 °C; and the lower the temperature, the faster the spindles are lost [14]. The motility of the oocyte organelles is reduced at room temperature, and, more importantly, the damage to the oocyte by the decrease in temperature appears irreversible. It has been shown that even when the temperature is restored, fertilization rates, embryo formation rates, and pregnancy rates of oocytes that have been exposed to low temperatures are still below normal [15]. Typically, a slight temperature increase stabilizes the meiotic spindle's morphology and enhances microtubule aggregation, allowing more microtubules to form spindles. However, when exposed to high temperatures above 40 °C, the spindle formation will be disrupted, and this disruption is irreversible and may inhibit cell division and lead to embryo death [16]. Also, high temperatures can introduce irreversible changes in the oocyte spindle by triggering the production of heat shock proteins [17].

2.2 Quality Management of Temperature in IVF Laboratory

The temperature of gametes and embryos during in vitro culture can be influenced by many factors, including the incubator, working bench, and microscope heating stage, culture dishes, the volume of culture medium, the volume of tissue culture oil used for covering the medium, in vitro operation time, airflow, and the list goes on. In vitro handling of gametes or embryos generally goes through three cycles with temperature differences: from a 37 °C incubator to room temperature; from room temperature to a heating microscope stage; and from the microscope stage to a 37 °C incubator. It is difficult to guarantee that embryos are always in a micro-environment at 37 °C. Still, we can maintain the stable func-

tion of all thermal devices through rigorous quality management to avoid the adverse effects of temperature fluctuations on embryos.

2.2.1 Quality Management of Incubators

Gametes and embryos are kept in the incubator for the majority of their in vitro development, making the stable performance of the incubator an essential determinant for a successful IVF. The incubator provides an incubation microenvironment with stable temperature, humidity, gas, pH, and osmolarity of the culture medium, making it an essential component of the culture system. Commonly used large incubators can be divided into water-jacketed heating incubators and gas-jacketed heating incubators. A water-jacketed incubator maintains the chamber temperature through a separate hot water compartment surrounding the chamber. In contrast, a gas-jacketed incubator heats the chamber gas directly through a heater inside the chamber. Regardless of the heating system used, there is always a temperature gradient inside a large incubator. Inside temperatures between the fronts and backs of incubators were significantly different (36.85 °C ± 0.15 °C in the front of the incubators versus 36.68 °C ± 0.08 °C in the back; $P < 0.001$) [18]. While it is unknown whether such temperature fluctuations would impact [10], recording temperatures at multiple sites within the incubator can provide more accurate temperature information and allow for the timely detection of temperature changes that may affect gamete and embryo development [18–20].

Although the incubator features the ability to maintain a stable temperature, it is still influenced by the external environment. For example, if the door of the incubator is frequently opened and closed, cold air from the outside will flow into the incubator, which will bring down the temperature inside. Therefore, in theory, each patient should be assigned a separate incubator to prevent the impact of opening and closing the door on other patients' gametes or embryos and to maintain a stable incubation environment to the greatest extent possible. However, this is unrealistic for fertility centers with an annual cycle volume of more than a thousand, which is why bench-top and drawer-type small incubators were developed. By applying multiple small incubators simultaneously, the number of patients sharing the same incubator can be reduced or even make it possible for each patient to have his or her own incubator. Large water-jacketed incubators utilize hot water to heat the walls of the chamber. It takes some time for the temperature inside the chamber to be restored after opening and closing the door. In contrast, small bench-top incubators are designed to allow effective heat exchange by directly heating the grooves in the incubator so that the surface of the culture dish is in direct contact with the heated internal surface of the incubator. A study compared the changes in temperature and oxygen concentration inside a small bench-top incubator and a traditional sizeable water-jacketed incubator following a 5-s door opening/closing procedure. The results showed that: the temperature of the chamber and culture dishes recovered in about 5 min after closing the door of the small bench-top incubator, while the conventional incubator needed about 30 min to restore the temperature inside the chamber and in the culture dish back to 37 °C. The researchers of this study then randomly assigned fertilized oocytes into the two incubators for culture and found that cleavage and blastocyst formation rates were significantly higher in the small bench-top incubator than in the conventional incubator (Table 2.1) [21]. What should also be noted is that the incubator should avoid being placed near

a vertical high-efficiency filter outlet, as the strong airflow can seriously impair the stability of the incubator, especially for small bench-top incubators.

The temperature in the incubator should be monitored and recorded daily. It is recommended that a real-time incubator temperature monitoring device be installed, which not only reduces the daily workload of laboratory personnel but also makes it easy to observe the temperature fluctuations inside the incubator and the impact of related influences (e.g., how frequently the incubator door is opened/closed and the change in room temperature). If it is found that the difference between the displayed temperature and the measured temperature is more than 0.2 °C, then a recalibration is required. However, except for the temperature setting and calibration, do not change any other factory settings and parameters (parameters for gas concentration and humidity also included) without permission. It is vital to ensure that the equipment operates in the best condition to provide a stable in vitro development environment for gametes and embryos.

In addition, the time-lapse culture system, which has been rapidly developed in recent years, allows embryos to be observed from inside the incubator without being exposed to the external environment, thus reducing temperature fluctuations, providing a stable micro-environment for embryo development while presenting comprehensive information on embryo developmental dynamics.

2.2.2 Quality Management of Thermostatic Equipment

Gametes and embryos are very sensitive to temperature changes in vitro. When in vitro manipulations are performed, the temperature of the culture medium (or microdroplets) in the culture dish is affected by multiple factors: room temperature, airflow, the material of the culture dish, whether the dish has a lid, the amount of medium in the dish and the amount of tissue culture oil covering the medium, whether there is heat radiated from the light source around the

Table 2.1 Key indicators of the two incubators

Key indicators	Small bench-top incubator	Conventional incubator
Early-stage embryo formation rate (%) (good embryos/ fertilized oocytes)	40.3* (75/186)	28.4 (42/148)
Blastocyst formation rate (%) (good blastocysts/total embryos)	15.1* (25/166)	7.2 (10/139)

*$P < 0.05$

dish (e.g., microscope), and the temperature of laboratory personnel's hands. Therefore, a heating plate or a thermostatic tube rack is necessary for manipulation of oocytes and embryos in vitro to maintain a stable temperature. The temperature inside the culture dish will be significantly lowered when it is taken out of the incubator, and it is impossible to keep the culture dish's temperature stable even if the dish is placed on a heating stage. It has been shown that when the culture dish was taken out of the incubator and placed on a 37 °C heating stage, the temperature of the culture medium would drop to 34.5 °C, and it would take up to 10 min for rewarming [10, 22]. Factors that affect the actual temperature of the culture medium in the dish on a heating plate include [23]: (a) The distance between the bottom of the culture dish and the heating stage; (b) the airflow around the culture dish; (c) the direct heat transfer efficiency between the surface of the heating stage and the medium in the culture dish; (d) volume of culture medium and tissue culture oil; (e) room temperature. Therefore, the heating plate temperature is usually set slightly higher than 37 °C to compensate for the heat loss caused by the above factors so that the actual temperature measured in the culture dish or test tube reaches 37 °C.

Laboratory staff should measure and record the temperature of the heating stage, heating plate, and thermostatic test tube rack daily and recalibrate immediately if any abnormalities are found. The laminar flow of the clean bench may interfere with the temperature measurement results, so an hour should be reserved for thermal equilibration before temperature measurements are made on the heating stage or heating plate installed within a laminar flow hood, and multiple measuring spots should be taken to compare the differences between them. The temperature of the microdroplets should also be monitored using a detection probe (e.g., a thermocouple). The temperature calibration of the heating stage or heating plate should refer to the actual temperature of the microdroplets. Otherwise, it will not be very sensible to simply measure the surface temperature of the heating

instruments. Meanwhile, the thermometric devices should also be calibrated annually to guarantee the accuracy of the measured temperature.

2.2.3 Quality Control of the Heating, Ventilation, and Air Conditioning System

The ambient temperature of the laboratory is controlled by the heating, ventilation, and air conditioning system. Changing airflow patterns during the heating and cooling cycles can produce cold and hot spots in the laboratory [24, 25]. There was a study in which room temperature was adjusted from 20 °C (±0.3) to 26 °C (±0.3) or 17 °C (±0.3), and the temperature variations of different devices before and after the adjustment were recorded with CIMScan probes. The results showed that the stability of the equipment temperature was directly associated with the room temperature; when the room temperature changed, the equipment temperature responded within 5 mins, and the temperature fluctuations of the microscope heating stage and slide warmer were greater than those of the heating block and incubator. This study suggests that fluctuations in ambient temperature can impact IVF equipment and that the ambient and equipment temperatures in IVF laboratories should be measured in real-time and adjusted as needed. Besides, the indoor ambient temperature of IVF laboratories is also affected by the outdoor temperature and seasonal changes, which is why special consideration should be given to factors such as the influence of the building's exterior walls and the temperature of the top floor when selecting a laboratory site.

Likewise, the temperature inside the culture room should be monitored and recorded daily. Generally, the temperature in the culture room should be controlled at about 24 °C. When the room temperature is too low, the temperature of oocytes and embryos will drop significantly and rapidly during in vitro manipulation, which will adversely affect the treatment outcome. At the same time, high room temperature will not only cause discomfort to laboratory staff but also adversely affect the regular operation, stability, and service life of electronic equipment in the laboratory.

2.3 Quality Management of the Transport and Storage Temperature of the Culture Media

In addition to the room, ambient temperature, and embryo culture temperature, temperature management of culture media transport and storage is also critical. Most culture media need to be stored in a refrigerator at 2–8 °C to maintain the long-term stability of the components and thus usually require cold chain transportation.

2.3.1 Impact of Low Temperature

If the temperature drops below 0 °C for a long time, it can lead to the formation of ice crystals in the culture media, and their homogeneity may be altered even after rewarming. Moreover, icing changes the culture media's osmolarity and pH, thus causing protein denaturation in the ready-to-use culture media (i.e., protein-containing culture media) [26]. Therefore, any frozen medium must be discarded instead of being used.

2.3.2 Impact of High Temperature

Delayed transportation or exposure to high temperatures may cause a break in the cold chain transport of the culture media. The main effects of high-temperature exposure on the culture media are oxidation and a decrease in the concentration of active ingredients. Amino acids and proteins in the culture medium are subject to spontaneous oxidation and deamination, resulting in the slow release of ammonium ions. Higher temperatures will accelerate this process [27, 28]. It has been demonstrated that ammonium release

and accumulation during culture affects blastocyst formation [29] and alters metabolism and subsequent gene expression in human embryos [30].

2.3.3 Selection of Refrigerators

Currently, there are no clear rules for refrigerators used to store culture media, so both medical refrigerators and household refrigerators can be found in IVF laboratories. Medical refrigerators used for drug preservation are more stable than home refrigerators in terms of temperature control. Still, even for home refrigerators, their internal temperature fluctuations can be well stabilized between 2–8 °C. What should be noted, however, is that medical refrigerators usually have light-transmitting doors, so appropriate measures (such as applying a film) should be taken to prevent the culture media from being exposed to light during storage. Furthermore, when using a household refrigerator, it should be prohibited to place culture media in the storage position on the refrigerator door.

2.3.4 Temperature Monitoring

1. Temperature monitoring during transportation: The cold chain transportation provided by the manufacturer is usually very professional, but particular attention should be paid to the transportation process from the domestic distributor to the hospital. We can request the distributor to put an electronic thermometer that can continuously record the temperature in the package (Fig. 2.1). The laboratory personnel should export and check the temperature data as soon as the delivery is made (Table 2.2). If the temperature exceeds the acceptable range (2–8 °C), the culture media should be returned decisively.
2. The temperature inside the refrigerator should be examined every day. Moreover, it is recommended to install a temperature monitoring sys-

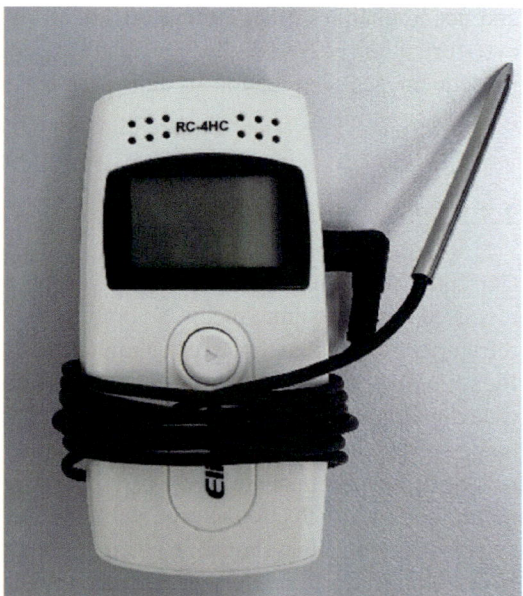

Fig. 2.1   Temperature and humidity recorder

Table 2.2   Data exported from temperature and humidity recorder

Indicator	Data
User information	RC-4HC Data Logger
Recording interval	5 min
Start-up delay time	2.0 h
Total data	495
Temperature max.	22.9 °C
Temperature min.	2.8 °C
Temperature average	4.3 °C
High-temperature alarm	8.0 °C
Low-temperature alarm	2.0 °C
Humidity max.	72.8% RH
Humidity min.	37.6% RH
Humidity average	51.6% RH
High humidity alarm	90% RH
Low humidity alarm	20% RH
Start time	2020-12-24 17:53:40
End time	2020-12-26 11:03:40
Time format	YYYY-MM-DD hh: mm: ss
Temperature unit	°C

RH relative humidity

tem with remote monitoring and automatic alarm functions (Fig. 2.2) so that refrigerators' abnormal temperature variations can be detected promptly during non-working hours, especially for the centers using household refrigerators.

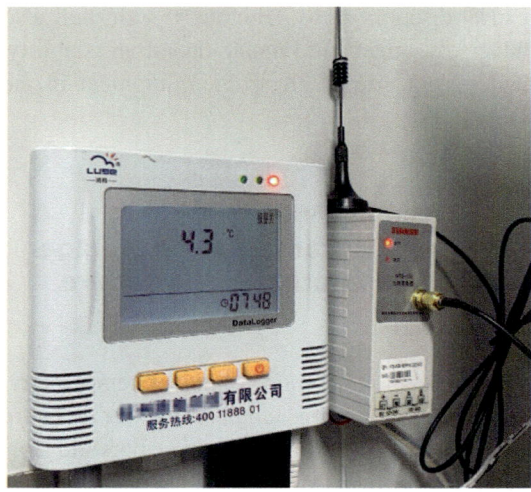

Fig. 2.2   Temperature monitoring system

In conclusion, the temperature is the most important among many influences on the quality of oocytes and embryos, and comprehensive quality management of temperature control should be implemented appropriately to avoid exposure of gametes and embryos to too high or too low temperatures. Each laboratory should establish an acceptable range of temperature variation. Any deviations outside the scope should be adjusted and recorded promptly, and all apparatus should be subject to regular maintenance and calibration.

References

1. Baak NA, Cantineau AE, Farquhar C, et al. Temperature of embryo culture for assisted reproduction. Cochrane Database Syst Rev. 2019;9(9):CD012192.
2. Mortimer D, Cohen J, Mortimer ST, et al. Cairo consensus on the IVF laboratory environment and air quality: report of an expert meeting. Reprod Biomed Online. 2018;36(6):658–74.
3. Swain JE. Optimal human embryo culture. Semin Reprod Med. 2015;33(2):103–17.
4. Bahat A, Tur-Kaspa I, Gakamsky A, et al. Thermotaxis of mammalian sperm cells: a potential navigation mechanism in the female genital tract. Nat Med. 2003;9(2):149–50.
5. Hunter RH, Bogh IB, Einer-Jensen N, et al. Preovulatory graafian follicles are cooler than neigh-

bouring stroma in pig ovaries. Hum Reprod. 2000;15(2):273–83.

6. Lopez-Gatiu F, Hunter R. Clinical relevance of pre-ovulatory follicular temperature in heat-stressed lactating dairy cows. Reprod Domest Anim. 2017;52(3):366–70.

7. Lopez-Gatius F, Hunter R. Pre-ovulatory follicular temperature in bi-ovular cows. J Reprod Dev. 2019;65(2):191–4.

8. Sherbahn R. Assessment of effect of follicular fluid temperature at egg retrieval on blastocyst development, implantation and live birth rates. Fertil Steril. 2010;94(4):S68–9.

9. Leese HJ, Baumann CG, Brison DR, et al. Metabolism of the viable mammalian embryo: quietness revisited. Mol Hum Reprod. 2008;14(12):667–72.

10. Swain JE. Decisions for the IVF laboratory: comparative analysis of embryo culture incubators. Reprod Biomed Online. 2014;28(5):535–47.

11. Sun XF, Wang WH, Keefe DL. Overheating is detrimental to meiotic spindles within in vitro matured human oocytes. Zygote. 2004;12(1):65–70.

12. Wang WH, Meng L, Hackett RJ, et al. Limited recovery of meiotic spindles in living human oocytes after cooling-rewarming observed using polarized light microscopy. Hum Reprod. 2001;16(11):2374–8.

13. Larman MG, Minasi MG, Rienzi L, et al. Maintenance of the meiotic spindle during vitrification in human and mouse oocytes. Reprod Biomed Online. 2007;15(6):692–700.

14. Gomes C, Merlini M, Konheim J, et al. Oocyte meiotic-stage-specific differences in spindle depolymerization in response to temperature changes monitored with polarized field microscopy and immunocytochemistry. Fertil Steril. 2012;97(3):714–9.

15. Wang WH, Meng L, Hackett RJ, et al. Rigorous thermal control during intracytoplasmic sperm injection stabilizes the meiotic spindle and improves fertilization and pregnancy rates. Fertil Steril. 2002;77(6):1274–7.

16. Huang GN, Sun HX. Laboratory techniques in in vitro fertilization and embryo transfer. Beijing: People's Medical Publishing House; 2012.

17. Mortensen CJ, Choi YH, Ing NH, et al. Heat shock protein 70 gene expression in equine blastocysts after exposure of oocytes to high temperatures in vitro or in vivo after exercise of donor mares. Theriogenology. 2010;74(3):374–83.

18. Walker MW, Butler JM, Higdon HL, et al. Temperature variations within and between incubators-a prospective, observational study. J Assist Reprod Genet. 2013;30(12):1583–5.

19. Higdon HR, Blackhurst DW, Boone WR. Incubator management in an assisted reproductive technology laboratory. Fertil Steril. 2008;89(3):703–10.

20. Anifandis G. Temperature variations inside commercial IVF incubators. J Assist Reprod Genet. 2013;30(12):1587–8.

21. Fujiwara M, Takahashi K, Izuno M, et al. Effect of micro-environment maintenance on embryo culture after in-vitro fertilization: comparison of top-load mini incubator and conventional front-load incubator. J Assist Reprod Genet. 2007;24(1):5–9.

22. Cooke S, Tyler JP, Deriscoll G. Objective assessments of temperature maintenance using in vitro culture techniques. J Assist Reprod Genet. 2002;19(8):368–75.

23. Korakaki D, Mouroutsos S, Tripsianis G, et al. Temperature decline in embryological culture dishes outside incubator. Int J Fertil Steril. 2020;14(1):63–7.

24. Butler JM, Johnson JE, Boone WR. The heat is on: room temperature affects laboratory equipment-an observational study. J Assist Reprod Genet. 2013;30(10):1389–93.

25. Bove R. Temperature measurement in the clinical laboratory. Med Lab Obs. 2011;43:36–9.

26. Cairo 2018 Consensus Group. 'There is only one thing that is truly important in an IVF laboratory: everything' Cairo Consensus Guidelines on IVF Culture Conditions. Reprod Biomed Online. 2020;40(1):33–60.

27. Lane M, Hooper K, Gardner DK. Effect of essential amino acids on mouse embryo viability and ammonium production. J Assist Reprod Genet. 2001;18(9):519–25.

28. Kleijkers SH, van Montfoort AP, Bekers O, et al. Ammonium accumulation in commercially available embryo culture media and protein supplements during storage at 2–8°C and during incubation at 37°C. Hum Reprod. 2016;31(6):1192–9.

29. Virant-Klun I, Tomazevic T, Vrtacnik-Bokal E, et al. Increased ammonium in culture medium reduces the development of human embryos to the blastocyst stage. Fertil Steri. 2006;85(2):526–8.

30. Gardner DK, Hamilton R, McCallie B, et al. Human and mouse embryonic development, metabolism and gene expression are altered by an ammonium gradient in vitro. Reproduction. 2013;146(1):49–61.

Gametes and embryos are highly sensitive to changes in culture media osmolality. Any fluctuation in culture media osmolality may adversely stress the gametes and embryos and obstruct their growth and development. Therefore, it is vital to understand the influence and regulatory mechanisms of culture media osmolality and effectively maintain its stability for quality control of embryo culture in IVF laboratories. In this chapter, we will introduce the osmolality of culture fluid from the viewpoint of its fundamental principles, regulatory mechanisms, and quality control of relevant experimental operations.

3.1   Basics of Osmotic Pressure

3.1.1   The Osmotic Pressure Concepts

Suppose the concentration of the solution on both sides of a semipermeable membrane is not equal, water molecules will diffuse freely from the side with a lower concentration to the side with a higher concentration—a phenomenon called osmosis. To prevent water molecule diffusion from the low- to high-concentration side, an additional pressure must be applied on the high-concentration side, with the minimum pressure required defined as the osmotic pressure (Fig. 3.1). In simple terms, osmotic pressure is the additional pressure exerted above the surface of a solution just enough to prevent osmosis. This is a requisite for osmosis in living organisms.

3.1.2   Factors Affecting Osmotic Pressure

1. Solution concentration: The value of the osmotic pressure of a solution is proportional to the concentration of the solution, that is, the number of solute particles per unit volume of solution that cannot pass through the semipermeable membrane. The osmotic pressure of a solution is correlated only with the total number of molecules or ions of the solute and not with their nature or size. In other words, as long as the solutions have the same number of molecules and ions, their osmotic pressure is the same regardless of whether the solute comprises small-molecule electrolytes or large-molecule proteins.

2. Solution temperature: At a given solution concentration, the osmotic pressure is proportional to the temperature of the solution, with higher temperatures indicating higher osmotic pressure of the solution and vice versa.

3. Formula for calculating osmotic pressure for dilute solutions of nonelectrolytes: $\pi = cRT$ ("π" is the osmotic pressure, "c" is the concentration of the solution, "R" is the gas constant, and "T" is the absolute temperature).

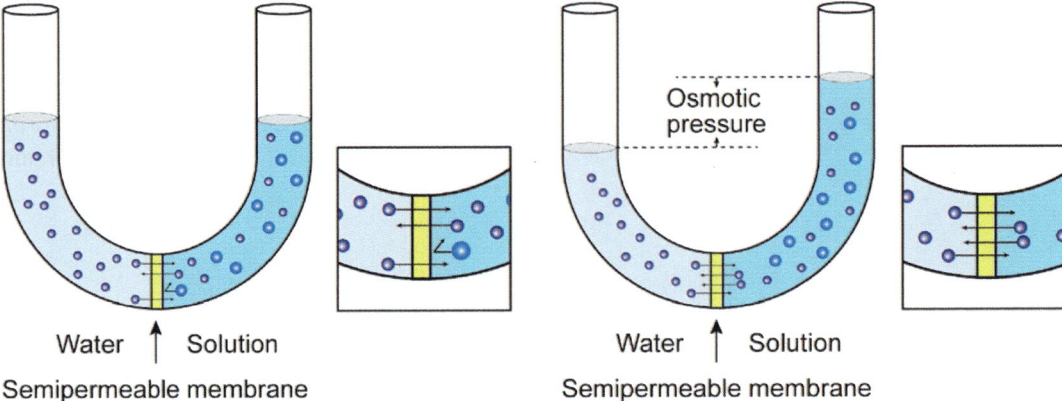

Fig. 3.1 Principle of osmotic pressure

3.1.3 Osmolarity/Osmolality

Solute particles in a solution capable of producing osmotic effects are collectively referred to as osmotically active substances, the concentration of which can be expressed using the term osmolarity/ osmolality. When the solute concentration is very low, the volume of the solute in the solution is negligible. For example, if a tiny amount of solute is dissolved in 1 kg of water, the total volume of the solution can be almost considered 1 L. This solution with a very low concentration is called a dilute solution. Embryo culture media used in IVF laboratories are usually dilute solutions. According to the osmotic pressure formula, the osmotic pressure of dilute solutions at a constant temperature is only associated with the concentration of osmotically active substances; thus, the osmotic pressure of the embryo culture medium can be measured by the osmolarity/osmolality.

3.1.4 Units of Osmolarity/ Osmolality

In the English context, different terms for osmolarity/osmolality have been used when expressed in different units: osmolarity in the volume unit "liter" and osmolality in the weight unit "kilogram" [1]. For dilute solutions, the osmolarity per unit volume is approximately equal to the osmolality per unit weight, given the negligible effect of the solute on the solvent volume. However, for concentrated solutions, a substantial difference exists between the two, and close attention should be paid to the unit conversion. The unit commonly used in clinical work is mOsm/kg, an expression commonly used for osmolality.

3.2 Culture Media and Osmolality

3.2.1 History of Culture Media Development

The development of embryo culture media has gone through a lengthy journey. Whitten culture medium had been the first culture medium exclusively used for mouse embryos, through which an 8-cell mouse embryo was successfully cultured to a blastocyst. Whitten culture medium is based on the Krebs-Ringer bicarbonate culture medium with the addition of glucose and calf serum albumin. Although the initial Whitten medium did not function very well for early embryo development, the addition of lactate considerably improved this medium's ability to support embryo development from the 2-cell stage to blastocyst. However, the culture outcomes were still underwhelming for earlier embryonic development (from fertilized oocyte to 2-cell embryo). Shortly after, Bigger confirmed that pyruvate was an essential nutrient required for fertilized oocytes to develop into

2-cell embryos [2]. Based on these findings, Whittingham published a report in 1971 on the M16 culture medium, a classic mouse embryo culture medium widely used in various studies since its availability. However, neither the Whitten culture medium nor the M16 culture medium could sustain the development of murine fertilized oocytes to blastocysts. More specifically, it is possible to develop fertilized oocytes into 2-cell embryos, and in vitro culture of 2-cell embryos developed in vivo to blastocysts using both culture media mentioned above. However, it is impossible to achieve continuous development of mouse fertilized oocytes to blastocysts in vitro. This phenomenon is called "2-cell arrest." After a prolonged exploration, media that can span the "2-cell arrest" in mouse embryos were developed. These media include Chatot-Ziomek-Bavister (CZB) medium, simplex optimized medium (SOM), and KSOM medium (this one was made based on SOM medium with the addition of K+ ions) [3]. They can be used for the whole in vitro culture, from fertilized oocytes to blastocysts. In 1985, Quinn reported the human tubal fluid (HTF) culture medium, the first culture medium specifically for human embryos [4]. The composition of the HTF culture medium was based on the ionic content of the human oviductal fluid. Subsequently, various culture media for human embryos were introduced, such as Global®, GM501, and G-1.

3.2.2 Osmolality of Culture Media

The total solute content determines the osmolality of a culture medium. The solutes of embryo culture media include inorganic salt ions, essential and nonessential amino acids, energy metabolizing substrates (glucose, lactate, and pyruvate), vitamins, antibiotics, antioxidants, and chelating agents. The concentration of inorganic salt ions is much greater than other solutes, making them the primary determinant of intra- and extracellular osmolality. Embryo culture media commonly contain the same inorganic salt ions, namely, Na^+, K^+, Ca^{2+}, Mg^{2+}, Cl^-, SO_4^{2-} (with Na^+ and Cl^- levels being the highest), most of which also contain PO_4^{3-} [5]. The osmolality of commercial

Table 3.1 Osmolality of commercial culture media

Brand	Culture medium	Culture stage	Osmolality (mOsm/kg)
Brand 1	Sydney IVF fertilization	Oocyte incubation, fertilization	285–295
	Sydney IVF cleavage	Cleavage stage embryo	285–295
	Sydney IVF blastocyst	8-cell embryo – Blastocyst, embryo transfer	285–295
Brand 2	Quinns advantage fertilization	Fertilization	257–273
	Quinns advantage cleavage	Cleavage stage embryo	257–273
	Quinns advantage blastocyst	8-cell embryo – Blastocyst	257–273
Brand 3	G-IVF PLUS	Oocyte incubation, fertilization	275–285
	G-1 PLUS	Cleavage stage embryo	275–285
	G-2 PLUS	8-cell embryo – Blastocyst, embryo transfer	275–285

culture media now available on the market is listed in Table 3.1 [5].

3.2.3 Effects of Changes in Culture Media Osmolality on Embryo Development

Both gametes and embryos are highly sensitive to changes in osmolality when cultured in vitro, and even small changes may significantly impair their developmental potential. The expected osmolality range of in vitro media for human embryos is approximately 250–290 mOsm/kg. Any osmolality exceeding this range is detrimental to embryo development.

1. Effects of elevated osmolality on gametes and embryos.
   (a) Elevated osmolality can induce developmental block in embryos: the term "2-cell

block" refers to the inability of a fertilized oocyte to continue its development after reaching the 2-cell stage in vitro. Similar phenomena have been observed in 8-cell stage bovine embryos [6] and 4- to 8-cell stage human embryos [7]. With the introduction of the KSOM culture medium, cell block during embryonic development has been significantly ameliorated. The KSOM culture medium features low osmolality (250 mOsm/kg) and low NaCl while supplemented with single amino acid glutamine and the divalent metal chelator EDTA. The effect of elevated osmolality on development block in mice was demonstrated in an experiment designed by Hadi, in which the incidence of 2-cell arrest in outbred mouse embryos was significantly higher when osmolality was increased from 250 to 310 mOsm/kg [8]. Moreover, when the osmolality was maintained at 310 and 330 mOsm/kg for more than 48 h, the development of 8-cell embryos and the formation of blastocysts slowed down significantly [9]. Furthermore, a high osmolality environment also exerts a detrimental effect on blastocysts. In a study by Xie et al., researchers added sorbitol to the blastocyst culture medium at different concentrations to simulate a series of culture environments with different osmolality levels. Their results showed that a hyper-osmolar environment could accelerate apoptosis and decelerate cell proliferation and blastocyst formation, and such effects were dose- and time-dependent [10].

(b) Elevated osmolality can lead to the activation of apoptosis-related signaling pathways. In response to elevated external osmolality, the embryo initiates regulatory mechanisms primarily dependent on MAPK signaling pathways. As osmolality increases, MAPK14/11 activation is enhanced, the apoptosis-related MAPK8 expression is increased, and the mRNA expression of aquaporin-3,9 is elevated [11]. Aquaporin can mediate the trans- membrane transport of water and small organic molecules [12]. In blastocysts, elevated osmolality promotes intracellular SAPK/JNK signaling pathway expression; however, such expression in early embryonic development remains to be further investigated.

2. Effects of reduced osmolality on gametes and embryos.

Reduced extracellular osmolality affects the concentration of inorganic ions in the cytoplasm, denaturing enzymes and thus affecting macro-molecular assembly. When exposed to a hypo-osmotic external environment, the cells will swell and eventually may either lyse or rupture. This mechanism is utilized in the hypo-osmotic swelling test to examine sperm membrane integrity and assess sperm viability. When placed in a hypo-osmotic solution, the sperm must re-establish equilibrium between intra- and extracellular fluids, and water molecules will enter the sperm through their membranes, causing varying degrees of swelling of the sperm tail. In this case, the entire sperm tail will swell when there is no damage to the cell membrane, whereas there will be only localized swelling or no swelling when the sperm tail membrane is damaged or incomplete.

3.2.4 Regulation of Culture Medium Osmolality

1. Inorganic ions: When the external osmolality increases and the cell crumples and shrinks, intracellular inorganic ion transporters act as the first responders. When the cell shrinks, the Na^+/H^+ exchangers are activated, transporting Na^+ into the cell and H^+ outside the cell. Subsequently, the pH rises due to the depletion of intracellular H^+. The increased pH will activate HCO_3^-/Cl^- exchangers, which transport Cl^- into the cell and HCO_3^- outside the cell. Finally, the net effect that results from the action of the Na^+/H^+ transporters and HCO_3^-/Cl^- transporters is an increase in intracellular Na^+ and Cl^- concen-

trations, an increase in intracellular osmolality, and restoration of cell volume. The process of cell volume regulation requires large amounts of Na^+ and Cl^- [5]. Moreover, high Na+ and Cl^- concentrations in the culture medium are required to ensure this process flows smoothly.

2. Organic osmolytes: Organic osmolytes are a series of small-molecule neutral organic compounds that can regulate cell volume and osmotic properties [3]. Since cells can only synthesize a small fraction of organic osmolytes, most organic osmolytes are provided by the culture medium and are taken up by cells via transport proteins. These transporter proteins are activated when the extracellular osmolality increases or when the cell volume decreases. The increase in intracellular organic osmolytes raises the intracellular osmolality and restores the cell volume. Unlike inorganic salt ions, organic osmolytes are biocompatible and do not disrupt cellular physiological or biochemical functions even when accumulated in cells at very high concentrations. The well-recognized organic osmolytes include glycine, proline, betaine, glutamine, taurine, and β-alanine.

(a) Glycine: Glycine is the most important organic osmolyte and is the basis for the biosynthesis of other organic osmolytes. Its transport system is currently the most intensively studied subject. In the early stages of embryonic development, the transport of glycine depends on the neurotransmitter transporter GLYT1. Supplementing glycine to the embryo culture medium prevents early developmental arrest caused by elevated osmolality and safeguards the embryo's continued development into a blastocyst. This is because glycine has an osmotic supporting effect on the embryo. When the extracellular osmolality is elevated, glycine acts as an organic osmolyte. It will be transported into the cell, thereby increasing the intracellular osmolality, regulating the cell volume, and helping the cell adapt to the hyperosmotic environment.

When the glycine accumulation inside the cell plateaus, the glycine concentration stops increasing, and its final intracellular concentration is proportional to the extracellular osmolality (i.e., the higher the extracellular osmolality, the higher the concentration of glycine accumulated inside the cell and vice versa). Unlike high concentrations of inorganic ions that can cause damage to cells, high concentrations of glycine have good compatibility, given that it does not affect the normal physiology of cells.

The glycine transporter GLYT1 exhibits different activities in oocyte and embryo development phases. In GV stage oocytes, GLYT1 activity is nearly undetectable. With the onset of ovulation induction, the content of activated GLYT1 increases rapidly and hits a peak, which may last until the 2-cell stage, followed by a gradual decrease. The level of activated GLYT1 is very low in morula and blastocysts. The activation of glycine transporter GLYT1 is of great importance as it indicates that the oocyte or embryo can regulate its volume independently. However, in preovulatory oocytes, the regulation of the oocyte's volume still relies on the tight adhesion of the oocyte to the zona pellucida.

Conversely, anion channels can help to excrete glycine when the cell swells, increases in volume and accumulates excessive amounts of glycine [13]. When glycine intake and excretion are balanced, the normal volume of the cell can be maintained.

(b) Betaine and proline: Betaine and proline also promote an osmotic supporting effect and can participate in the regulation in response to changes in cell volume caused by altered osmolality [14]. Betaine and proline are transported by SIT1, the transport process of which requires the participation of inorganic ions Na^+ and Cl^-. Activated SIT1 is expressed briefly, only at the 1-cell and 2-cell stage [15].

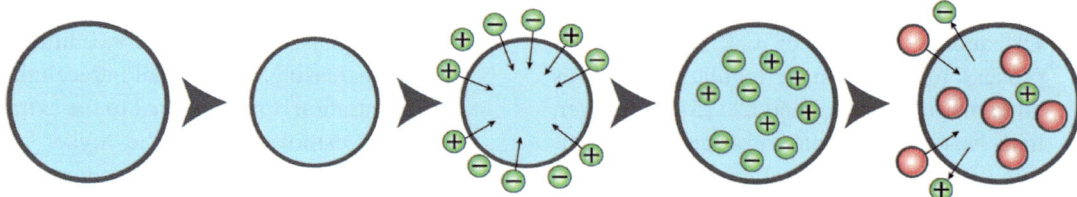

Fig. 3.2 Regulation of cell volume. Note: Green spheres represent inorganic ions, and red spheres represent organic osmolytes

3. Interaction between the two: Inorganic ions and organic osmolytes jointly regulate intracellular osmolality and interact with each other. Inorganic ions can respond rapidly and vigorously to changes in cell volume. However, excess intracellular inorganic ions may impair the physiological functions of the cell, for example, by disrupting enzyme activity and interfering with macromolecular assembly. In the long term, cells tend to replace some inorganic ions with organic osmolytes (Fig. 3.2). These organic osmolytes (e.g., glycine) serve to not only reduce intracellular inorganic ions but also maintain osmolality and prevent intracellular ion concentration from reaching levels that might hinder development. Early culture media lacked components that can serve as organic osmolytes, allowing preimplantation embryos to develop only at lower osmolality and salt concentrations. In contrast, when organic osmolytes are present, embryos can be cultured in a higher osmolality environment.

4. Regulatory mechanisms of embryonic cell volume at different stages: Changes in the extracellular fluid osmolality promote a reduction or swelling of the cell volume. Baltz and Tartia proposed a model of cell volume regulation in oocytes and early embryos with a timeline depicting the active transport of glycine and betaine via transporter proteins [3]. First, the oocyte within the follicle cannot regulate its volume autonomously, given that the surrounding zona pellucida restricts its size with strong physical adhesive properties. Shortly after ovulation, adhesions between the oocyte and the zona pellucida are released. From post-ovulation to the 4-cell stage embryo, early embryogenesis-specific cell

volume regulation mechanisms are activated, initiating GLYT1-mediated glycine transport to maintain normal embryo size. Moreover, from fertilization to the 2-cell stage, mechanisms regulating cell volume via betaine transport and accumulation contribute to cell volume homeostasis. Studies have been inconclusive regarding how volume is controlled in late embryonic stages. However, there is currently an intriguing hypothesis, which suggests that as blastocyst cells approach the size of typical adult somatic cells, there is a shift to more conventional volume homeostasis approaches.

3.3 Quality Management of Microdroplet Osmolality in Culture Dishes

Commercial culture media come with standard osmolality. However, during actual practice in IVF laboratories, inadvertent or unconscious manipulation by staff may impose artificial effects on the osmolality of the culture medium. Although embryos can tolerate changes in external osmolality to a certain extent, a steep increase in medium osmolality can still harm the embryos. Therefore, avoiding osmolality changes in medium microdroplets is essential to prevent embryo injury.

3.3.1 Preparation of Culture Dishes

Water evaporation is a critical determinant that alters the culture medium osmolality during the preparation of culture dishes, which should be minimized. The microdroplet volume in embryonic culture dishes is quite small, usually around

Fig. 3.3 Two methods for preparing microdroplets in culture dishes

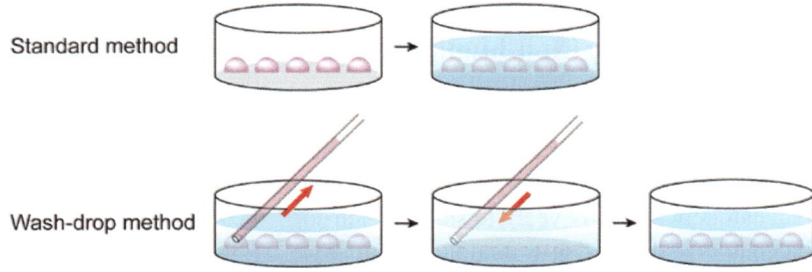

Standard method

Wash-drop method

15–100 µL. Timely covering with tissue culture oil is a practical approach for preventing water evaporation and alteration of osmolality. Other significant influences on water evaporation from culture dishes include staff proficiency, exposure time of microdroplets, the volume of microdroplets, temperature of environment and working bench, ambient humidity, workstation airflow, and whether culture oil is applied for coverage.

There are two methods for preparing microdroplets in culture dishes: the standard method and the wash-drop method (Fig. 3.3). The standard method for microdroplet preparation involves applying microdroplets into a culture dish and subsequently covering the dish with oil. In contrast, the wash-drop method involves pipetting the microdroplets out of the dish after preparing them using the standard method and replenishing them with a fresh culture medium. Swain compared the osmolality changes of microdroplets at 5 mins and 24 h after preparation using two methods under different conditions [9]. The results showed that at 5 mins, the standard method, increased temperature and reduced microdroplet volume, resulting in a more significant increase in osmolality. In contrast, after 24 h, the above factors no longer significantly impacted osmolality.

3.3.2 Key Points for Maintaining Stable Osmolality of the Culture Microdroplets [1]

1. Be aware of the osmolality of the culture medium used and avoid mixing media with different osmolalities. If there is a risk that the osmolality will increase during the preparation, consider using a culture medium with a lower osmolality.

2. Prepare culture dishes at room temperature immediately after taking the culture media out of the refrigerator.

3. Microdroplets should not be at least 20 µL.

4. Pay attention to the expiration date of the culture medium and document the opening date. The osmolality of the culture medium in the vial may change after repeated opening. The remaining culture medium should be sealed immediately with sealing film and returned to the refrigerator.

5. Microdroplets should be prepared quickly. Preparing too many dishes and microdroplets at one time should be avoided to reduce the exposure time of the microdroplets and thus reduce the water evaporation.

6. Culture dishes should be prepared by two laboratory personnel: one prepares the microdroplets, and the other immediately covers the microdroplets with tissue culture oil.

7. After covering the culture dish with culture oil, the oil surface should be checked to ensure that the microdroplets are completely covered.

8. Do not prepare culture dishes on a bench that is too warm: high temperatures will lead to accelerated evaporation and may affect the osmolality of the culture medium.

9. The humidity inside the incubator can affect the osmolality, and the water volume in the water tank of the incubator should be checked regularly.

10. The airflow of the clean bench should be turned off during the preparation of the culture dishes.

11. Laboratory operation protocols should be rigorously followed, and aseptic operation ensured.

3.3.3　Key Points of Working with a Dry (Non-humidified) Incubator

Over recent years, incubators of various brands have constantly been optimized, from large incubators in the early years to small bench-top incubators and time-lapse imaging culture systems today, to maintain the best development environment for embryos. Some small bench-top incubators and most time-lapse imaging culture systems today utilize dry incubation. This is because evidence suggests that one significant disadvantage of humidified incubators is the potential for microbial overgrowth, which can negatively affect embryo development. Although oil-covered culture is commonly used today, it remains unclear whether prolonged exposure to a dry environment alters the osmolality of microdroplets and impairs embryo development.

Keitaro et al. found that 50 μL and 200 μL microdroplets showed a significant linear increase in osmolality over a 5-day incubation in a dry bench-top incubator, with a maximum increase of 20 mOsm/kg [16]. Moreover, they found that the extent of the increase was influenced by the volume of the microdroplets and possibly also by the type of tissue culture oil covering them (higher viscosity oils are more effective in preventing evaporation). In contrast, no significant change in microdroplet osmolality was observed after a 5-day incubation in a humidified incubator. The authors concluded that tissue culture oil coverage as a single means is inadequate to prevent gradual changes in the osmolality of low-volume microdroplets when performing in vitro culture in a dry incubator and thus would adversely affect clinical outcomes. Another prospective randomized controlled trial that included 297 women undergoing in vitro fertilization found that humidified culture was significantly preferable to dry culture [17]. Their results showed that humidified culture delivered a better high-quality embryo rate on day 3, a better high-quality blastocyst rate on day 5, a higher clinical pregnancy rate, a higher sustained pregnancy rate, and a higher implantation rate. Similarly, the investigators of the mentioned trial suggested that the altered osmolality of the culture microdroplets due to the dry culture approach, which compromised the development of embryos, was the main reason for the above results.

However, in both studies, the incubation was performed from day zero to day five without renewing the culture medium. In contrast, in clinical practice, most reproductive centers employ sequential incubation, which indicates that the culture medium is renewed on day 3, thereby reducing the adverse effects caused by osmolality changes. This practical approach probably is why many centers utilizing dry culture still achieve excellent pregnancy outcomes. Another prospective cohort study compared the clinical outcomes of applying a single culture medium without (one-step method) and with renewal during incubation (two-step method with culture medium renewal on day 3) [18]. This study was performed using a dry time-lapse imaging culture system. The results revealed no significant differences between the two groups concerning dynamic parameters of embryo development, clinical pregnancy rate, implantation rate, live birth rate, and neonatal weight. This result indicates that although prolonged incubation causes an increase in microdroplet osmolality, it is likely to remain within the physiological fluctuation range and therefore does not adversely affect clinical outcomes.

Therefore, finding the right volume of culture microdroplets, covering them with sufficient culture oil, mastering the abovementioned key points of culture microdroplet preparation, and performing a culture medium renewal on the third day of incubation can minimize the impact of osmolality fluctuations and can protect embryos even when using a dry incubator.

References

1. Elder K, Van den Bergh M, Woodward B. Troubleshooting and problem-solving in the IVF laboratory. Cambridge: Cambridge University Press; 2017.
2. Huang GN, Sun HX. Laboratory techniques in in vitro fertilization and embryo transfer. Beijing: People's Medical Publishing House; 2012.

3. Baltz JM, Tartia AP. Cell volume regulation in oocytes and early embryos: connecting physiology to successful culture media. Human Reprod Update. 2010;16(2):166–76.

4. Quinn P, Kerin JF, Warnes GM. Improved pregnancy rate in human in vitro fertilization with the use of a medium based on the composition of human tubal fluid. Fertil Steril. 1985;44(4):493–8.

5. Baltz JM. Media composition: salts and osmolality. Methods Mol Biol. 2012;912:61–80.

6. Camous S, Heyman Y, Meziou W, et al. Cleavage beyond the block stage and survival after transfer of early bovine embryos cultured with trophoblastic vesicles. J Reprod Fertil. 1984;72(2):479–85.

7. Bolton VN, Hawes SM, Taylor CT, et al. Development of spare human preimplantation embryos in vitro: an analysis of the correlations among gross morphology, cleavage rates, and development to the blastocyst. J In Vitro Fert Embryo Transf. 1989;6(1):30–5.

8. Hadi T, Hammer MA, Algire C, et al. Similar effects of osmolarity, glucose, and phosphate on cleavage past the 2-cell stage in mouse embryos from outbred and F1 hybrid females. Biol Reprod. 2005;72(1):179–87.

9. Swain JE, Cabrera L, Xu X, et al. Microdrop preparation factors influence culture-media osmolality, which can impair mouse embryo preimplantation development. Reprod Biomed Online. 2012;24(2):142–7.

10. Xie Y, Zhong W, Wang Y, et al. Using hyperosmolar stress to measure biologic and stress-activated protein kinase responses in preimplantation embryos. Mol Hum Reprod. 2007;13(7):473–81.

11. Bell CE, Lariviere NM, Watson PH, et al. Mitogen-activated protein kinase (MAPK) pathways mediate embryonic responses to culture medium osmolarity by regulating aquaporin 3 and 9 expression and localization, as well as embryonic apoptosis. Hum Reprod. 2009;24(6):1373–86.

12. Edashige K, Ohta S, Tanaka M, et al. The role of aquaporin 3 in the movement of water and cryoprotectants in mouse morulae. Biol Reprod. 2007;77(2):365–75.

13. Sonoda M, Okamoto F, Kajiya H, et al. Amino acid-permeable anion channels in early mouse embryos and their possible effects on cleavage1. Biol Reprod. 2003;68(3):947–53.

14. Anas MK, Hammer MA, Lever M, et al. The organic osmolytes betaine and proline are transported by a shared system in early preimplantation mouse embryos. J Cell Physiol. 2007;210(1):266–77.

15. Anas MK, Lee MB, Zhou C, et al. SIT1 is a betaine proline transporter that is activated in mouse eggs after fertilization and functions until the 2-cell stage. Development. 2008;135(24):4123–30.

16. Yumoto K, Iwata K, Sugishima M, et al. Unstable osmolality of microdrops cultured in non-humidified incubators. J Assist Reprod Genet. 2019;36(8):1571–7.

17. Fawzy M, Abdelrahman MY, Zidan MH, et al. Humid versus dry incubator: a prospective, randomized, controlled trial. Fertil Steril. 2017;108(2):277–83.

18. Costa-Borges N, Bellés M, Meseguer M, et al. Blastocyst development in single medium with or without renewal on day 3: a prospective cohort study on sibling donor oocytes in a time-lapse incubator. Fertil Steril. 2016;105(3):707–13.

Hydrogen Ion Concentration Index of Culture Media

4

The hydrogen ion concentration index, commonly referred to as "pH," with "p" derived from the German word "Potenz" and "H" for hydrogen ion. The pH is the ratio of the total count of hydrogen ions to the total amount of substance in a solution. Its value depends on the binding of compounds in the solution and various factors that affect the hydrogen ion equilibrium. The pH value is dynamic, and the process of pH change in a particular aqueous solution during in vitro culture can be roughly divided into three phases: equilibration, set value, and stabilization (Fig. 4.1) [1]. It is worth noting that pH results from a logarithmic calculation, and a slight change in pH means a considerable change in H^+ concentration. The acceptable pH range for an embryo culture medium is between 7.2 and 7.4, and there is a 60% difference in H^+ concentration between the two—a difference could result in dramatic effects on oocytes and embryos. Therefore, pH changes in the culture system should be minimized and continuously monitored, and pH stability is essential to quality management in the IVF laboratory.

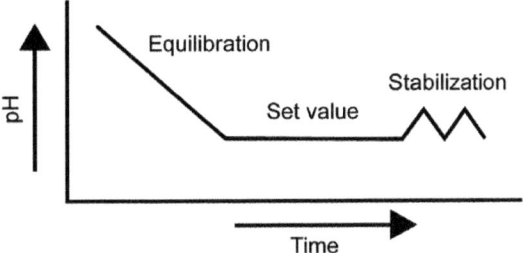

Fig. 4.1 The three phases of pH change

4.1 Regulation of Hydrogen Ion Concentration Index in Cells and the Influencing Factors

4.1.1 Intracellular pH and its Importance

A stable intracellular pH (pH_i) is one of the vital influences of cellular homeostasis. Intracellular pH regulates many physiological processes, such as protein conformation, cell division and differentiation, glycolysis, cytoskeleton dynamics, and other critical metabolic, cellular transport, and epigenetic functions [2]. As such, a slight change in pH_i can compromise embryonic development. The embryo primarily utilizes pyruvate and lactate as the primary energy source during early development in culture, which are metabolized through oxidative phosphorylation in the mitochondria. In order to produce adenosine triphosphate (ATP), a proton gradient must be formed across the inner mitochondrial membrane, with a high concentration of H^+ in the intermembrane space and a low concentration of H^+ in the mitochondrial matrix [3]. H^+ is free to pass through the outer mitochondrial membrane but not the inner mitochondrial membrane. When mitochondria are exposed to a low pH environment, ATP can be produced by the action of ATP synthase. Changes in pH_i values will cause variations in the basic biochemical metabolic pathways that rely on mitochondria for ATP supply, thus exerting significant influences on cellular metabolism.

For the pH_i of mammalian oocytes and embryos in an in vitro culture environment (Table 4.1), values provided by different research teams slightly vary, which may be due to differ-

ences in culture media, CO_2 setting values, maternal age, and ovarian function. Furthermore, in vivo measurement of the pH_i of mammalian oocytes and embryos is difficult.

4.1.2 pH_i Regulation in Oocytes and Embryos

1. Classical pH_i Regulating Ion Channels
    Stable pH_i values in mammalian gametes and embryos are mainly achieved through a variety of ion channels, with classical regulatory systems including HCO_3^-/Cl^- exchangers (to relieve alkalosis), Na^+/H^+ exchangers (to relieve acidosis), and Na^+-dependent HCO_3^-/Cl^- exchangers (to relieve acidosis) (Fig. 4.2) [13].
    (a) HCO_3^-/Cl^- exchangers: They can relieve alkalosis. In human embryos, a pH_i value higher than 7.2–7.3 will activate HCO_3^-/Cl^- exchange, allowing Cl^- to enter the cell while moving HCO_3^- out of the cell, thereby reducing the pH_i.
    (b) Na^+/H^+ exchangers: They can relieve acidosis. In human embryos, as the pH_i value

Table 4.1 pH_i values of human and mouse oocytes and embryos cultured in vitro

Species	Oocyte or embryo stage	Mean pH_i	Authors (year of publication)
Human	GV	7.30	Dale et al. (1998) [4]
		7.04	Phillips et al. (2000) [5]
	MI	7.03	Phillips et al. (2000)
	MII	7.40	Dale et al. (1998)
		6.98	Phillips et al. (2000)
	Fertilized oocytes	7.40	Dale et al. (1998)
	Cleavage stage	7.12	Phillips et al. (2000)
Mouse	GV	6.96	Phillips and Baltz (1996) [6]
		~7.11	FitzHarris and Baltz (2006) [7]
	MII	7.13	House (1994) [8]
		7.00	Phillips and Baltz (1996)
	Fertilized oocytes	7.02	Phillips and Baltz (1996)
	1-cell	~7.10	Zhao et al. (1995, 1996) [9, 10]
	2-cell	~7.10	Zhao et al. (1995, 1996)
		7.19	Edwards et al. (1998a, b) [11, 12]
	8–16 cell	7.21	Edwards et al. (1998a, b)
	Morula	~7.10	Zhao et al. (1995, 1996)
		7.22	Edwards et al. (1998a, b)
	Blastocyst	~7.10	Zhao et al. (1995, 1996)

GV germinal vesicle, *MI* metaphase I, *MII* metaphase I

Fig. 4.2 Classical pH_i regulatory systems

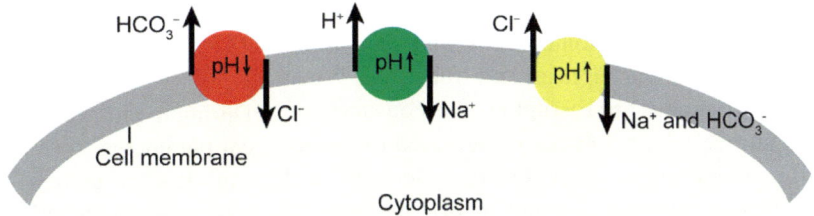

drops below 6.8, Na⁺/H⁺ exchange will be activated, allowing Na⁺ to enter the cell while moving H⁺ out of the cell, with the effect of elevating the pH_i.

(c) Na⁺-dependent HCO_3^-/Cl^- exchangers: They can relieve acidosis. In human embryos, when the pH_i value drops below 7.0, the Na⁺-dependent HCO_3^-/Cl^- exchangers will be activated, allowing HCO_3^- and Na⁺ to enter the cell while moving Cl^- out of the cell, with the effect of elevating the pH_i.

2. pH_i regulation in oocytes and embryos at various stages.

   Oocytes exhibit a relatively weak ability to regulate pH_i. Their pH_i regulating ability gradually improves as they develop into cleavage stage embryos and becomes better refined as they develop into morulas and blastocysts.

(a) Oocytes: Right now, there are few studies on the pH_i regulation function of human oocytes, while most research results were obtained from animal experiments. Dale et al. used human eggs that had failed fertilization as study subjects and showed that they could recover to physiological pH_i after being subjected to alkaline stress (pH = 8.0); however, they could not recover to physiological pH_i after being subjected to acidic stress [4].

   The oocyte of mice initiates its pH_i regulation when the oocyte in the follicle develops to 80% of its normal volume. Before that, the pH_i regulation of the oocyte rested only on the granulosa cells [7]. When the oocyte matures, its internal pH_i regulation is deactivated and then reactivated the following fertilization.

   HCO_3^-/Cl^- exchangers in mice germinal vesicle (GV) phase oocytes are highly active. However, their activity is inhibited during the meiotic maturation of the oocytes (conversion from MI to MII). The activity change pattern of Na⁺/H⁺ exchangers is basically the same as that of HCO_3^-/Cl^- exchangers. The activity of Na⁺-dependent HCO_3^-/Cl^- exchangers changes in the opposite direction from the previous two, with the activity in MII oocytes and zygotes being greater than that in GV-phase oocytes.

(b) Cleavage stage embryos: Human cleavage stage embryos can maintain their pH_i stability to some extent. They can alleviate alkalosis with the help of HCO_3^-/Cl^- exchangers, and acidosis with the help of Na⁺/H⁺ exchangers.

(c) Morulas and blastocysts: Mammalian morulas and blastocysts have more refined pH_i regulating capabilities. On the one hand, mouse morulas can adapt well to a weak acid environment. This pH_i regulation ability is associated with the tight junctions between morula cells. This adaptive capacity is compatible with the physiological state. When the embryo develops into a morula and then a blastocyst, it is in the relatively acidic uterine cavity (compared to the oviduct). On the other hand, morulas and blastocysts can also maintain pH_i stability in a weak alkaline environment. However, their HCO_3^-/Cl^- exchangers are inactive, so other mechanisms likely mediate this stabilizing effect.

4.1.3   Extracellular pH and Its Importance

Although embryos can maintain their intracellular homeostasis before implantation, extracellular pH (pH_e) changes may cause cellular stress responses. The pH_e and pH_i gradients are essential for ion homeostasis and can affect cells' molecular uptake and function. When such gradients are disrupted, the consumption of intracellular resources is increased to restore the homeostatic equilibrium. Oocytes and embryos can only respond to pH_e fluctuations within a specific range. For example, pH_i can stay relatively stable when pH_e is between 7.0 and 7.4. When pH_e exceeds this range, pH_i will shift and impair critical cellular functions, thus compromising fertilization and embryonic development. A slight increase in culture medium pH_e can significantly affect the development of mouse blastocysts and alter their gene expression profile [14]. Therefore, it is vital to maintain pH_e in an optimal range to minimize the adverse effects on embryos before implantation.

The pH of the human oviductal fluid and intra-uterine fluid may vary at different stages of the menstrual cycle and in different locations from the proximal to the distal part of the oviduct. Moreover, the pH_e values vary among species [13] (Table 4.2).

4.1.4 Recommended pH Range of Commercial Culture Media

During in vitro fertilization, some physicochemical parameters specific to the culture conditions can alter the embryo's pH_i and may change its requirements and adaptability. The physiological pH in the oviduct or uterus may not be optimal for the culture medium. The culture media manufacturers' recommendation is to maintain pH_e slightly above pH_i to compensate for acidification associated with cell metabolism. Therefore, commercial culture media generally recommend a pH_e range of 7.2–7.4 for embryo culture (Table 4.3).

4.1.5 Factors Influencing the pH of Culture Medium

During IVF culture, the pH_e of gametes and embryos equals the pH in the culture medium. The stability of culture medium pH is influenced by multiple factors, such as its pH buffer system, CO_2 concentration in the incubator, preparation

Table 4.2 The pH_e values of follicular fluid, oviductal fluid, and uterine secretions in mammals

Species	Part	pH_e value	Authors (year of publication)
Human	Follicles	7.27	Shalgi et al. (1972)
		7.34	Fraser et al. (1973)
		7.26	Imoedemhe et al. (1993)
	Uterus	6.50 to 6.70	Sedlis et al. (1967)
		7.12	Yedwab et al. (1976)
Cow	Oviduct	7.60	Hugentobler et al. (2004)
		6.40 to 6.70	Olds and VanDemark (1957)
	Uterus	6.96	Hugentobler et al. (2004)
Monkey	Oviduct (follicular phase)	7.20	Maas et al. (1977)
	Oviduct (ovulatory phase)	7.60	Maas et al. (1977)
Rabbit	Oviduct	7.80 to 8.20	Hamner and Williams (1965)
		7.90	Vishwakarma (1962)
	Isthmus	~7.24	Beier (1974)
	Infundibulum	~7.67	Beier (1974)
	Uterus	7.90	Iritani et al. (1971)
		7.40 to 7.80	Beier (1974)
		7.80	Vishwakarma (1962)
Sheep	Oviduct	7.40	Iritani et al. (1969)
		6.80 to 7.00	Hadek (1953)
	Uterus	7.00	Iritani et al. (1969)

Table 4.3 Recommended pH ranges for commercial culture media

Brand	Culture medium	Culture stage	Recommended CO_2 concentration	Recommended pH range
Brand 1	Sydney IVF fertilization	Oocyte incubation, fertilization	6%	7.30 to 7.50
	Sydney IVF cleavage	Cleavage stage embryo	6%	7.30 to 7.50
	Sydney IVF blastocyst	8-cell to blastocyst, embryo transfer	6%	7.20 to 7.40
Brand 2	Quinns advantage fertilization	Oocyte incubation, fertilization	5%	7.20 to 7.40
	Quinns advantage cleavage	Cleavage stage embryo	5%	7.10 to 7.30
	Quinns advantage blastocyst	8-cell to blastocyst	5%	7.20 to 7.40
Brand 3	G-IVF	Oocyte incubation, fertilization	6%	7.20 to 7.40
	G-1	Cleavage stage embryo	6%	7.20 to 7.34
	G-2	8-cell to blastocyst, embryo transfer	6%	7.20 to 7.34

The recommended CO_2 concentrations are applicable to low-altitude areas

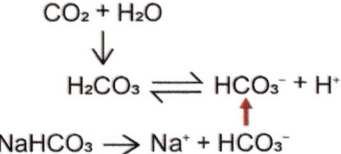

Fig. 4.3 Bicarbonate buffer system

protocol of the culture system, culture method, and altitude. It is therefore imperative to understand how pH changes under the influence of the above factors to ensure stable operation of the IVF culture system.

1. pH buffering system of culture medium

   The pH buffering system helps maintain a stable pH in the culture medium. Culture media can be broadly divided into main media and handling media, which require different buffer systems.

   (a) Main culture medium

   The main culture medium is used for the routine culture of gametes and embryos in the incubator, with bicarbonate as its pH buffering system. The pH level of the main culture medium is primarily maintained by sodium bicarbonate along with in-incubator CO_2 (Fig. 4.3). The concentration of sodium bicarbonate is determined by the commercial culture medium, while the CO_2 concentration in the incubator is set by the laboratory staff. The bicarbonate buffer system reduces the pH fluctuations caused by embryo metabolism and keeps the culture medium pH within the recommended range.

   (b) Handling medium for gametes and embryos.

   The handling medium is used for out-of-incubator manipulation of gametes and embryos, such as sperm washing, oocyte pick-up, ICSI, embryo transfer, freezing, and thawing (Table 4.4). Common pH buffer systems include phosphate-buffered saline (PBS), 4-(2-hydroxyethyl)-1-piperazineethanesulfonic acid (HEPES) buffer system, and 3-(N-morpholino)-propanesulfonic acid (MOPS) buffer system, all of which can maintain the physiological pH in the atmosphere.

   The PBS buffer system was more commonly used in IVF laboratories in the early days and can maintain a stable pH in the handling medium. However, a wealth of evidence from further studies suggests that the PBS buffer system is detrimental to embryonic development [15], for example, by disrupting cellular metabolic processes, altering organelle distribution,

Table 4.4 Application range of buffer solutions [15]

Buffer solution	Sperm washing	Oocyte pick-up	ICSI	Embryo transfer	Cryopreservation
PBS	?	×	?	?	Vitrification of blastocysts
HEPES	√	√	√	√	Slow freezing and vitrification of gametes and embryos
MOPS	√	√	√	√	Vitrification of oocytes and embryos, slow freezing of sperms

"√" means applicable, "?" means not yet known, "×" means not recommended

and affecting intracellular ion homeostasis. As a result, the PBS buffer system is rarely used in embryo laboratories and has been replaced by HEPES and MOPS.

HEPES is a zwitterionic organic buffer, which can react with both H^+ and OH^- in solution. The effects of the HEPES buffer system on gamete and embryo development have been quite intensively studied, with both supporting and opposing evidence. It is worth noting that the confounding effects of relevant factors such as osmolality, ion concentration, pH, CO_2 level, and exposure time should all be fully considered when discussing HEPES cytotoxicity. The judicious use of HEPES does not affect the developmental outcome of the embryo when the above conditions are properly addressed. The pH of the HEPES buffer will be reduced when exposed to an incubator with a CO_2 concentration of 6%, making it acidic. Therefore, it is important to secure the lid when placing vials with HEPES buffer into a 6% CO_2 incubator [16].

MOPS has the same properties as HEPES and is also a zwitterionic buffer, which can better maintain pH stability in response to environmental changes. Moreover, MOPS has yielded favorable outcomes for its application in IVF laboratories. However, the effects of MOPS on cellular physiological activities remain controversial. It can interfere with taurine uptake by tumor cells and alter the electrical conductivity of chloride in neuronal cells [17, 18]. Whether these impacts can

be present in germ cells is still subject to further study.

Furthermore, it has been found that the pH in HEPES or MOPS buffer systems increases as the temperature decreases. Given the above-mentioned inconclusive evidence of their embryotoxicity, exposing gametes or embryos in vitro for an extremely long period is not recommended. This is especially true for denuded oocytes, which are highly sensitive to pH changes.

2. CO_2

During the in vitro culture of fertilized embryos, CO_2 in the incubator dissolves in the culture medium and forms carbonic acid. As a result, the pH_e will depend on the equilibration between the in-incubator CO_2 concentration and the bicarbonate concentration in the culture medium, which is also the main premise for adjusting the pH of the culture medium. The bicarbonate concentration is predetermined by the manufacturer of the commercial culture medium, which means that the pH adjustment is primarily achieved by changing the CO_2 concentration in the incubator. The CO_2 concentration inside the incubator is usually set between 5% and 6%. The specific set concentration value can refer to the recommended CO_2 concentration in the commercial media manual and can be fine-tuned according to the measured pH in the culture medium—increase the CO_2 concentration to lower the pH, and decrease the CO_2 concentration to elevate the pH. The understanding of pH_e is based on Fig. 4.1, where the time required to reach equilibration is related to the time taken for CO_2 to diffuse into the culture medium and the time of the above reaction. The frequency of opening and closing the incubator door, the duration of the door opening, or other events that would disturb the CO_2 concentration can also cause pH_e fluctuations. Therefore, small or mini benchtop incubators are more advantageous than large incubators for rapidly restoring CO_2 stability inside the incubator. However, they also have the disadvantage of a more significant drop in CO_2 concentration at the moment of opening the door.

3. In vitro culture system for embryos

   Like osmolality and temperature, the pH equilibration of the culture medium is directly related to the culture system used. The volume of the medium in the culture dish, whether it is covered with tissue culture oil, and the time of equilibration can all affect the pH of the culture medium. The pH change of the culture medium in a culture dish without oil coverage is very sensitive to the different environments inside and outside the incubator. 1 mL of medium in a four-well dish takes 2 h to reach a stable pH in a 5% CO_2 environment, while 0.5 mL of medium is much faster to reach equilibrium under the same conditions. When a culture dish containing 1 mL of culture medium is removed from the incubator and placed at 37 °C, the pH of the culture medium will soon rise to a non-physiological state. The pH in a 1 mL medium can increase to 7.52 after 5 mins of exposure to air, while the pH in a 0.5 mL medium can increase to 7.77 under the same conditions [19]. Covering the medium with oil mitigates the rapid pH changes but also greatly increases the time required to reach equilibrium in the incubator. CO_2 diffuses very slowly in the oil, and when 0.5 mL of culture medium is covered with 0.5 mL of oil, it takes 12 h to reach a stable pH in the incubator [16]. In addition, the source and concentration of protein also affect pH_e.

4. Culture time

   There was a significant difference between the pH in the culture medium on day one and day four in continuous 4-day culture. However, despite the change in pH, the values still fell within the acceptable range for embryos (7.2 to 7.4). The reason for this pH change could be the accumulation of metabolites of amino acids (e.g., NH_4^+) in the culture medium coupled with the evaporation of water.

5. Altitude

   The altitude at which the laboratory is located and the corresponding atmospheric pressure may also be one of the factors influencing pH. Even with the same CO_2 concentration provided and the same culture medium, laboratories at different altitudes may yield different equilibration times or different pH values. Theoretically, higher CO_2 concentrations should be adopted in incubators at high altitudes to get the optimal pH of the culture medium. More specifically, a CO_2 concentration of 6% can be applied in plain areas to maintain culture medium pH in the range of 7.2–7.4, and it should be increased by 0.6% for every 1 km of elevation gain.

4.2   Effect of Hydrogen Ion Concentration Index on Gametes and Embryos

The pH regulates many cellular physiological processes, such as the stability of the meiotic spindle of the oocyte, cell division and differentiation, embryonic enzyme activity, and blastocoel formation [20]. There is growing evidence that culture conditions during in vitro fertilization play a decisive role in favorable fertilization outcomes and that a quick change in pHi may impair the embryo's development. Culture conditions are critical not only for pre-implantation embryo development but also for post-implantation embryo development and its long-term health [21, 22].

4.2.1   Oocyte

The ability of the oocyte to regulate its pH_i is not yet well established, and hence the stability of the pH_e value is very important for the oocyte.

Spindle disturbance may lead to the formation of aneuploidy and stalled maturation. pH_e can also affect the oocyte fertilization process. In conventional in vitro fertilization, when pH_e increases from 7.0 to 7.5, the rate of oocyte fertilization and the rate of oocyte cleavage are significantly improved [20]. Furthermore, the pH_i of oocytes may also be influenced by maternal age, which is up to 7.6 in older mice. An elevated pH_i can affect the action of adhesion proteins and may increase the incidence of aneuploidy.

4.2.2   Cleavage Stage Embryos

It was demonstrated in animal experiments that acidification or alkalinization of embryonic pH_i during cleavage would impair the outcome of embryonic development with a temporal effect. Embryonic damage is irreversible when cells are acidified or alkalinized for more than 12 h, whereas it is partially reversible if it does not exceed 12 h. Lowering the pH_i of mouse 1-cell stage embryos from 7.25 to 7.10 and sustaining it for 19 h can result in a significant decrease in the number of blastocyst cells, an increase in the level of apoptosis, and a significant decrease in fetal top-rump length and weight [23].

Either acidification or alkalinization of embryonic pH_i during cleavage will compromise organelle distribution. When the pH_i of a hamster embryo is increased from 7.2 to 7.4 or decreased to 6.8 for 3 h, the localization of cytoskeletal actin microfilaments will be disrupted, and the distribution of mitochondria will change (from an initial distribution mainly around the nucleus to a uniform distribution throughout the cytoplasm) [24].

Acidification or alkalinization of embryonic pH_i during cleavage will impair the metabolic processes of the embryo. pH_i can also affect enzyme activity—for example, pH_i above 7.2 stimulates the activity of phosphofructokinase (PFK), and even very mild changes in pH (0.2) can affect PFK activity. Increased PFK activity may prematurely activate the glycolytic process and reduce aerobic metabolism, possibly contributing to developmental arrest. Furthermore, a weakly acidic extracellular medium reduces pH_i in early mouse embryos, decreasing glycolytic activity. This effect was not found in mouse morulas, suggesting that the morula may have a more efficient pH regulation system [12].

4.2.3   Blastocysts

pH regulation is also important for mammalian blastocyst development. The blastocoele formation is driven by the osmolality gradient caused by the accumulation of sodium ions inside the cavity. The activity of Na^+/H^+ exchange contributes to the passage of Na^+ through the trophectoderm and is required for blastocoele expansion [25, 26].

4.3   Monitoring of Hydrogen Ion Concentration Index

4.3.1   Methods of pH Measurement

Common methods of pH measurement include an acid-base indicator, pH test strips, pH meter, and blood gas analyzer.

1. Acid-base indicator: Most acid-base indicators are organic pigments. After adding a pH indicator to the solution to be measured, different indicators will change color according to different pH values, and the pH range can be determined according to the color of the solution. For example, the color change interval of methyl orange is from pH 3.1 to 4.4. The solution is red when the pH is <3.1 and yellow when the pH is >4.4 after adding methyl orange.

2. pH test strips: The pH of the solution can be measured by dipping a small amount of the solution onto the test strip with a glass rod and then comparing the strip's color with the standard colorimetric card after the test strip has finished changing color. It is worth noting that the pH test strip relies on hydrogen ions for its action, but oil does not contain hydrogen ions. Thus, pH test strips cannot indicate the pH level of oil.

3. pH meter: pH meter is a more economical instrument to measure the pH value of a solution, and the pH value is measured through a pH selective electrode (such as a glass electrode), which can be accurate to two decimal places.

4. Blood gas analyzer: It is an instrument that utilizes electrodes to measure pH, partial pressure of carbon dioxide, partial pressure of oxygen, and other related indexes in a relatively fast manner. It is quick and easy to operate but relatively expensive.

4.3.2 pH Measurement in IVF Laboratories

1. pH meter: IVF labs mostly use pH meters to measure pH. The pH meters used in IVF laboratories usually have dual-composite (glass and reference electrodes) or tri-composite electrodes (integrating a temperature compensated probe) and need to be calibrated with reference samples before each use. There are two points to note when using such devices:

    (a) pH measurement with a pH meter is highly dependent on temperature, so calibration and sample measurement should be performed and recorded at the same temperature. Temperature affects the detection result in two major ways: a. by slightly changing the conductivity of the hydrogen ion; b. by causing a temperature effect on the electrode, resulting in a slight measurement error (0.01 to 0.02 pH unit/°C). A good pH meter should be equipped with a probe that compensates for temperature.

    (b) Proteins in the medium can cause pH measurement errors, because proteins tend to adhere to the electrode's glass membrane and block it. The electrode can be cleaned with detergent or regenerated with fluorine or hydrochloric acid, but there is a risk of damage to the electrode. When using a detergent, one may place the electrode in a 60 °C water bath for

30 min. However, regeneration and cleaning are not always effective; the best method is replacing the electrode.

2. Tips for using pH meters: IVF laboratories must have standard operating procedures for pH measurement, calibration, and pH meter maintenance. pH measurement is considered one of the basic operations IVF lab personnel must master with proficiency. However, many lab technicians are unfamiliar with the operating instructions to use pH meters properly. They are not systematically trained after purchase, do not have sufficient understanding of the device's performance, or do not keep detailed records during use. Laboratory personnel should read the manual carefully and follow the manufacturer's instructions for handling, cleaning, storage, and calibration of the electrodes. The following are some tips for measuring pH in IVF laboratories with pH meters [16]:

    (a) Immerse the new electrode in a 1:1 saturated potassium chloride solution and a pH = 4 buffer solution.

    (b) The porous glass film must be kept clean to ensure that molecules can pass freely.

    (c) Use a fresh buffer solution.

    (d) Keep the temperature constant.

    (e) Mix the sample thoroughly while reading the data.

    (f) Keep the filling hole on the reference electrode open during the measurement.

    (g) Recalibration is required after 2 h of use, or after testing 20–30 samples.

3. Blood gas analyzer: The calibration and maintenance of the electrodes limit the application of pH meters, as well as the inability to directly detect the pH of culture medium microdroplets, so a portable blood gas analyzer (BGA) can be applied instead. It is operated by adding a small amount of culture medium onto a special pH test card with a syringe or pipette and inserting it into the machine. Moreover, the result can be read within 2 min. It is convenient, fast, and suitable for testing culture medium microdroplets that are equilibrated in various incubators, but it also has the drawback of being more costly.

It is still controversial whether BGA can replace pH meters or not. Because the calibration buffer used for the pH meter (pH electrode) conforms to the metrological traceability standard, indicating more accurate and reliable measurement results. Furthermore, since the BGA is not designed to test IVF culture media, its accuracy can only be verified by comparing the results with a pH meter or by analyzing the CO_2 response curve (i.e., the correlation between CO_2 and pH). Juan D. et al. concluded that although the BGA offers fairly good precision, a comparison with the pH meter revealed that it was not as accurate [27], probably because some particular components of the culture medium can interfere with the BGA. A study by Swain et al. showed that a portable BGA and a pH meter gave essentially the same results at 37 °C but showed a large difference at 23 °C. The authors, therefore, concluded that any pH testing device should be fully validated before being applied in clinical IVF laboratories [28].

References

1. Swain JE. Optimizing the culture environment in the IVF laboratory: impact of pH and buffer capacity on gamete and embryo quality. Reprod Biomed Online. 2010;21(1):6–16.
2. Swain JE, Pool TB. New pH-buffering system for media utilized during gamete and embryo manipulations for assisted reproduction. Reprod Biomed Online. 2009;18(6):799–810.
3. Jovin IS. The cell: a molecular approach. Yale J Biol Med. 2003;76(3):139–40.
4. Dale B, Menezo Y, Cohen J, et al. Intracellular pH regulation in the human oocyte. Hum Reprod. 1998;13(4):964–70.
5. Phillips KP, Léveillé MC, Claman P, et al. Intracellular pH regulation in human preimplantation embryos. Hum Reprod. 2000;15(4):896–904.
6. Phillips KP, Baltz JM. Intracellular pH change does not accompany egg activation in the mouse. Mol Reprod Dev. 1996;45(1):52–60.
7. Fitzharris G, Baltz JM. Granulosa cells regulate intracellular pH of the murine growing oocyte via gap junctions: development of independent homeostasis during oocyte growth. Development. 2006;133(4):591–9.
8. House CR. Confocal ratio-imaging of intracellular pH in unfertilised mouse oocytes. Zygote. 1994;2(1):37–45.
9. Zhao Y, Chauvet PJ, Alper SL, et al. Expression and function of bicarbonate/chloride exchangers in the preimplantation mouse embryo. J Biol Chem. 1995;270(41):24428–34.
10. Zhao Y, Baltz JM. Bicarbonate/chloride exchange and intracellular pH throughout preimplantation mouse embryo development. Am J Phys. 1996;271(5 Pt 1):C1512–20.
11. Edwards LJ, Williams DA, Gardner DK. Intracellular pH of the mouse preimplantation embryo: amino acids act as buffers of intracellular pH. Hum Reprod. 1998a;13(12):3441–8.
12. Edwards LJ, Williams DA, Gardner DK. Intracellular pH of the preimplantation embryo: effects of extracellular pH and weak acids. Mol Reprod Dev. 1998b;50(4):434–42.
13. Swain JE. Is there an optimal pH for culture media used in clinical IVF? Hum Reprod Update. 2012;18(3):333–9.
14. Koustas G, Sjoblom C. Epigenetic consequences of pH stress in mouse embryos. Hum Reprod. 2011;26:i78.
15. Will MA, Clark NA, Swain JE. Biological pH buffers in IVF: help or hindrance to success. J Assist Reprod Genet. 2011;28(8):711–24.
16. Elder K, Van den Bergh M, Woodward B. Troubleshooting and problem-solving in the IVF laboratory. Cambridge: Cambridge University Press; 2015.
17. Wersinger C, Rebel G, Lelong-Rebel IH. Characterisation of taurine uptake in human KB MDR and non-MDR tumour cell lines in culture. Anticancer Res. 2001;21(5):3397–406.
18. Schmidt J, Mangold C, Deitmer J. Membrane responses evoked by organic buffers in identified leech neurones. J Exp Biol. 1996;199(Pt 2):327–35.
19. Conaghan J. Culture media, solutions, and systems in human ART: pH control in the embryo culture environment. Cambridge: Cambridge University Press; 2014.
20. Gatimel N, Moreau J, Parinaud J, et al. Need for choosing the ideal pH value for IVF culture media. J Assist Reprod Genet. 2020;37(5):1019–28.
21. Dumoulin JC, Land JA, Van Montfoort AP, et al. Effect of in vitro culture of human embryos on birthweight of newborns. Hum Reprod. 2010;25(3):605–12.
22. Nelissen EC, Van Montfoort AP, Coonen E, et al. Further evidence that culture media affect perinatal outcome: findings after transfer of fresh and cryopreserved embryos. Hum Reprod. 2012;27(7):1966–76.
23. Zander-Fox DL, Mitchell M, Thompsonet JG, et al. Repercussions of a transient decrease in pH on embryo viability and subsequent fetal development. Reprod Fertil Dev. 2008;20(9):84.
24. Squirrell JM, Lane M, Bavister BD, et al. Altering intracellular pH disrupts development and cellular

organization in preimplantation hamster embryos. Biol Reprod. 2001;64(6):1845–54.

25. Barr KJ, Garrill A, Jones DH, et al. Contributions of Na$^+$/H$^+$ exchanger isoforms to preimplantation development of the mouse. Mol Reprod Dev. 1998;50(2):146–53.

26. Watson AJ, Barcroft LC. Regulation of blastocyst formation. Front Biosci. 2001;6:D708–30.

27. Diaz de Pool JDN, Van Den Berg SAA, Pilgram GSK, et al. Validation of the blood gas analyzer for pH measurements in IVF culture medium: prevent suboptimal culture conditions. PLoS One. 2018;13(11):e0206707.

28. Swain JE. Comparison of three pH measuring devices within the IVF laboratory. Fertil Steril. 2013;100(3):S251–1.

Gas Supplies of Incubators, Air Quality, and Volatile Organic Compounds Management of the Laboratory Environment

5

A safe and stable environment for gamete and embryo culture is essential for assisted reproductive treatment, but this environment is influenced by multiple factors, one of which is gas. Regardless of ambient air or medical grade gas in an incubator, the cleanliness, purity, concentration, and the level of volatile organic compounds (VOCs) will directly affect gamete function, embryo development, and pregnancy outcomes [1, 2].

5.1 Quality Management of Gases

5.1.1 Types of Gases and Their Preparation

1. Types of gases: High-purity CO_2, high-purity N_2, and a standard gas mixture (6% CO_2, 5% O_2, and 89% N_2) are commonly used in IVF laboratories. High-purity CO_2 is mainly used to balance the culture medium containing the bicarbonate buffer system to reach the physiological pH (7.2–7.4) [3]. CO_2 is also an essential element for protein and nucleic acid synthesis during development. High-purity N_2 is mainly used to dilute the air to form a low-oxygen environment. The standard gas mixture is used for the same purpose as high-purity gases, except that it has been premixed in a fixed proportion before being delivered. High-

purity gases are compatible with all medium and large incubators, some benchtop incubators, and time-lapse culture systems on the market. Among those, the two-gas incubators mix high-purity CO_2 and air in proportion to stabilize the CO_2 concentration inside the incubator at 5–6% (at low altitude). In contrast, the three-gas incubators mix high-purity CO_2, high-purity N_2, and air in proportion to finally make the CO_2 concentration in the incubator range from 5% to 6% and O_2 concentration at 5%. Meanwhile, the standard gas mixture applies to some small benchtop incubators.

2. Purity and preparation: The gas purity is usually expressed as a percentage, and different purity is applied to various fields (Table 5.1). Indeed, the lower the gas purity, the higher the impurity components it contains. For example, food grade CO_2 is 99.9%; however, its impurities can still contain embryotoxic substances, such as benzene, methanol, and acetaldehyde [4]. Therefore, IVF laboratories should use high-purity gases with a purity of $\geq 99.999\%$, and an inline filter should usually be added to further refine the gas supply. Although gases with even higher purity ($\geq 99.9995\%$–99.9999%) are also used in some laboratories, such gases are expensive. The production of commercial high-purity gases and standard gas mixtures should comply with the standards promulgated and implemented by the local quality supervision

department. Relevant standards in China include ① *High-purity Carbon Dioxide* (GB/T 23938-2009); ② *Pure, High-purity, and Ultra-purity Nitrogen* (GB/T 8979-2008); and ③ *Gas Analysis—Preparation of Calibration Gas Mixtures—Part 1: Gravimetric Method for Class I Mixtures* (ISO 6142-1:2015). Among them, the industrial manufactured high-purity CO_2 mainly comes from the tail gas of hydrogen plants, ammonia plants, iron, and steel plants, petrochemical plants, cement plants, and brewing industries, and a small portion comes from natural gas CO_2 gas wells, which then recovered by physical absorption, chemical absorption, variable pressure adsorption, membrane separation, and distil-lation separation. The recovered CO_2 raw gas is purified through acid washing, water washing, dehydration, desulfurization, drying, adsorption, and distillation, and then liquefied and filled. High-purity N_2 is generally produced by the deep-cooled air separation method, which characterizes high-product purity ($\geq 99.999\%$) output without further purification, making high-purity N_2 relatively inexpensive. The standard gas mixture is made of high-purity gases in specific proportions in the first place and then combined with an inline filter; thus, impurities are not much concerning. However, gases from major manufacturers should be preferred as much as possible to ensure the proportion accuracy of each gas component.

3. Inline gas filter (Fig. 5.1): Activated carbon combined with a high-efficiency particulate air filter (HEPA) or poly tetra fluoroethylene microporous membrane can adsorb VOCs, bacteria, and other impurities in the gas, thus improving embryonic development and pregnancy outcome [5]. It should be noted that the activated carbon may become saturated, which is dependent on the quality of the gas, so the in-service date of the filter should be recorded, and the filter should be replaced regularly while taking into account both the manufacturer's requirements and the actual culture results.

Table 5.1 Application fields of CO_2

Purity (V/V)	Grade	Application fields
$\geq 99\%$	Industrial grade	Chemical raw material production, refrigerant, and metal smelting
$\geq 99.9\%$	Food grade	Food additives, raw materials, preservation, and storage
$\geq 99.998\%$	Electronic grade	Semiconductor manufacturing, and instrument analysis
$\geq 99.99\%$–99.999%	Medical grade	Surgery, pharmaceutical, scientific research, and cell culture

V/V volume fraction

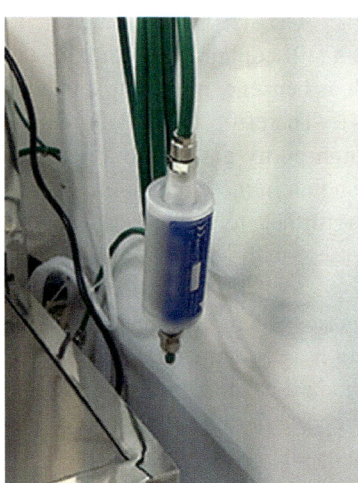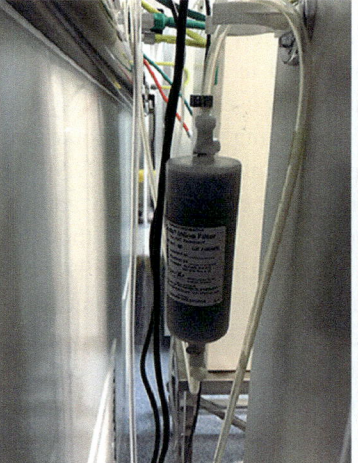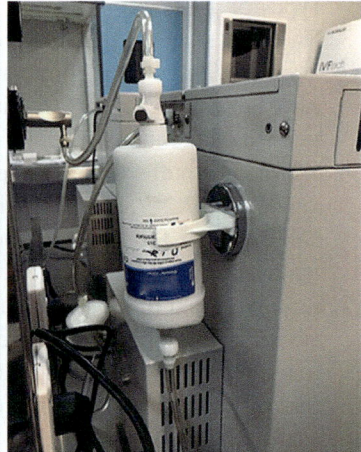

Fig. 5.1 Inline filters of different brands for VOCs removal

5.1.2 Safety Management of Gas Cylinders

Gas cylinders should adhere to the quality standard promulgated and implemented by the local quality supervision department. Cylinders for different gases should have their exclusive colors for identification [6], such as aluminum white for carbon dioxide cylinders and black for nitrogen cylinders. A quality certificate should be attached to each gas cylinder, containing the product name, manufacturer, production date, and purity information.

For safety concerns, gas cylinders should be stored in a dedicated room outside the main building [7]. In IVF laboratories, a dedicated, separate gases supply room from the culture room should be available, considering that the cylinders can be the source of contamination. A safe and stable gas supply is a fundamental component of an IVF laboratory, which makes the design of the gas supply room and the safety management of the storage and use of gas cylinders particularly important:

1. The gas supply room, in which gas cylinders were located, is strictly prohibited from being near fire, heat sources, and corrosive environment.
2. The gas supply room must be equipped with explosion-proof switches and lamps, and the use of an open flame is prohibited around such rooms.
3. The gas supply room should be thoroughly ventilated, especially for the room where nitrogen is stored. At least three air exchanges per hour should be ensured, and it is recommended to install low O_2 monitoring devices and keep the room cool and shaded.
4. No miscellaneous items are allowed in the gas supply room.
5. Gas cylinders must be placed upright when stored and used, and it is strictly prohibited to put them down when used. The connection part of the gas cylinder and pipeline is at the upper end, which should be under special protection (such as partitions and chains) to prevent the cylinder from tipping over and pulling off the pipeline (Fig. 5.2).
6. Empty cylinders and full cylinders should be partitioned, and some manufacturers' cylinders are equipped with "full," "in use," and "empty" labels to facilitate identification (Fig. 5.3).
7. When the gas is delivered, the quality certificate of each cylinder should be checked, the types and quantities of each delivery should be recorded, and the cylinders should be wiped clean and placed in the gas supply room.
8. Always maintain adequate full gas cylinders for backup.
9. Avoid bumping during gas cylinder transportation and/or relocation, as violent bumping may lead to cylinder damage. If there is any sign of damage or gas leakage, contact the supplier immediately for a replacement.
10. Recording the gas cylinder pressure loss daily is recommended to predict the service life of a gas cylinder or a group of gas cylinders. A shorter usage duration is found to significantly indicate a gas leak, and the cylinder should be inspected promptly. To examine for leaks, one may apply soap, water, or hand sanitizer solution to the suspected leak site, and the presence of bubbles that gradually

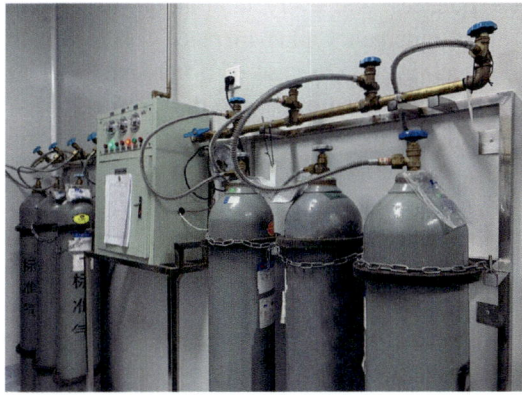

Fig. 5.2 Gas pipeline manifold: alternate gas supply between the left and right groups, with an automatic gas switching device in the middle (containing a level 1 pressure reducing valve), and the cylinders are partitioned and secured by chains

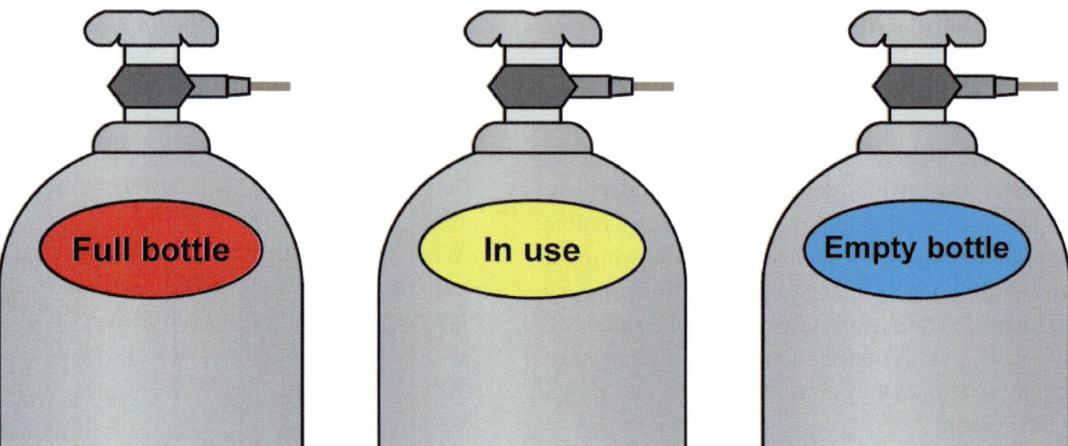

Fig. 5.3 Gas usage labels: full cylinder (red); in use (yellow); empty cylinder (blue)

become bigger indicates a leak. However, with only a slight leakage, very careful observation is required. If a leak does exist or cannot be located, a professional person should be contacted in time for inspection and repair. Leaking sites are commonly located at the cylinder valve, the connection between the cylinder and pipeline and/or the pressure reducing valve.

11. Develop emergency plans for gas leaks. Gas leaks in laboratories are mostly slight leaks at the joints of gas lines, while leaks in the middle of the pipe body are rare. Massive pipeline gas leaks pose very serious consequences, and every laboratory should have an emergency plan in place to prepare for such events. In case of a massive gas leak, the gas pressure alarm in the room will be set off; the incubator will also set off an alarm alert due to the cessation of the gas supply. At this time, the gas cylinder valve should be switched off immediately, a backup gas cylinder should be directly connected to the incubator to secure the embryos, and professionals should be contacted in time for inspection and repair of the pipeline. A significant gas leak can also threaten the lives of those working on site. A large amount of inhaled carbon dioxide will combine with hemoglobin to form carboxyhemoglobin, causing red blood cells to lose the ability to carry oxygen, which will trigger dizziness,

vomiting, and other symptoms arising from brain cell hypoxia, so personnel should be quickly evacuated in the event of a carbon dioxide leak. A nitrogen leak can cause suffocation of a person due to lack of oxygen, which can lead to the so-called nitrogen narcosis and even coma and death in severe cases. Therefore, in addition to evacuation, the leaking area should also be isolated with strict access restrictions. The asphyxiated person should be rescued from the scene to fresh air as soon as possible and ensure that he or she can breathe freely. In case of massive gas leakage, professionals should be contacted to handle the situation on the premise of ensuring their own safety.

5.1.3   Gas Output and Pressure Adjustment

1. Gas output: Since the gas supply room is separated from the culture room, a robust piping system is required to deliver gases to incubators within the culture room. The following pipe-laying standards should be considered [7]: (a) Gas pipelines for gas purity of ≥99.99% should be made of stainless steel, copper, or seamless steel pipes. The gas pipeline in our center is made of molybdenum-containing stainless steel, commonly known as 316 stainless steels. (b) The connections

between high-purity gas pipes should be socket welded. (c) Flanges or threaded connectors should be used to connect the gas pipeline to the equipment, valves, and other accessories. These pipe-laying standards are designed to make the pipeline system resistant to high-temperature, corrosion, and leakage, thereby safeguarding a safe and stable gas output.

Centers with high gas consumption usually use manifolds for gas supply which are fitted with automatic switching devices and two groups of gas cylinders (Fig. 5.2), thus enabling an alternate supply of gas from two groups of cylinders. In this case, when the pressure of one group of gas cylinders drops to the set lower limit, the system will automatically switch to the other group of full cylinders. The empty group should be replaced with full cylinders as soon as possible. Moreover, it is recommended against setting the lower pressure limit of automatic switching to 0 to avoid completely exhausting the gas in the cylinder. The reasons are as follows: (a) The gas in the cylinder shall not be completely used up, and the residual pressure of a permanent gas cylinder shall be not less than 0.05 megapascal (MPa); the cylinder of liquefied gas should have residual gas not less than 0.5%–1.0% of the specified filling volume [8]. The "base gas" left in the cylinder can maintain a certain level of pressure to prevent outside air or impurities from entering the cylinder. For example, oxygen entering the bottle will corrode the inner wall, while the entry of impurities will compromise the purity of the re-filled gas. (b) Some scholars also believe that high-pressure liquefied gases (such as CO_2) may also be a source of VOCs, such as acetaldehyde, isovaleraldehyde, benzaldehyde, and formaldehyde, which can be dissolved in liquid carbon dioxide without transforming to the gaseous phase. When the pressure in the gas cylinder becomes low, these aldehydes will turn into gas and get into the incubator [9]. All the gases used in our center are of 99.999% purity, and inline filters

Table 5.2 Gas input pressures of incubators in our center

Incubator	Model	Gas input pressure
Brand 1	3131	0.1034 MPa
Brand 2	APM-30D	0.03–0.05 MPa
Brand 3	K-MINC-1000	0.15 ± 0.015 MPa
Brand 4	C200	0.08 MPa, must not exceed 0.1 MPa
Brand 5	MRI-TL8	0.06 MPa

are installed in the pipeline for VOCs removal to minimize such risks.

2. Gas pressure control: Different incubators require specific gas input pressures (Table 5.2), and the cylinder output pressure is much higher than the input pressure required by the terminal equipment. For a more precise adjustment of the gas pressure and to protect the equipment, the gases will go from the cylinder into the pipeline at various levels before they get into the incubator, with a three-level pressure reduction achieved by adjustable pressure reducing valves (Fig. 5.4). Take the standard gas mixture output as an example: the output pressure of the cylinder is around 12 MPa, which will be reduced to about 0.8 MPa after the first level of pressure reduction, then reduced to about 0.4 MPa after the second level of pressure reduction, and finally enters the incubator after the third level of pressure reduction. The pressure after the third level of pressure reduction is adjusted according to the requirements of the incubator.

5.1.4 Incubator Gas Setting, Testing, and Calibration

1. Gas setting: A stable internal gas environment is crucial for an incubator. In particular, the CO_2 concentration (%), primarily used for balancing the pH of the culture medium, is an important variable affecting gamete function and embryo development. The CO_2 concentration should be set according to the manufacturer's instructions for the culture medium

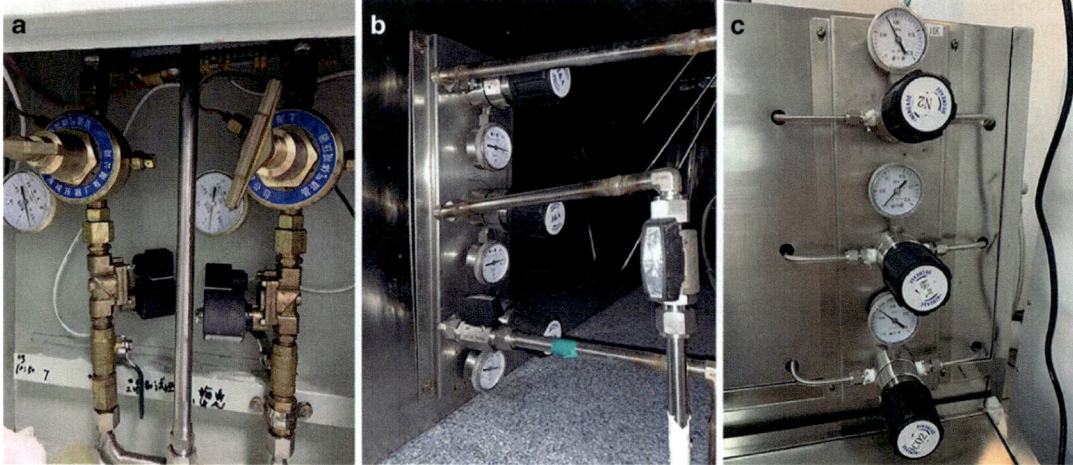

Fig. 5.4 Pressure reducing valves. (**a**) Level 1 pressure reducing valve (located in the gas supply room); (**b**) level 2 pressure reducing valve (located in a hidden spot, such as the roof or under the table/bench); (**c**) level 3 pressure reducing valve (located near the incubator for easy adjustments)

(usually 5–6% for zero or low altitude) and fine-tuned according to the actual pH value tested to achieve the optimal pH range for the culture medium. The maintenance of pH at a fixed temperature does not depend solely on the proportion of CO_2 in the gas mixture but the actual amount of CO_2 dissolved in the culture medium. The CO_2 solubility decreases with the increase of altitude (the higher the altitude, the lower the air pressure), so a higher concentration may be needed at high altitudes to compensate for the decrease in solubility (Fig. 5.5). This is particularly important for incubators that use a standard gas mixture, in which case it is necessary to customize the gas with the required concentration ratio from the supplier. However, some researchers in China found that at high altitude (3650 m), if the in-incubator CO_2 concentration required was projected according to the above theory, it should be set between 8.16% and 10.50% [10]. Yet, the research results showed that when CO_2 was set at 4.5%, it could satisfy the pH range recommended by the culture medium manufacturer and the best culture results. Therefore, the CO_2 setting must be adjusted with the actual pH test results.

In addition, the setting and detection of O_2 concentration (%) in three-gas incubators is critical for embryo development. Hundreds of studies on the effects of low-oxygen (5–10%) or high-oxygen (~20%) culture environments on embryonic development in mammals, including humans, have confirmed that the actual O_2 concentration in the female reproductive tract is much lower than that in ambient air. Some studies suggest that embryo culture with high-oxygen can increase the reactive oxygen species concentration, which may affect embryo development and pregnancy outcomes [11, 12]. To date, no studies have shown that high-oxygen (~20%) positively affects the development of human preimplantation embryos [13]; in contrast, many animal and human embryo studies have confirmed that low-oxygen is more beneficial for embryo development (especially in the blastocyst stage) and improves pregnancy outcomes [14–17]. Although the optimal O_2 concentration for embryo development is unknown, 5% is currently the recommended concentration for human embryo culture [18].

The CO_2 concentration in the incubator should be measured daily, and the O_2 concentration should also be checked regularly. The

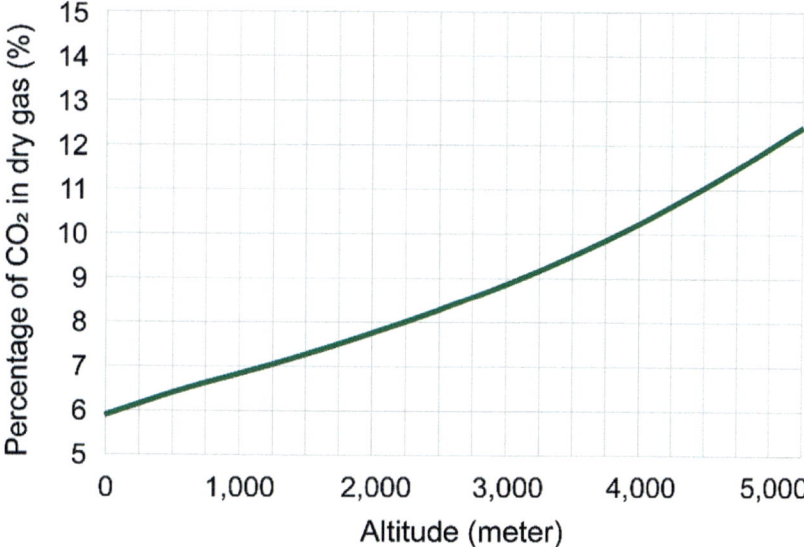

Fig. 5.5 Relationship between CO_2 setting value and altitude. The percentage of CO_2 required to maintain a pH of 7.3 varies with altitude

fluctuation range of CO_2 concentration should be controlled within ±0.2% of the set value [19]. Once the gas concentration in the incubator fluctuates abnormally, the cause should be identified promptly—check the connection of the gas pipe and the gas pressure, and take actions to solve the problem, such as recalibration or contacting an engineer.

2. CO_2 detection: Most incubators used for in vitro fertilization cycles are equipped with CO_2 sensors (except for incubators using standard gas mixtures) to regulate and detect the CO_2 concentration. There are two main types of sensors: thermal conductivity (TC) sensors and infrared (IR) sensors [20].

(a) TC sensor: Thermal conductivity sensors function through measurement of resistance between two thermistors, with one enclosed and the other exposed to the incubator chamber. The presence of CO_2 in the incubator chamber changes the resistance between the two thermistors and permits elucidation of gas concentrations. But since humidity and temperature can affect the thermistor of the TC sensor, and the detection is only accurate under saturated humidity (>90%), readings or adjustments can only be made when the temperature and humidity return to stable after each door opening. The water tank

Table 5.3 Advantages and disadvantages of the two types of CO_2 sensors

Type	Advantages	Disadvantages
Thermal conductivity sensor	Good stability, long lifespan, and low-price	Temperature- and humidity-dependent, the reading can only be taken after the temperature and humidity have stabilized after opening and closing the door
Infrared sensor	It is sensitive, accurate, and does not depend on temperature and humidity	Relatively short lifespan, and high price, may be affected by impurities in the incubator

of incubators with TC sensor must be replaced regularly to avoid false detection of CO_2 concentration.

(b) IR sensor: It detects CO_2 levels through an optical sensor system that includes an infrared emitter and a sensor. When the CO_2 in the incubator absorbs some of the infrared light radiated by the emitter, the sensor can detect the amount of absorption, which is proportional to the CO_2 concentration.

Either sensor has its advantages and disadvantages (Table 5.3). Early conventional incubators mostly used TC sensors, and some manufacturers now offer incubators with both types of sensors. On the other hand, most three-gas (non-premixed gas) benchtop incubators and time-lapse imaging incubation systems utilize IR sensors.

3. O_2 detection: Two main types of sensors are used to detect O_2 concentrations: galvanic/fuel cell or zirconium sensors.

   (a) Galvanic/fuel cell type: Oxygen diffuses through the outer barrier of the sensor to reach the inner cathode where it is reduced to hydroxyl ions which, in turn, oxidize the metal anode. A current, proportional to the O_2 consumption rate, is generated when the cathode–anode circuit is completed. The O_2 diffusion rate to reach the cathode and cell current is a direct function of this diffusion rate, which in turn directly functions as the O_2 concentration in the sample. Such sensors have a certain service life. Incubator manufacturers have provided specific replacement cycles. However, the actual service life may be longer than the recommended replacement cycle, depending on the factory battery voltage, and the user's use habits, among others. The prolonged absence of a three-gas mixture (high-oxygen state) in the incubator would shorten the battery life. Therefore, daily monitoring is warranted. Once the O_2 detection value appears to dramatically change or the calibration value rapidly changes, the sensor may have expired or is faulty, and an engineer should be promptly contacted for replacement.

   (b) Zirconia sensor: A zirconium sensor is an impervious tube with a zirconia element with a closed end and is coated externally and internally with porous metal electrodes. At elevated temperatures, the element becomes an O_2-ion conductor, which results in a voltage being generated between the electrodes. The value of the voltage is dependent upon the differences between the partial pressures of the O_2 in the sample and the O_2 in a reference gas (generally air). Zirconia sensor has the advantages of rapid response and long service life. Meanwhile, it is a high-temperature sensor, whether its accuracy is affected by the temperature in the incubator (37 °C) is still controversial, plus its comparatively high price, so most of the incubators on the market are equipped with galvanic/fuel cell sensors.

When the power to an incubator with saturated humidity is turned off, condensation will likely appear inside the chamber, affecting the sensor's function. Therefore, the power should not be turned off when the incubator is in saturated humidity. Humidification should be turned off, or the water tank should be removed before shutting down the incubator to prevent causing sensor and circuit damage. If the power is accidentally turned off at saturation humidity, the incubator door must be left open for at least 1 h.

4. Third-party detector: No matter how stable the sensors are, they must be recalibrated after a certain period. Given the inconvenience of disassembling the sensors in the incubator, IVF labs should be routinely equipped with a third-party portable CO_2/O_2 detector, which can test CO_2/O_2 daily and calibrate the sensors in the incubator regularly. Such devices would only need to be sent to the local metrology institute for annual calibration.

Older manual CO_2/O_2 detectors based on chemical methods were cumbersome, error-prone, and used toxic, corrosive chemicals that can generate VOCs. IVF laboratories nowadays commonly use electronic detectors that integrate CO_2, O_2, and temperature sensors, which work on much the same principle as the incubator sensors. Their advantages include ease of use, accuracy, and repeatability (Fig. 5.6).

5. Calibration of incubator CO_2: The CO_2 concentration inside the incubator will deviate after the incubator is cleaned and restarted or after a long period of operation, especially for incubators with TC sensors, which are more

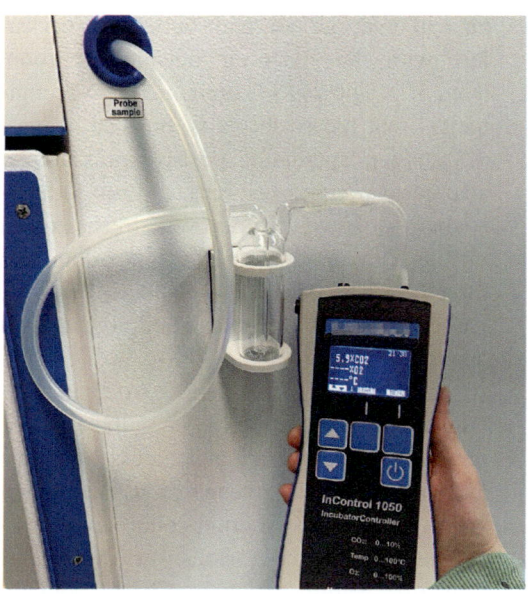

Fig. 5.6 Electronic detector

susceptible to changes in temperature and humidity, and therefore need to be calibrated periodically. The calibration procedure includes two main steps: zero-adjustment and concentration calibration.

(a) Zero-adjustment: a. Change the CO_2 concentration setting of the incubator to 0.0% with the power on. Close the cylinder gas pressure reducing valve and keep the incubator door and glass door open for 3–5 min to ensure all the residual CO_2 inside the incubator is discharged. b. Close the door and leave it for more than 24 h for equilibration. Especially for incubators with TC sensors, make sure that the temperature inside the incubator is stable at 37 °C and the humidity is close to saturation. At this time, the CO_2 concentration should be displayed as 0.0%. If not, manually change the display value to 0.0% according to the instruction manual.

(b) Concentration calibration: (a) After the zero point is adjusted and stabilized for some time (2 h is recommended), change the CO_2 concentration setting to the expected value, e.g., 5.0%. Turn on the cylinder gas supply, and when the concentration display value rises to 5.0%, test the CO_2 concentration with a portable detector. (b) If the measured value does not match the set value, say if it is 4.7%, then change the display concentration to the measured value (4.7%) via the incubator calibration program. Repeat the above steps after the displayed concentration value is restored to the set value (5%). If the deviation between the measured and displayed values is within ±0.2%, it is considered qualified; otherwise, it is considered unqualified and must be recalibrated.

It is generally recommended that the zero-adjustment of CO_2 concentration be performed once every 2 months and at the initial switch-on and that the concentration calibration be carried out once per year.

5.2 Quality Management of Indoor Air

The assessment of air quality in IVF laboratories usually include the size and number of suspended particles in the air, the number of pathogenic microorganisms, inorganic substances harmful to humans, and the level of VOCs. IVF laboratories have strict demand for air quality, and many adverse factors such as PM10 (particulate matter <10 µm in diameter), PM2.5 (particulate matter <2.5 µm in diameter), CO, NO_2, SO_2, and VOCs in the air may interfere with the outcome of IVF. It is therefore crucial for IVF laboratories to eliminate harmful ingredients from the air. Currently, IVF laboratories mainly utilize heating, ventilation, and air conditioning (HVAC) systems, IVF workstations in culture rooms, and VOCs removal filtration equipment to decontaminate the air and to make sure that the indoor environment, the surroundings for gamete/embryo manipulation, and the interior microenvironment of the incubator meet the requirement for healthy embryo development.

5.2.1 Heating, Ventilation, and Air Conditioning System

1. Working principle: HVAC consists of control systems for temperature, humidity, air decontamination, and air circulation. It is fitted with a series of filters with increasing filtration efficiency [21, 22] (Table 5.4) to reduce suspended particles and microorganisms in fresh air (microorganisms typically take suspended particles as transmission carriers) and decontaminates the indoor air through the air circulation control system, making it an effective, safe, and convenient method to eliminate microorganisms. Outside air goes through the coarse filter first and then through the medium efficiency filter. After regulating the temperature and humidity, the air finally flows through the HEPA into the IVF laboratory, a process allowing full dynamic control of bacteria. Although it cannot completely filter viruses, most HEPA can eliminate a portion of particles with viruses attached, greatly reducing the risk of contamination and creating a clean and comfortable environment. A small portion of the air entering the room is discharged from the exhaust vent or via the positive pressure mechanism to the surrounding rooms of lower cleanliness levels. The majority of the air will enter the return air outlet and recirculate with the fresh air outside the room (Fig. 5.7). The *2018 Cairo Consensus* recommends that the fresh air volume be at least >20% to maintain the positive pressure by also ensuring the fresh air supply to the personnel [9]. However, too much fresh air will increase the burden on the generator unit; therefore, a good trade-off should be made based on the actual climate conditions and air quality.

2. Air cleanliness classification: After decontamination by the HVAC system, the environment is graded for air cleanliness based on airborne particle concentrations in cleanrooms and zones. Different countries or institutions have issued various versions of the standard cleanliness levels. The air cleanliness classification of each room/area in our IVF laboratory is as follows (Table 5.5):

    The specific cleanliness levels of each room can be achieved by setting air exchange times per hour (air exchange times/hour)—the higher the purification level, the more air exchange times. Because the volume of the room is fixed, the number of air exchanges can be adjusted by changing the total air supply volume to the room, which is calculated as follows:

Table 5.4 Classifications and functions of particulate air filters

Classification	Efficiency at a rated air volume	Function
Coarse filters	The efficiency of removing particles with a diameter of $\geq 2.0\ \mu m$: $\geq 50\%$ (highest level of coarse filters)	As pre-filters to filter fresh air
Medium efficiency filters	The efficiency of removing particles with a diameter of $\geq 0.5\ \mu m$: 60–70% (highest level of medium efficiency filters)	Filter fresh air and returned air; reduce the load on the high-efficiency filters and protect the accessories within the HVAC system, extending their functional life
High-efficiency filters	The efficiency of removing particles with a diameter of $\geq 0.5\ \mu m$: $\geq 99.999\%$ (highest level of high-efficiency filters)	Terminal filters for high-level cleanrooms

The rated air volume refers to the maximum air volume flow rate per unit of time under guaranteed filter efficiency. Efficiency refers to the ability of air filters to remove particulate matter from the circulating air under the rated air volume. The particle size refers to the geometric diameter of the particulate matter.

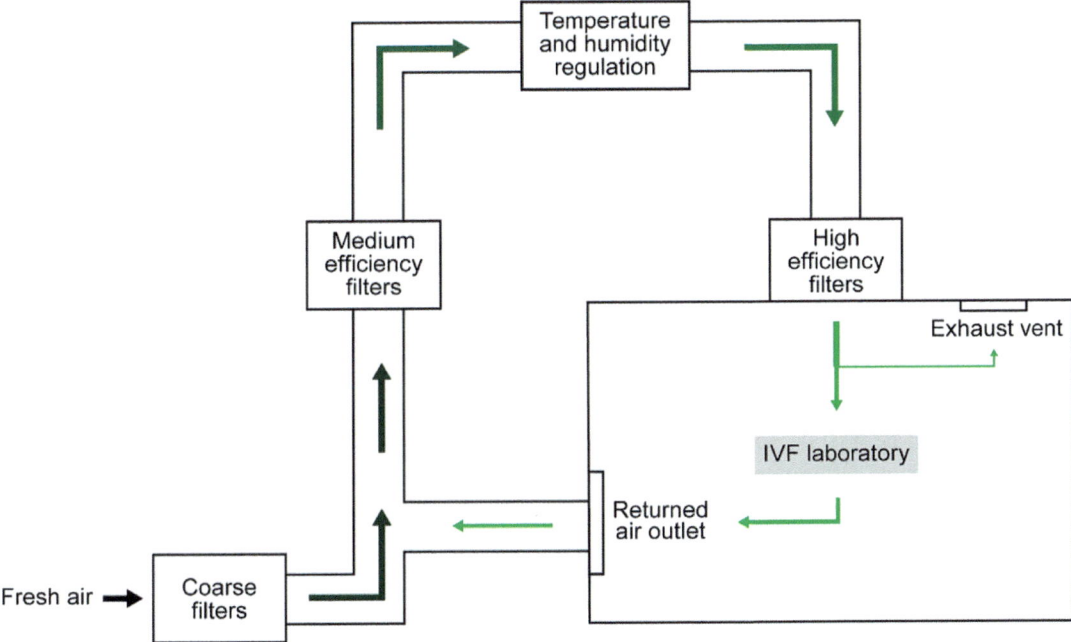

Fig. 5.7 The HVAC system in IVF laboratory (arrows represent the direction of airflow)

Table 5.5 Air cleanliness classification of each room/area based on specific standards in our IVF laboratory

Different areas in the IVF laboratory	US FS209D (1988)	China GMP (2010)	ISO-14644-1 (2002) Classification	Particle concentration[b] (particles/m³)
Gamete and embryo manipulation area[a]	Class 100	Class A	IOS Class 5	3520
Embryo culture room	Class 1000	Class B	IOS Class 6	35,200
Oocyte retrieval room, embryo transfer room, artificial insemination room, male surgery room, semen processing room, and cryopreservation room	Class 10,000	Class C	IOS Class 7	352,000
Hand washing room, dressing room, gas cylinder room, and sperm retrieval room	Class 100,000	Class D	IOS Class 8	3520,000

US FS209D refers to *Federal Standard 209D* issued by the United States in 1988 (repealed), from which the commonly-referred Class 100, Class 1000, and other classification levels are derived. GMP refers to good manufacturing practices according to the *"Quality Management Standards for Drug Production (2010 Revision),"* which was considered and adopted by the former Ministry of Health of the People's Republic of China. ISO-14644-1 (Second Edition, 2015) refers to the *"Cleanrooms and Associated Controlled Environments, Part 1: Classification of Air Cleanliness by Particle Concentration"* issued by the International Organization for Standardization. [a]The air cleanliness level of the gamete/embryo manipulation area is achieved through dedicated IVF workstations. [b]Data shown in this column was derived from the international standard (ISO-14644-1), and the particle concentration includes particles ≥0.5 μm. All concentrations mean the maximum allowable particle concentration for the class considered

$$\text{Air exchange times / hour} = \frac{\text{total room air supply}\left(m^3\right)/\text{hour}}{\text{room volume}\left(m^3\right)}$$

$$= \frac{\text{air delivery speed}\left(\dfrac{m}{s}\right) \times \text{area of single air supply outlet}\left(m^2\right) \times 3{,}600\,s \times \text{no. of outlets}}{\text{room volume}\left(m^3\right)}$$

In addition, according to the *"Architectural technical code for hospital clean operation department"* [23]: (a) Between two interconnected rooms with different cleanliness levels, the higher cleanliness room should maintain a relative positive pressure toward the lower cleanliness room, with the minimum static pressure difference ≥ 5 Pa and the maximum static pressure difference <20 Pa, to avoid the discomfort of personnel caused by the whistling sound generated by the differential pressure. (b) The minimum static pressure difference between the clean and outdoor areas should be ≥10 Pa. (c) There should be a proper pressure difference between interconnected rooms of the same cleanliness level to maintain the required airflow direction. For example, when the embryo culture room is at the same cleanliness level as the adjacent operation room, normally, a positive pressure of about 5 Pa from the culture room toward the operation room is maintained to ensure that the air always flows toward the operation room when the transfer window is opened, thereby avoiding the flow of embryotoxic disinfectants or patient-derived potential contaminants from the operation room into the embryo culture room. Suppose excessive noise or opposite direction airflow is found in the room. In that case, an electronic differential pressure meter should be taken for testing, and HVAC maintenance personnel should be contacted in time for adjustment. The main technical parameters corresponding to operation rooms of different cleanliness levels are shown in Tables 5.6 [23]. Further requirements also include: IVF laboratory personnel should have a fixed route in and out of a clean room; the laboratory should be equipped with a differential pressure gauge or electronic differential pressure meter to monitor the differential static pressure between different areas; if the differential pressure is found to be abnormal, the laminar flow maintenance personnel should be contacted promptly to adjust.

3. Filter maintenance and cleaning: The coarse, medium, and high-efficiency filters work merely by inter-particle impact, interception, adsorption, and other physical means to filter harmful particles. When their filtration capacities reach saturation, with the change of temperature or unit airspeed, the adsorbed particles and pathogenic microorganisms may free out. In this case, the HVAC system itself becomes a source of contamination. Therefore, it should be secured that the responsible maintenance personnel clean and/or replace the coarse and medium- efficiency filters and replace the high-efficiency filters regularly, and a third-party professional company be called upon to conduct laminar flow level testing after replacing the high-efficiency filters. Meanwhile, the air return vents and ceiling exhaust filters should also be cleaned regularly to safeguard the air exchange effect. The cleaning and replacement cycles of various filters and vents in our center are given in Table 5.7. In addition, the laminar flow clean rooms should be tested for settling bacteria every three months—that is, to assess the cleanliness level of the clean room based on the principle of natural sedimentation as per the *"Test Method for Settling Microbe in Clean Room (zone) of the Pharmaceutical*

Table 5.6 Technical parameters concerning operation rooms of different cleanliness levels

Operation room grade	Cleanliness level		Indoor pressure	Minimum air exchange times per hour	Average airflow speed in the working area (m/s)	Temperature (°C)	Relative humidity (%)	Noise dB (A)
	Operation zone	Surrounding zone						
I	Class 5	Class 6	Positive	–	0.20 to 0.25	21 to 25	30 to 60	≤51
II	Class 6	Class 7	Positive	24	–	21 to 25	30 to 60	≤49
III	Class 7	Class 8	Positive	18	–	21 to 25	30 to 60	≤49
IV	Class 8.5		Positive	12	–	21 to 25	30 to 60	≤49

Table 5.7 Cleaning and replacement cycles of particulate air filters in our center

Filters	Cleaning cycle	Cleaning method	Replacement cycle
Coarse filter	Every week	Water washing	2 months
Medium efficiency filter	Every week	Vacuum cleaner	3 months
High-efficiency filter	–	–	2–3 years
Filter screen at return air outlet	Every week	Water washing	–
Filter screen at exhaust vent	Every week	Water washing	–

Industry (GB/T 16294-2010)" [24] and "*Cleanrooms and Associated Controlled Environments—Biocontamination Control. Part 1: General Principles and Methods* (ISO 14698-1)" [25]. This test is easy to perform, causes little damage to the air environment, and does not interfere with airflow direction, making it widely used for environmental monitoring in clean areas.

4. Management system: The control of air cleanliness in IVF laboratories cannot rely solely on HVAC systems, as personnel is also a potential source of contamination, making it necessary to establish a corresponding embryo laboratory management system to prevent human-induced contamination (see Chap. 7 for details).

5.2.2 IVF Workstation

Generally, the highest cleanliness level of the embryo culture room is class 1000, which is equivalent to class 6 according to the international standard (ISO-14644-1), as given in Table 5.5. An IVF workstation (clean bench) designed specifically for IVF laboratories can be used to achieve a higher level of cleanliness (ISO class 5) required by gamete/embryo manipulations. Such equipment works by drawing room air from a pre-filter film using a fan at the top of the workstation, further purifying the air through

the main filter with a higher filtration efficiency, and finally discharging decontaminated air vertically into the cabinet chamber. IVF workstations are not biosafety cabinets. Their primary purpose is to maintain a clean environment for gamete/embryo manipulations while also considering the operators' biosafety. The airflow in the IVF workstation is vertical laminar flow, which will not blow directly toward the operator; some workstations of certain brands are equipped with return vents or exhaust vents, which can further reduce the airflow toward the personnel (Fig. 5.8). The primary indicators of the decontamination capacity in IVF workstations are the main filter efficiency and laminar air velocity: (a) The main filter efficiency refers to the ability to retain particles of the most-penetrating particle size (MPPS), which is normally at 0.12–0.25 μm [26]. The main filters of most imported IVF workstations refer to and comply with class H14 (air cleanliness efficiency of >99.995%) of the European Standard EN 1822–1. (b) Laminar air velocity: "*Technical Specification for the Construction of Clean Surgical Departments in Hospitals*" [23] indicated the average air velocity in an ISO class 5 area should be 0.20–0.25 m/s.

Then there are also closed IVF workstations that can regulate CO_2, temperature, and humidity in the operating area. Such workstations were originally modified by Testart et al. in the early 1980s based on neonatal incubators [27]. Although this workstation also has air decontamination capabilities, its primary purpose is main-

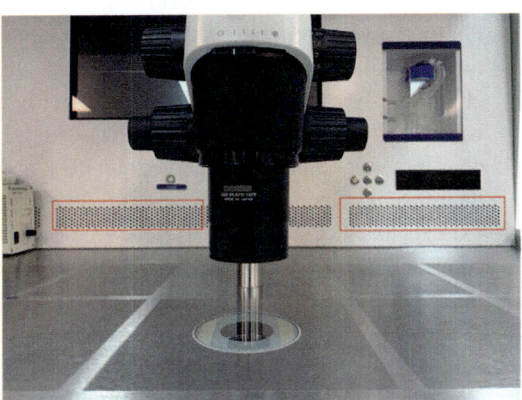

Fig. 5.8 Multi-hole design for air return on IVF workstation backplane (red box)

taining a constant temperature, humidity, and pH in the in vitro environment for gamete/embryo manipulations. They are not commonly applied because of their high price, but they should be a good backup in case of HVAC system failure.

5.2.3   VOCs-Filtering Equipment

HVAC systems, HEPA in IVF workstations, or HEPA in incubators can only filter limited amounts of suspended particles (microorganisms) of certain sizes. However, they cannot effectively trap toxic and harmful gases such as VOCs much smaller than their effective pore size of the filters [28]. Gametes will be exposed to air (without tissue culture oil covering) during oocyte pick-up and semen processing. The incubation process in incubators other than those using standard gas mixtures will rely on room air to provide oxygen. Therefore, effective removal or reduction of VOCs from room air can significantly improve the outcome of in vitro fertilization [29].

1. The working principle of VOCs-filtrating equipment: (a) Activated carbon/activated carbon combined with potassium permanganate: It absorbs toxic and harmful substances via micro-pores on the surface of activated carbon and decomposes harmful gases (formaldehyde as the main part) through the strong oxidizing property of potassium permanganate. (b) Photocatalytic oxidation (PCO): Photocatalysts generate photocatalytic reactions similar to photosynthesis under the effect of short-wave ultraviolet light with a wavelength of 200–280 nm (this wavelength does not decompose oxygen molecules and therefore does not produce ozone), which can oxidize and decompose a variety of organic compounds and some inorganic substances into water and carbon dioxide, and can also destroy the cell membrane of bacteria and solidify the proteins of viruses [30, 31]. Current air cleaners with a PCO function are also usually equipped with an activated carbon filter.

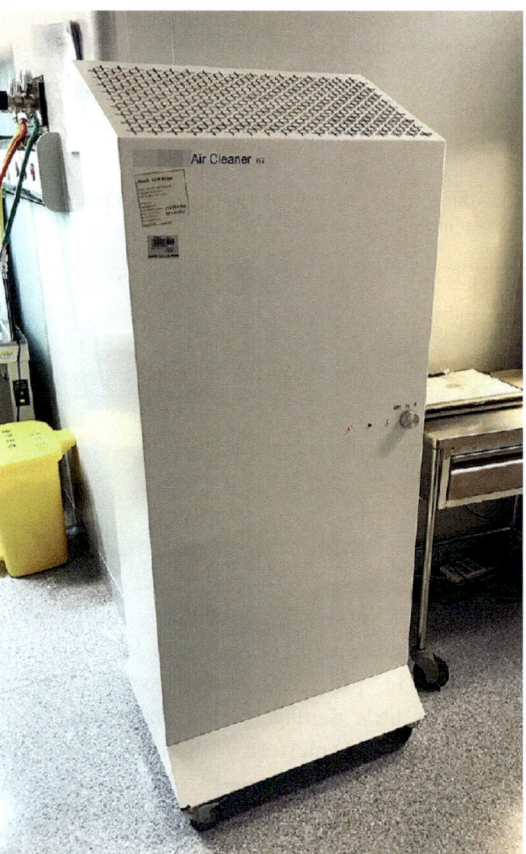

Fig. 5.9 An activated carbon air cleaner in our IVF laboratory

2. VOCs-filtrating equipment for IVF laboratories: VOCs-filtering equipment for IVF laboratories includes inline gas filters applied to gas cylinders (see Sect. 5.1 of this chapter for details) and VOCs-filtering equipment for room or incubator air decontamination.

  (a) Portable air cleaner: It is the most common VOCs removal equipment in IVF labs and works similarly to IVF workstations, except that it has a more efficient VOCs removal filter (activated carbon or PCO system), which can be combined with HEPA for air decontamination (Fig. 5.9). It is important to note that the air cleaner is mobile and can be placed anywhere in the culture room, but its clean capacity (space) is limited. Therefore, the number of air cleaners and their placement should be determined by the size of the culture room and the location of the centralized area for embryo manipulation/culture, e.g., small portable air cleaners can be placed near the IVF workstations. And again, the pre-filter membrane, the activated carbon filter, and the HEPA of the air cleaner should be replaced regularly according to the manufacturer's instructions.

(b) Decontamination system installed inside the HVAC: This equipment works based on photocatalytic oxidation and should be constructed and installed at the same time as HVAC in new laboratories. If an old laboratory is retrofitted with this system, the air supply pipelines need to be restructured. It has been reported that by the installation of a positive pressure, in-duct air filtration system, the level of VOCs in the laboratory can be reduced from 0.3 parts per million (ppm) to 0.0 ppm compared to freestanding air filtration units, which can significantly improve embryo quality and pregnancy outcomes [32]. However, VOCs in IVF laboratories do not only originate from the outside air. Some studies have even shown that the concentration of VOCs in the laboratory can be higher than that in the outside air [33]. So, while air circulation systems can effectively reduce the concentration of VOCs, the removal of indoor VOCs cannot be entirely dependent on such systems, and more important is the prevention and control of multiple sources that generate VOCs (see Sect. 5.3 of this chapter for details).

(c) Built-in air cleaner in the incubator: Regardless of two- or three-gas incubators, the oxygen inside a medium or large incubator is derived from the in-house air of the laboratory; plus incubators and culture dishes can also release VOCs after heating [34], while the HEPA filter that comes with the incubator can only filter particles—which is why a filter for removing VOCs from the inside of the incubator was introduced in the late 1990s. Similar to the way HEPA works, the gas inside the incubator is circulated through this filter to remove VOCs. Some studies have shown that incubators retrofitted with built-in VOCs filters can benefit blastocyst formation [19]. However, there is no further or more robust evidence of their benefits in improving treatment outcomes. The fact that the air in the laboratory room has already been decontaminated in multiple ways to a good cleanliness level, along with the promotion of small drawer incubators, benchtop incubators, and time-lapse imaging incubation systems, resulting in such built-in VOCs filters not being utilized much.

5.3 Management of Volatile Organic Compounds of Laboratory Environment

Volatile organic compounds have different forms of definition in different countries, organizations, or industries. In China, VOCs are defined as organic compounds with saturated vapor pressure >70 Pa at room temperature, a boiling point below 260 °C at atmospheric pressure, or organic compounds with vapor pressure $\geq$ 10 Pa and volatile under 20 °C. VOCs include hydrocarbons, oxygenated compounds, halides, and other carbon compounds, which are widely present in the atmosphere in the form of gas [35]. VOCs resulting from production activities and daily life pose a great threat to human health. Long-term exposure to high concentrations of VOCs can cause acute poisoning, malignant tumors (such as leukemia), acute and chronic neurological impairment, deterioration of the reproductive system, and diseases involving the heart, lungs, kidneys, and many other organs [36].

5.3.1 The Hazard of VOCs to IVF

The hazard of VOCs has been confirmed in animal experiments, with acrolein severely affecting embryonic development in mice and formaldehyde being the most toxic to mouse embryonic stem cells [33, 37]. An unpublished data suggest that elevated levels of formaldehyde, acetaldehyde, and high-molecular-weight aldehydes are associated with poor, delayed, or absent embryonic development (in mice and humans); and that embryonic development improves as aldehyde content decreases [9]. Numerous studies have also shown that improved air quality in IVF laboratories can significantly increase the fertilization rate, oocyte cleavage rate, high-quality embryo rate, blastocyst formation rate, implantation rate, and live birth rate while reducing the incidence of miscarriage [38–41].

5.3.2 Sources and Types of VOCs in IVF Laboratories

The main sources of VOCs in IVF laboratories are fresh air from outside (outdoor air can be heavily polluted), decoration materials, disinfectants and cleaning agents, devices and equipment along with their power cords (especially newly purchased), gas cylinders, various plastic consumables and their outer packaging, electronic products (computers, printers, etc.) and personnel themselves (accessories, cosmetics, clothing, etc.). Common VOCs in IVF laboratories include ethanol, isopropyl alcohol (2-propanol), acetone, propene (from plastic), hexamethylcyclotrisiloxane (from silicone pads), acetonitrile (from plastic), formaldehyde, acetaldehyde, limonene, and α-pinene (from cologne and detergents) [9]. Of these, ethanol and isopropyl alcohol (2-propanol) are the most frequently encountered (with the highest concentration). They can be metabolized to acetaldehyde and formaldehyde, which can cause serious biological damage to gametes and embryos.

5.3.3 Detection of VOCs in IVF Laboratories

Abnormal odors are perhaps the easiest to notice, but there are often individual differences in olfactory perception. More critically, when harmful gases reach the threshold of olfactory perception, their concentrations may be already well above the acceptable range for gametes/embryos. In fact, the concentration of each VOC component in the air is rather low and would need sophisticated instruments to detect them. Photoionization detectors (PID) are commonly used in IVF laboratories to detect VOCs. However, they can only detect total volatile organic compounds (TVOCs) in the environment and have a poor detection capability for aldehydes. There is currently no detection tool that can be routinely applied in IVF laboratories with the ability to identify and quantify each VOC component. The measurement units for VOC concentrations vary depending on the detection means. The common measurement units include: (a) mg/m^3 or ug/m^3 for methods that can identify specific components; (b) PID sensors usually use ppm or parts per billion (ppb). Compared to older laboratories, new laboratories built with multiple decontamination and air purification means can reduce TVOCs from $819.4\ \mu g/m^3$ to $32\ \mu g/m^3$, delivering significant improvements in treatment outcomes [41]. The *"Indoor Air Quality Standard"* GB/T 18883–2002 implemented in China stipulates that the concentration of TVOCs in residential and office buildings must be $<0.60\ mg/m^3$ and the concentration of formaldehyde must be $<0.10\ mg/m^3$ [42]. There is not yet a national standard for VOCs concentration thresholds in IVF laboratories, and the recommendation from domestic scholars for IVF laboratories is TVOCs <0.5 ppm (ideally <0.2 ppm). The *2018 Cairo Consensus* recommends that IVF laboratories have TVOCs $<500\ \mu g/m^3$ (~400–800 ppb) and aldehydes $<5\ \mu g/m^3$. A PID detector can be used to regularly inspect the culture room, especially when new equipment or large quantities of consumables are introduced. If the concentration of TVOCs exceeds 500 ppb (0.5 ppm), the relevant professional department should be consulted to identify and quantify the specific components to find the contamination source. Since the concentration of VOCs in the laboratory must be controlled at a ppb level (0–500 ppb), a more sophisticated detector with higher accuracy (with ppb as the measurement unit) should be preferred.

5.3.4   Prevent and Reduce the Generation of VOCs in IVF Laboratories

The presence of VOCs and aldehydes in IVF laboratories is unavoidable. Therefore, VOCs generation should be considered, avoided, and controlled as much as possible in aspects such as laboratory site selection, design, building construction, and material selection. Measures should be taken in daily work so that the VOCs concentration in IVF laboratories can be maintained at a low level.

1. Laboratory site selection and design: IVF laboratories set up within general hospitals should be as far away as possible from roads, cafeteria exhausts, and parking lots and should be in places with relatively fewer people moving around, and are usually situated on relatively independent floors, e.g., avoid sharing a floor with other departments. IVF laboratories should be separated from the diagnostic andrology lab and should not share decontamination units with other clean rooms, such as research labs, animal labs, etc.

2. Construction: Use environmentally friendly materials. Avoid using paint and medium-density fiberboards (which have adhesives and water repellents containing VOCs). Stainless steel should be employed to make benchtops or lockers, but be aware that stainless steel items are often coated with oil during the production process, which should be thoroughly cleaned. New laboratories should be fully ventilated before use, which can effectively reduce the level of VOCs. Off-gassing is a time-dependent reaction, and a higher temperature (33 °C) can accelerate the release of formaldehyde [9].

3. When replacing the medium- or high-efficiency air filter, the package should be opened in advance, and the new filter should be maintained in a well-ventilated, clean area for about 1 week. Typically, highly efficient air filters are replaced when the clinical treatment cycle is stopped/finished, i.e., in the absence of ongoing embryo culture. Again, at least a one-week interval is recommended after the replacement before resuming the embryonic culture. Some studies have recommended that filter membranes be pretreated in a dry heat oven at 40–50 °C for 3–4 h to remove VOCs before replacement [43]. If such a measure is unavailable, at least ensure adequate ventilation to release odor at pre- and post-installation.

4. VOCs can be released from the internal components of a new incubator or from the sealing gasket attached to the door. It has been reported that the concentration of VOCs in a new incubator can be more than 100 times higher than in a used same model incubator [34]. To address this problem, a new incubator may first be placed in a clean and well-ventilated room (such as a class 100,000 clean area: scrubbing area, preparation room, etc.) for pre-treatment before use. For example, it can be done in this way: set the incubator temperature to 37–40 °C without installing the water tank, partitions, and filters and without ventilation; and open the door of incubator at least twice a day during the pre-treatment period (1–2 months). This means the incubator will run dry for a while before moving into the culture room. Similarly, a new IVF workstation should be left running (powered on, with laminar flow and heating turned on) for some time before moving into the culture room. It is worth noting that new parts used for replacement during equipment repair or regular maintenance can also generate VOCs.

5. Plastic products, such as various culture tubes, culture dishes, and their outer packaging, are the main source of styrene, which is why plastic consumables should not be stored in the culture room, but in a special sterile preparation room. In our center, the standard procedure is to unpack the culture dishes or culture tubes 24–48 h in advance and place them on a clean bench to release potential VOCs. This clean bench is located in a class 10,000 clean room next to the culture room to avoid contamination of consum-

ables and prevent VOCs from being released into the culture room. The personnel should avoid putting unnecessary plastic products into the incubator as much as possible in their daily work.

6. If there is painting or construction work near the fresh air vent or during heavy atmospheric pollution days, the HVAC system may be switched to 100% internal circulation to avoid seriously polluted fresh air from entering the lab, and a record should be made. However, it should be noted that this may cause changes in temperature and humidity, loss of positive pressure, and discomfort to personnel.

7. Smoking is prohibited in the vicinity of the IVF lab (smoking is prohibited inside all medical facilities). Even non-smoking laboratory personnel can bring "thirdhand smoke" into the laboratory through clothing, skin, hair, etc., which can cause damage to cells [44].

8. The use of alcohol-based products for laboratory cleaning is prohibited. Sterilized injection water or special commercial VOCs-free products designed for IVF laboratories may be purchased for cleaning and disinfection.

9. The use of alcohol lamps in embryo culture rooms should be avoided. When self-made modified glass pasteurized pipettes are required, use the alcohol lamp to prepare the required number of pipettes collectively when there is no embryo manipulation.

10. The number of people accessing the laboratory every day should be restricted. Lab personnel should not wear perfume, hair gel, or nail polish. Surgical gowns and caps should not be washed with strong smelling laundry, and patients should be reminded of this before the operation day.

11. Using a marker with low VOCs content or using an engraver when marking culture tubes or dishes is recommended.

12. Minimize the use of electronic devices: For example, laser printers can release formaldehyde and ozone; desktop computers will release VOCs as power consumption increases, and a variety of hazardous substances (such as phenol, toluene, 2-ethylhexanol, formaldehyde, and styrene) can be detected especially when new desktop computers are introduced. Computers should be kept off as much as possible when not in use, and newly purchased desktop computers should also be operated first outside the IVF lab for some time. The power cords that come with electronic devices are also a source of VOCs.

13. Use indoor air cleaners or install VOCs removal devices in HVAC systems (see Sect. 5.2 of this chapter for details).

14. The gas pipeline should be installed with inline filters (see Sect. 5.1 of this chapter for details). It is worth noting that apart from the incubators using standard gas mixtures, other incubators still source part of the gas from the room air, and there will be air entering when the incubator door is opened, making the decontamination of the room air a top priority.

15. Incubators using standard gas mixtures (usually benchtop incubators) coupled with inline filters are very likely to be effective in reducing VOCs inside the incubator. Moreover, this incubator constantly emits gas to the outside environment, so the air that enters when the door is opened will soon be expelled. However, the VOCs generated by the culture dishes and the incubator will remain. Therefore, IVF-specific culture dishes (that have passed the mouse embryo test and the endotoxin quality control test) should be selected whenever possible.

16. Cover with tissue culture oil. Tissue culture oil can not only block external VOCs from entering the culture medium but can also adsorb hydrophobic VOCs from the culture medium, thus reducing the VOCs concentration during the culture process. Tissue culture oil can adsorb VOCs not only from the culture medium but also from the outside air, so the concentration of VOCs dissolved in the oil might be better diluted by applying more tissue culture oil as appropriate (i.e., to thicken the oil layer).

References

1. Morbeck DE. Air quality in the assisted reproduction laboratory: a mini-review. J Assist Reprod Genet. 2015;32(7):1019–24.
2. Esteves SC, Varghese AC, Worrilow KC. Clean room technology in ART clinics: a practical guide. Boca Raton: CRC Press; 2016.
3. Swain JE. Is there an optimal pH for culture media used in clinical IVF? Hum Reprod Update. 2012;18(3):333–9.
4. Elder K, den Bergh MV, Woodward B. Troubleshooting and problem-solving in the IVF laboratory. Cambridge: Cambridge University Press; 2015.
5. Esteves SC, Junior SV, Gomes AP. Comparison between International Standard Organization (ISO) type 5 and type 6 cleanrooms combined with volatile organic compounds filtration system for micromanipulation and embryo culture in severe male factor infertility. Fertil Steril. 2006;86(3-supp-S):S353–4.
6. GB/T 7144-2016. Coloured cylinder mark for gases. Former General Administration of Quality Supervision, Inspection and Quarantine of the People's Republic of China. Standardization Administration of the People's Republic of China; 2016.
7. JGJ91-93. Scientific Laboratory Building Design Code. Institute of Architecture Design and Research, Chinese Academy of Sciences. Former Ministry of Construction of the People's Republic of China; 1993.
8. TSG R0006-2014. Regulations for safety and technical supervision of gas cylinders. Former General Administration of Quality Supervision, Inspection and Quarantine of the People's Republic of China; 2014.
9. Mortimer D, Cohen J, Mortimer ST, et al. Cairo consensus on the IVF laboratory environment and air quality: report of an expert meeting. Reprod Biomed Online. 2018;36(6):658–74.
10. Meng XQ, He J, Tang G, et al. Pilot study of optimal CO_2 concentration in culture condition for assisted reproductive technology at high altitude in Tibet. J Reprod Med. 2016;25(12):1083–8.
11. Bedaiwy MA, Falcone T, Mohamed MS, et al. Differential growth of human embryos in vitro: role of reactive oxygen species. Fertil Steril. 2004;82(3):593–600.
12. Bedaiwy MA, Mahfouz RZ, Goldberg JM, et al. Relationship of reactive oxygen species levels in day 3 culture media to the outcome of in vitro fertilization/intracytoplasmic sperm injection cycles. Fertil Steril. 2010;94(6):2037–42.
13. Gardner DK. The impact of physiological oxygen during culture, and vitrification for cryopreservation, on the outcome of extended culture in human IVF. Reprod Biomed Online. 2016;32(2):137–41.
14. Karagenc L, Sertkaya Z, Ciray N, et al. Impact of oxygen concentration on embryonic development of mouse zygotes. Reprod Biomed Online. 2004;9(4):409–17.
15. Kelley RL, Gardner DK. In vitro culture of individual mouse preimplantation embryos: the role of embryo density, microwells, oxygen, timing and conditioned media. Reprod Biomed Online. 2017;34(5):441–54.
16. Waldenström U, Engström AB, Hellberg D, et al. Low-oxygen compared with high-oxygen atmosphere in blastocyst culture, a prospective randomized study. Fertil Steril. 2009;91(6):2461–5.
17. Bontekoe S, Mantikou E, van Wely M, et al. Low oxygen concentrations for embryo culture in assisted reproductive technologies. Cochrane Database Syst Rev. 2012;7:CD008950.
18. Consensus Group C. 'There is only one thing that is truly important in an IVF laboratory: everything' Cairo Consensus Guidelines on IVF Culture Conditions. Reprod Biomed Online. 2020;40(1):33–60.
19. Higdon HL 3rd, Blackhurst DW, Boone WR. Incubator management in an assisted reproductive technology laboratory. Fertil Steril. 2008;89(3):703–10.
20. Swain JE. Decisions for the IVF laboratory: comparative analysis of embryo culture incubators. Reprod Biomed Online. 2014;28(5):535–47.
21. GB/T 13554-2020. High efficiency particulate air filter. State Administration for Market Regulation of the People's Republic of China. Standardization Administration of the People's Republic of China; 2020.
22. GB/T 14295-2019. Air Filter. State Administration for Market Regulation of the People's Republic of China. Standardization Administration of the People's Republic of China; 2019.
23. GB50333-2013, Architectural technical code for hospital clean operation department. Ministry Of Housing and Urban-Rural Development of The People's Republic of China, Former General Administration of Quality. Supervision, Inspection and Quarantine of the People's Republic of China; 2013.
24. GB/T 16294-2010. Test method for settling microbe in clean room (zone) of the pharmaceutical industry. Former General Administration of Quality Supervision, Inspection and Quarantine of the People's Republic of China. Standardization administration of the People's Republic of China; 2010.
25. ISO 14698-1. Cleanrooms and associated controlled environments—biocontamination control. Part 1: general principles and methods. International Organization for Standardization; 2003.
26. EN 1822-1-2009. High efficiency air filters (EPA, HEPA and ULPA)—part 1: classification, performance testing, marking. European Committee for Standardization; 2009.
27. Testart J, Lassalle B, Frydman R. Apparatus for the in vitro fertilization and culture of human oocytes. Fertil Steril. 1982;38(3):372–5.
28. Esteves S, Bento F, Agarwal A. Quality management in ART clinics: a practical guide. New York: Springer; 2013.
29. Agarwal N, Chattopadhyay R, Ghosh S, et al. Volatile organic compounds and good laboratory practices

in the in vitro fertilization laboratory: the important parameters for successful outcome in extended culture. J Assist Reprod Genet. 2017;34(8):999–1006.

30. Liou JW, Chang HH. Bactericidal effects and mechanisms of visible light-responsive titanium dioxide photocatalysts on pathogenic bacteria. Arch Immunol Ther Exp. 2012;60(4):267–75.

31. Varghese AC, Sjoblom P, Jayaprakasan K, et al. A practical guide to setting up an IVF Lab, Embryo Culture Systems and Running the Unit. Jaypee Brothers Medical Pub; 2013.

32. Meyer LR, Hazlett WD, Schorsch K, et al. Let's clear the air. In-duct versus freestanding air filtration: does it make a difference in viable blastocyst development and pregnancy outcome in an urban, multistory IVF laboratory setting? Fertil Steril. 2015;104(3):e316–7.

33. Hall J, Gilligan A, Schimmel T, et al. The origin, effects and control of air pollution in laboratories used for human embryo culture. Hum Reprod. 1998;13(Suppl 4):146–55.

34. Cohen J, Gilligan A, Esposito W, et al. Ambient air and its potential effects on conception in vitro. Hum Reprod. 1997;12(8):1742–9.

35. World Health Organization Regional Office for Europe. Air quality guidelines-global update 2005: particulate Matter, ozone, nitrogen dioxide and sulfur dioxide. Germany: WHO; 2006.

36. Tsai WT. An overview of health hazards of volatile organic compounds regulated as indoor air pollutants. Rev Environ Health. 2019;34(1):81–9.

37. Shen S, Yuan L, Zeng S. An effort to test the embryotoxicity of benzene, toluene, xylene, and formaldehyde to murine embryonic stem cells using airborne exposure technique. Inhal Toxicol. 2009;21(12):973–8.

38. Esteves SC, Gomes AP, Verza S Jr. Control of air pollution in assisted reproductive technology laboratory and adjacent areas improves embryo formation, cleavage and pregnancy rates and decreases abortion rates: comparison between a class 100 (ISO5) and a Class 1000 (ISO6) clean-room for micromanipulation and embryo culture. Fertil Steril. 2004;82(Suppl 2):S259–60.

39. Esteves SC, Bento FC. Implementation of air quality control in reproductive laboratories in full compliance with the Brazilian Cells and Germinative Tissue Directive. Reprod Biomed Online. 2013;26(1):9–21.

40. Khoudja RY, Xu Y, Li T, et al. Better IVF outcomes following improvements in laboratory air quality. J Assist Reprod Genet. 2013;30(1):69–76.

41. Heitmann RJ, Hill MJ, James AN, et al. Live births achieved via IVF are increased by improvements in air quality and laboratory environment. Reprod Biomed Online. 2015;31(3):364–71.

42. GB/T 18883-2002. Indoor Air Quality Standard. Former General Administration of Quality Supervision, Inspection and Quarantine of the People's Republic of China. Former Ministry of Health of the People's Republic of China, Former State Environmental Protection Administration of the People's Republic of China; 2002.

43. Huang GN, Sun HX. Laboratory techniques in in vitro fertilization and embryo transfer. People's Medical Publishing House; 2012.

44. Hang B, Sarker AH, Havel C, et al. Thirdhand smoke causes DNA damage in human cells. Mutagenesis. 2013;28(4):381–91.

Light of Microscopes and Laboratory Environment

Oocytes development, ovulation, fertilization, and embryo development occur without exposure to light under physiological conditions in vivo. Although in vitro fertilization-embryo transfer technology is becoming more sophisticated and the IVF operation process replicates this environment to some extent, it does not yet fully simulate the physiological environment in vivo. When performing in vitro manipulations, including oocyte pick-up, denudation, ICSI, morphological evaluation of embryos, and embryo transfer, gametes and embryos are inevitably exposed to light. Although a low level of light exposure does not entirely impede fertilization and embryo development, such unnatural light exposure may potentially affect gametes or embryos. Coupled with the fact that the threshold for the intensity of light that produces an effect is not fully known, it is still necessary to understand the impacts of light in daily practice and minimize them during ART treatment.

6.1 The Effects of Light and Its Mechanism

6.1.1 Types of Light, Their Effects on Gametes and Embryos, and Underlying Mechanisms

The effect of light on gametes and embryos is related to the light wavelength (the first and fore-most influencing factor) and the duration and intensity of light exposure. IVF laboratory-related light can be classified into three types by wavelength: ultraviolet (UV), visible light, and infrared light (Fig. 6.1).

1. UV light: The wavelength range of UV light is about 10–380 nm. Gametes and embryos are extremely sensitive to UV light exposure. This is because the absorption peak of DNA (260 nm) lies right in the wavelength range of UV light, with the result that UV light can induce DNA strand breaks and therefore alter the integrity of the genome. UV light can also damage cells by triggering the production of oxygen free radicals through multiple pathways. For example, brief exposure of sperm to UV light can result in decreased sperm motility and reduced fertilization and cleavage rates [1]. Studies indicated that UV radiation at 290–320 nm can cause DNA damage, and oxidative stress in sea urchin embryos [2]. Among them, DNA damage can cause the cells to stay in the G1/S phase of the meiotic cycle to repair their damaged DNA, which results in delayed cell division and development. Moreover, if DNA repair fails, these sea urchin cells will undergo apoptosis and programmed cell death.

2. Visible light: The wavelength range of visible light is about 380–760 nm. Many studies have demonstrated that visible light can adversely

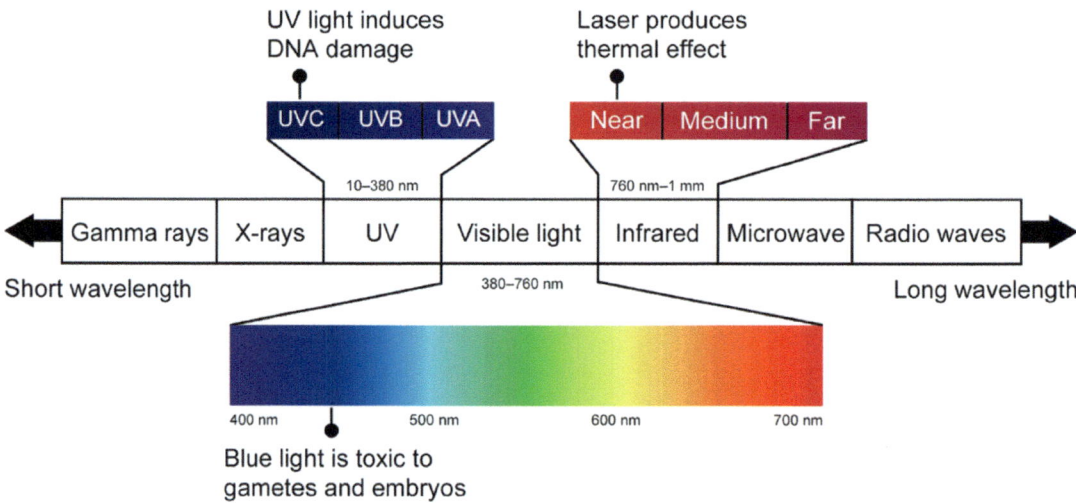

Fig. 6.1 Types of light relevant to IVF laboratories and their wavelength ranges

affect the early development of animal and human embryos [3], and visible light of different wavelengths has different effects on gametes and embryos. In 1964, Daniel first reported the effects of light exposure on mammalian embryos [4]. His findings showed that rabbit oocytes exposed to light for up to 12 h had a reduced oocyte cleavage rate; and that the oocyte cleavage rate was affected to varying degrees using different filters, with the red filter causing the slightest impact. Studies on mouse embryos have confirmed that exposure to white light can interfere with implantation potential, and these effects can be partly corrected by a red filter [5]. Takenaka et al. investigated the effect of cool white light versus warm white light on the development of mouse embryos, and the results indicated that the implantation rate of embryos exposed to warm white light sources (58%) was higher than that exposed to cool white light sources (44%) [6]. Cool white light consists of more short wavelength visible light, while warm light contains more long-wavelength visible light. The influences of visible light of various colors on the blastocyst formation rate of mouse embryos were investigated. The results, expressed as blastocyst formation rates, were 49% for blue light (445–500 nm), 72% for green light (500–575 nm), 71% for

yellow light (575–585 nm), and 84% for red light (620–750 nm). Within visible light, blue light, which has a shorter wavelength, is several orders of magnitude more harmful than those of other colors. Gametes and embryos are less sensitive to green and red light (with longer wavelengths)—the time-lapse imaging culture system utilizes red or green light with reduced light intensity.

The cytotoxicity of light to embryos is associated with an increase in the production of reactive oxygen species (ROSs). ROSs are oxygen-derived molecules that act as powerful oxidants. Some of the ROS members, such as superoxide (O_2^-), hydrogen peroxide (H_2O_2) and the hydroxyl radical (OH^-), are an intrinsic outcome of cellular metabolism. ROSs can react with any molecule and modify it oxidatively, resulting in structural and functional alterations [7]. Low flux ROSs can trigger the release of cellular transcription factors and activate gene expression, muscle contraction, and cell growth. Evidence shows that trace amounts of ROSs may engage in sperm capacitation and acrosome reaction [8]. In contrast, excessive ROSs may damage DNA, protein, and lipid molecules, cause gene mutations, impaired mitochondrial function, and even cell death. Germ cells are susceptible to ROSs, and increased intra- and extracellular

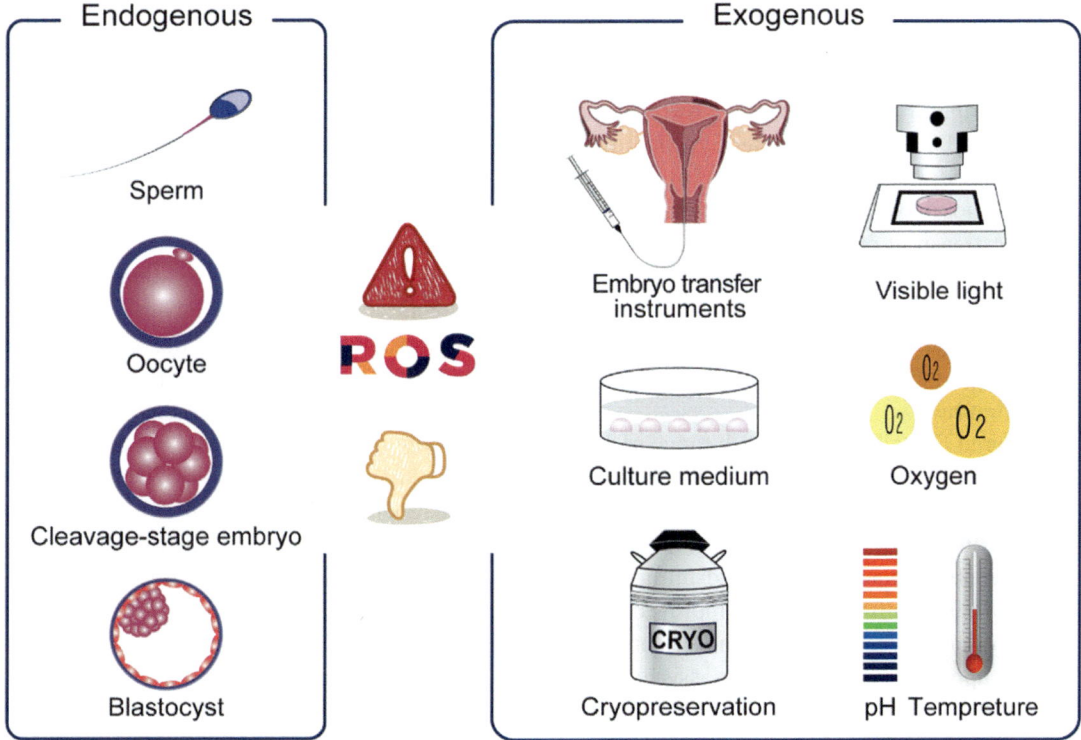

Fig. 6.2 Sources of ROSs during IVF

ROSs may cause damage to the reproductive potential, with ROSs that may originate from every aspect of IVF (Fig. 6.2). Both endogenous and exogenous ROSs can eventually lead to oxidative stress, negatively affecting fertilization rates and pregnancy outcomes [9]. Prevention of oxidative stress is critical for maintaining normal reproductive capacity. The lack of physiological defense mechanisms and the multiple sources of ROSs lead to a greater risk of developing oxidative stress in vitro than in vivo [7, 10]. Although exogenous ROSs are unavoidable in real situations, the damage they cause can be reduced by appropriate preventive measures. The inherent antioxidant capacity of the culture medium and embryos may counteract the adverse effects of ROSs [11]. The intrinsic antioxidant capacity powered by supplemented exogenous antioxidants (e.g., ascorbic acid) may also counteract the damaging effects of ROS exposure. Moreover, some technical means,

such as lowering the incubator oxygen concentration, can reduce ROSs production. However, the lowered oxygen concentration's impact on embryo development must be adequately considered.

Single-cell RNA sequencing can reveal a more comprehensive picture of how light affects embryonic development [12]. A significant decrease in blastocyst formation rate can be observed when the light was applied to 2-cell stage mouse embryos under the light intensity of 3000 lux for 6 h (the control group was not exposed to light). Differential expression gene level is much higher in 2-cell stage embryos exposed to light, with differential genes mainly enriched in mitochondrial translation termination and mRNA splicing-related pathways via spliceosomes. Meanwhile, differentially expressed genes in 4-cell and 8-cell embryos are mainly found in apoptotic pathways; differential gene expression in morulas and blastocysts is associated with DNA damage repair. Also, light exposure can interfere with the maternal-to-zygotic transition process, when the zygotic genome begins transcription and maternal mRNAs are degraded. The associated differentially expressed genes are involved in oxidative phosphorylation, metabolic pathways, and RNA transport processes. Light exposure can cause persistent damage to subsequent embryo development, affecting gene expression in multiple pathways, which may explain the light-induced decrease in blastocyst formation rate.

3. Infrared light: The wavelength range of infrared light is about 760 nm–1 mm. Due to the extensive range of wavelengths, infrared light is further divided into three categories by wavelength: near-infrared, mid-infrared, and far-infrared. Infrared light is employed in IVF laboratories where laser techniques are used, with applications such as laser-assisted hatching and artificial shrinkage. The introduction of laser technology has effectively shortened the in vitro operation time on embryos and increased the stability and reproducibility of various techniques. The laser's three parameters are important when considering its effect on gametes or embryos: wavelength, power, and pulse duration (duration of action). Current commercial laser systems often use relatively safe non-contact lasers at 1460 nm or 1480 nm wavelength (both long-wave near-infrared). The operator must set the appropriate power and pulse duration for the specific operation. The output power of lasers of different brands ranges from 110 to 400 mW, and although the power can be adjusted, people usually set it to 100% output habitually. Therefore, in daily operation, the adjustment of the ablation aperture size after a single excitation is mainly achieved by adjusting the pulse duration (the longer the pulse duration, the larger the aperture size).

The infrared laser produces a thermal effect when it strikes the embryo because of the heat it carries. There has been controversy regarding the influence of laser thermal effect on embryos. One study used a 1480 nm non-contact laser to remove the entire zona pellucida of mouse 8-cell embryos and showed that the laser did not induce elevated expression of the oocyte heat shock protein hsp70i, even in the blastomere closest to the laser beam [13]. This result suggests that embryo manipulation with laser is reasonably safe. Similarly, Uppangala et al. found in their study on human embryos using high resolution nuclear magnetic resonance (NMR) and time-lapse imaging culture technology that laser-assisted hatching did not affect the morphology and metabolism of blastomeres and embryos in the vicinity of the laser strike for at least 24 h after laser treatment [14]. However, the impacts of the laser thermal effect on human embryos are still unclear due to a lack of relevant studies, leaving room for further long-term follow-up and research.

In addition, it has also been demonstrated that high-intensity short-wavelength near-infrared laser radiation (<800 nm) can cause cell damage, and trapping sperm with this light for 1 min can result in UVA-like autofluorescence modifications (oxidative stress) and lead to sperm death [15].

6.1.2 Effects of Light Exposure Duration and Intensity on Gametes and Embryos

The damage caused by light exposure is proportional to the duration and intensity (in lux) with respect to the same wavelength. A dramatic increase in DNA fragmentation was recorded after 5 min UV irradiation but no significant changes in sperm motility were observed at this time. Longer irradiation (10 and 15 min) resulted in a decrease in motility parameters and further increase of DNA fragmentation [16]. In hamsters, exposure of fertilized oocytes to visible light for 10 min can decrease the cleavage rate, and the oocyte cleavage can be blocked entirely after 30 min of exposure [3]. The blastocyst formation rate of embryos exposed to light at 900 lux is significantly lower than that of embryos exposed to 200 lux light [17].

6.1.3   Effects of Light on Tissue Culture Oil and Mechanisms Involved

In IVF culture procedures, tissue culture oil is usually utilized to cover the culture medium microdroplets, maintaining a stable pH and osmolality. However, improper transport and storage conditions can compromise the quality of tissue culture oil and generate components that are detrimental to gamete and embryo development. Light can indirectly affect cells by oxidizing the medium or specific components in the tissue culture oil and turning them into cytotoxic substances. In 2007, Otsuki reported a vivid case in which the quality of embryo development declined significantly in the laboratory [18]. Following assessment and analysis, they were convinced that the culture techniques, the embryo culture environment, the quality of the culture media, and the storage conditions of the tissue culture oil were all intact in the laboratory. This finding led them to strongly suspect that there was a problem with the quality of a specific batch of tissue culture oil (which had not expired). They tested the tissue culture oil for endotoxin and bacterial contamination, and both returned clean. They tested the tissue culture oil from the suspicious batch for peroxide value. The result was 2.97 mEq/kg, much higher than other batches of tissue culture oil from the same manufacturer (0.00 mEq/kg). What caused the elevated peroxide levels in these tissue culture oils? They compared the effects of high temperature (50 °C, protected from light), sunlight, and UV light on tissue culture oil. The results showed that either sunlight exposure for seven weeks or UV light exposure for 120 h could increase the peroxide level in tissue culture oil from 0 to 3.0 mEq/kg. In contrast, when stored at a high temperature while protected from light (equivalent to the temperature in a car in summer) for 20 days, only a slight increase in the peroxide value in the tissue culture oil was observed (from 0 to 0.04 mEq/kg). It is therefore evident that the peroxides produced by tissue culture oil exposure to light can significantly influence the quality of embryos.

Peroxides in the tissue culture oil can get into the embryo culture media, altering the concentration of peroxides. The albumin supplemented in the culture media mediates this process, and free radicals can bind to albumin, affecting the embryos [19]. Several studies have confirmed the cytotoxic effects of peroxides and oxygen free radicals on embryonic development [20, 21]. Martinez et al. studied the effect of peroxidized mineral oil (peroxide content: 638.4 µmol/L) versus normal quality mineral oil (peroxide content: 6.4 µmol/L) on porcine embryo development [21], and found that the cleavage rates were 25.0% and 59.6%, and blastocyst formation rates were 0 and 33.1%, respectively. After covering the culture medium microdroplets with mineral oil and co-incubating for 22 h, peroxidized mineral oil-covered microdroplets had a total oxidant content of 9.4 mol/L. In contrast, normal quality mineral oil-covered culture medium microdroplets had a very low (non-detectable) total oxidant level. In conclusion, peroxidized mineral oil impairs embryonic development by accelerating the oxidation of the culture media. Therefore, the storage of oil used for tissue culture should be strictly protected from light, avoid using oil that has been stored for too long, and keep the oil at 2–8 °C as much as possible.

6.1.4   Effects of Light on Culture Media

Studies have revealed that the good-quality blastocyst rate drops when the culture media are exposed to daylight or fluorescent light for 1, 4, or 24 h and then used for embryo culture [22]. This manifestation is probably because certain contents of the culture medium are sensitive to light, and light exposure alters the composition of the medium, thus compromising the development of the embryos. For example, it is well known that UV light can accelerate the breakdown of proteins in culture media. Even if the exposure to light is only for a short time on each occasion, it will have an effect after many accumulations. There is no definite conclusion about the threshold value of acceptable light exposure for the culture media, making it necessary to schedule the operation process properly and minimize the light exposure of the culture media.

6.2 Sources of Light

Light in the IVF laboratory can be divided into natural and artificial light. Typically, gametes and embryos are exposed to artificial light in IVF laboratories. The primary sources of light are the laboratory ambient light and the light source of the microscope. Since the intensity of light is inversely proportional to the square of the distance between the light source and the embryo, and the microscope light source is closer to the embryo, so the embryos will be exposed to light intensity from the microscope light source that significantly exceeds that of the ambient light.

6.2.1 Ambient Light

In the early days of IVF technology, laboratories were converted from rooms used for other purposes. IVF laboratories have evolved from dressing rooms without lighting to operating rooms with variable light sources, then to rooms equipped with incandescent lamps with variable intensity control, and rooms only with standard fluorescent lamps. The type, quality, and intensity of lighting vary greatly from laboratory to laboratory, and there is a lack of consistent standards regarding lighting. Noda et al. observed an increased blastocyst formation rate when using a low-intensity ambient light [23]. Another study investigated the spectral composition and light intensity in an IVF laboratory and calculated the light radiation dose to embryos during handlings and manipulations. The researchers found that ambient light in their laboratory had an illumination intensity of 0.1–0.5 w/m^2 (200–400 lux), typically much lower than a microscope's light source [24]. Ambient light has a lower light intensity in the short wavelength spectrum than microscope light—despite this, ambient light still adversely affects embryos.

Ambient lighting may influence the embryos even during embryo transfer, as the surgeon must apply a bright light to the cervix during the operation. The embryos are exposed to that same light when implanted into the uterine cavity. However, it is unknown whether and to what extent the embryos are affected in this scenario.

6.2.2 Microscopic Light

It is reported that 95% of the total light exposure to embryos during in vitro fertilization comes from the microscope [24], and that ambient light's effect on embryos is insignificant if the room's lighting is soft enough. Since microscope light intensity accounts for the vast majority of total light exposure to embryos, it is essential to minimize the length of time embryos are observed under the microscope. The illumination intensity of the microscope lamp is about 20–30 W/m^2 (2500–5000 lux). Meanwhile, embryologists should be aware that light in the 400–500 nm (blue light) range is most likely to affect gametes and embryos and that most light sources encompass this wavelength spectral range (Fig. 6.3). Installing a blue light filter can effectively eliminate light at wavelengths below 490 nm, and culture dishes can also absorb a small fraction of the light.

6.2.3 Common Types of Light Sources in IVF Laboratories and Relevant Light Parameters

6.2.3.1 Common Types of Light Sources
Incandescent lamp: also known as "tungsten lamp," was the most common light source in the early days. Its luminescent mechanism is that heat will be generated when the current passes through the tungsten wire. When the temperature rises to about 2000 °C, it reaches the incandescent state, and light can be emitted. The spectrum emitted by incandescent lamps is continuous and uniform, with excellent color rendering (the color

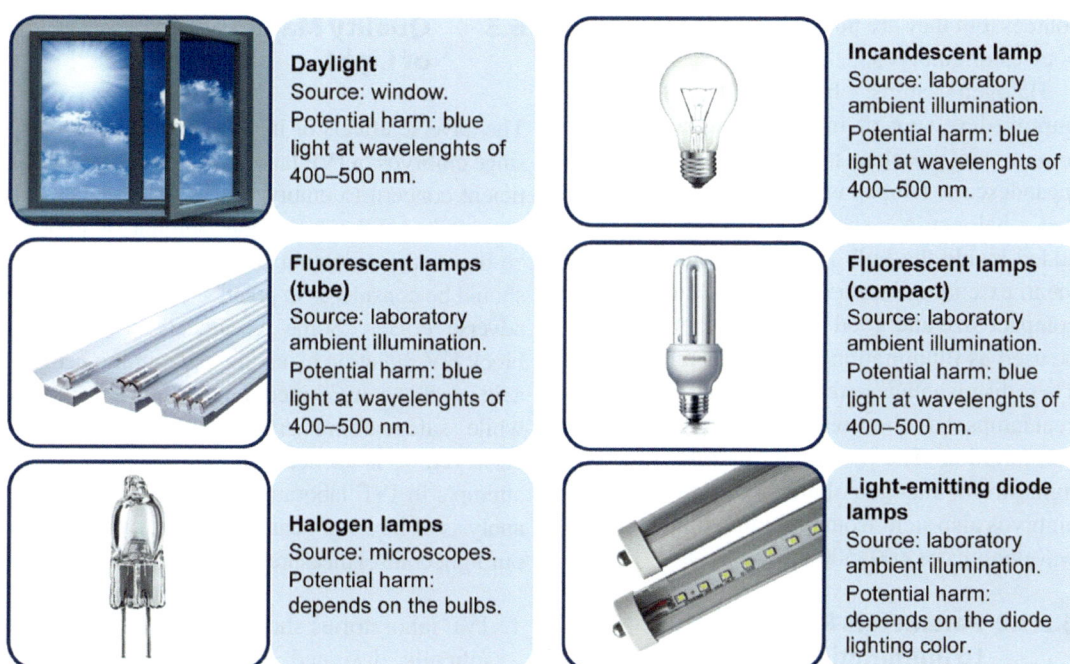

Daylight
Source: window.
Potential harm: blue light at wavelenghts of 400–500 nm.

Incandescent lamp
Source: laboratory ambient illumination.
Potential harm: blue light at wavelenghts of 400–500 nm.

Fluorescent lamps (tube)
Source: laboratory ambient illumination.
Potential harm: blue light at wavelenghts of 400–500 nm.

Fluorescent lamps (compact)
Source: laboratory ambient illumination.
Potential harm: blue light at wavelenghts of 400–500 nm.

Halogen lamps
Source: microscopes.
Potential harm: depends on the bulbs.

Light-emitting diode lamps
Source: laboratory ambient illumination.
Potential harm: depends on the diode lighting color.

Fig. 6.3 Common sources of light in IVF laboratories

rendering index can be up to 99–100). Nevertheless, the disadvantages of incandescent lamps include high-power consumption, short life span, and being potentially harmful to gametes and embryos because they contain blue light at wavelengths of 400–500 nm.

Fluorescent lamps: their luminescent mechanism is to utilize ultraviolet light released by low-pressure mercury vapor after being energized, which irradiates the fluorescent powder on the lamp to emit visible light. The radiation spectrum of fluorescent powder consists of three base colors: red (peak wavelength 611 nm), green (peak wavelength 541 nm), and blue (peak wavelength 450 nm). Fluorescent powders of these three colors are filled in the fluorescent lamp at a specific ratio. The potential hazard of fluorescent lamps is that their emission spectrum contains blue light. Fluorescent lamps can be divided into cool white and warm white light, and the latter is recommended for IVF laboratories. Fluorescent lamps are now mostly installed in IVF workstations and clean benches, so it is important to make sure they are turned off when performing in vitro operations on oocytes or embryos.

Light-emitting diode (LED) lamps: LED lamps are solid-state semiconductor devices that convert electrical energy into visible light. LED lamps feature the advantages of high luminous efficiency and long service life. However, their color rendering index is not as good as incandescent and halogen lamps. LED lamps are available in a variety of colors, allowing users to choose the right color according to their needs. Currently, most clean rooms such as surgery rooms and laboratories are equipped with flat-panel LED clean lamps, which have the advantages of a giant illuminated area and extremely uniform light and allow sterilization and air decontamination. In our center, for example, there are two types of LED lamps: (a) warm white flat-panel LED clean lamps for daily operation lighting, with four sets in each of the two culture rooms (55 m² and 49 m² respectively), with a color temperature of about 3000 K and an average illuminance of about 100 lux; and (b) cool white flat-panel LED clean lamps for lighting during non-embryo activities (such as equipment maintenance, cleaning, and sanitation). It is important to note that some microscopes utilize LED lamps as their light sources, but they are not well suited for observing oocytes or embryos.

Halogen lamps: Halogen lamps are an improved version of incandescent lamps. Their luminescent mechanism is similar to that of incandescent lamps, with the difference being that a halogen gas such as iodine or bromine is added inside the bulb housing the tungsten filament, extending its service life. Because of their compact size and good color rendering, they can be used as illumination sources for microscopes. Their disadvantages are also similar to incandescent lamps, i.e., short service life, and high-power consumption. The potentially harmful effects of light from halogen lamps on gametes and embryos also stem from including blue light with wavelengths of 400–500 nm.

6.2.3.2 Parameters Related to Illumination

Luminous flux: It indicates the brightness of the light source itself and is measured in lumens (lm). And it is not necessarily proportional to power consumption, for example, a 100-Watt old-fashioned incandescent lamp may be as bright as a 12-Watt LED lamp.

Illuminance: It indicates the effectiveness of lighting and is measured in lux. For example, a lamp looks brighter when held closer and less bright when held farther. The lamp's brightness (luminous flux) does not change; instead, the illuminance we receive is changed. Notably, illuminance is called light intensity in some studies, which is easily, but not rigorously, understood.

Color rendering index: It is an indicator of color fidelity. Generally, the higher the color rendering index of light, the closer the color of an object under this light to its actual color. The full score of the color rendering index is 100, that is, the color rendering index of sunlight.

Color temperature: It is a measurement that indicates the color component contained in the light and is expressed in Kelvins (K). For example, warm white light (white light with a touch of red), color temperature <3000 K; intermediate color light (white light), color temperature 3000–5000 K; cool white light (white with a touch of blue), color temperature >5000 K.

6.3 Quality Management of Light

The adverse effects of light on gametes and early-stage embryos in IVF laboratories should be of sufficient concern to embryologists. Although we do not yet know the acceptable amount of light for embryos, the reduction of embryo light exposure should be considered in practice due to the possible adverse effects. Some researchers have tried to block UV radiation by adding para-amino benzoic-acid to the culture medium for mouse embryos while safeguarding embryo development [25]. However, it is difficult for us to make similar attempts in IVF laboratories. But instead, with an analysis of how light causes damage, we can focus our light control measures on the following aspects:

1. IVF laboratories should be carefully and specifically designed, no longer be converted from rooms initially used for other purposes, and be protected from sunlight, preferably without windows.
2. Apply the right light source: Use adjustable light sources better to control the light intensity in the IVF laboratory, and avoid using any light sources with UV radiation.
3. Filters can be installed on the microscope to reduce light at wavelengths below a certain level. For example, the green filter blocks light at wavelengths below 500 nm. Moreover, warm white flat-panel LED clean lights can be used for laboratory lighting.
4. Light does not only affect the embryo. As previously elaborated, light may worsen the quality of culture media and tissue culture oil, so it is crucial to put the prepared media back into the refrigerator for light-proof storage as soon as possible and avoid leaving them on the bench for a long time. If a medical refrigerator with a glass door is used, be sure to cover the refrigerator door with light-proof film.
5. Schedule the embryo observation process appropriately, avoid unnecessary microscopic observations, and minimize the time embryos are exposed to light.
6. Time-lapse imaging culture systems usually use low-intensity red (or green) visible light for illumination and, therefore, radiant lower energy.

This protective setup, together with the short exposure time (even if consecutive images are superimposed over several days), should be beneficial in reducing the stress on the embryo and can be applied where appropriate in practice.

In addition, it is worth noting that the light conditions in the IVF laboratory are related to the staff's productivity. Too much light tends to make people tired and stresses gametes and embryos, while too little light interferes with the concentration of the staff, which is unfavorable for observing the markings on the culture dishes and prone to errors. Therefore, laboratory light intensity should be minimized, and the time gametes and embryos are exposed to light should be reduced while enabling room lighting to be adequate for work.

References

1. Zan-Bar T, Bartoov B, Segal R, et al. Influence of visible light and ultraviolet irradiation on motility and fertility of mammalian and fish sperm. Photomed Laser Surg. 2005;23(6):549–55.
2. Lesser MP, Kruse VA, Barry TM. Exposure to ultraviolet radiation causes apoptosis in developing sea urchin embryos. J Exp Biol. 2003;206(Pt 22):4097–103.
3. Umaoka Y, Noda Y, Nakayama T, et al. Effect of visual light on in vitro embryonic development in the hamster. Theriogenology. 1992;38(6):1043–54.
4. Daniel JC Jr. Clevage of mammalian ova inhibited by visible light. Nature. 1964;201:316–7.
5. Bognar Z, Csabai TJ, Pallinger E, et al. The effect of light exposure on the cleavage rate and implantation capacity of preimplantation murine embryos. J Reprod Immunol. 2019;132:21–8.
6. Takenaka M, Horiuchi T, Yanagimachi R. Effects of light on development of mammalian zygotes. Proc Natl Acad Sci U S A. 2007;104(36):14289–93.
7. Lampiao F. Free radicals generation in an in vitro fertilization setting and how to minimize them. World J Obstet Gynecol. 2012;1(3):29–34.
8. Hammadeh ME, ALHasani S, Rosenbaum P, et al. Reactive oxygen species, total antioxidant concentration of seminal plasma and their effect on sperm parameters and outcome of IVF/ICSI patients. Arch Gynecol Obstet. 2008;277(6):515–26.
9. Du Plessis SS, Makker K, Desai NR, et al. Impact of oxidative stress on IVF. Exp Rev Obstret Gynecol. 2008;3:539–54.
10. Agarwal A, Gupta S, Sharma R. Oxidative stress and its implications in female infertility a clinician's perspective. Reprod Biomed Online. 2005;11(5):641–50.
11. Guerin P, Mouatassim EL, S, Menezo Y. Oxidative stress and protection against reactive oxygen species in the pre-implantation embryo and its surroundings. Hum Reprod Update. 2001;7(2):175–89.
12. Lv B, Liu C, Chen Y, et al. Light-induced injury in mouse embryos revealed by single-cell RNA sequencing. Biol Res. 2019;52(1):48.
13. Hartshorn C, Anshelevich A, Wangh LJ. Laser zona drilling does not induce hsp70i transcription in blastomeres of eight-cell mouse embryos. Fertil Steril. 2005;84(5):1547–50.
14. Uppangala S, D'Souza F, Pudakalakatti S, et al. Laser assisted zona hatching does not lead to immediate impairment in human embryo quality and metabolism. Syst Biol Reprod Med. 2016;62(6):396–403.
15. Konig K, Tadir Y, Patrizio P, et al. Effects of ultraviolet exposure and near infrared laser tweezers on human spermatozoa. Hum Reprod. 1996;11(10):2162–4.
16. Dietrich GJ, Szpyrka A, Wojtczak M, et al. Effects of UV irradiation and hydrogen peroxide on DNA fragmentation, motility and fertilizing ability of rainbow trout (Oncorhynchus mykiss) spermatozoa. Theriogenology. 2005;64(8):1809–22.
17. Oh SJ, Gong SP, Lee ST, et al. Light intensity and wavelength during embryo manipulation are important factors for maintaining viability of preimplantation embryos in vitro. Fertil Steril. 2007;88(4 Suppl):1150–7.
18. Otsuki J, Nagai Y, Chiba K. Peroxidation of mineral oil used in droplet culture is detrimental to fertilization and embryo development. Fertil Steril. 2007;88(3):741–3.
19. Otsuki J, Nagai Y, Chiba K. Damage of embryo development caused by peroxidized mineral oil and its association with albumin in culture. Fertil Steril. 2009;91(5):1745–9.
20. Hughes PM, Morbeck DE, Hudson SB, et al. Peroxides in mineral oil used for in vitro fertilization: defining limits of standard quality control assays. J Assist Reprod Genet. 2010;27(2–3):87–92.
21. Martinez CA, Nohalez A, Ceron JJ, et al. Peroxidized mineral oil increases the oxidant status of culture media and inhibits in vitro porcine embryo development. Theriogenology. 2017;103:17–23.
22. Li R, Liu Y, Pedersen HS, et al. Effect of ambient light exposure of media and embryos on development and quality of porcine parthenogenetically activated embryos. Zygote. 2015;23(3):378–83.
23. Noda Y, Goto Y, Umaoka Y, et al. Culture of human embryos in alpha modification of Eagle's medium under low oxygen tension and low illumination. Fertil Steril. 1994;62(5):1022–7.
24. Ottosen LD, Hindkjaer J, Ingerslev J. Light exposure of the ovum and preimplantation embryo during ART procedures. J Assist Reprod Genet. 2007;24(2–3):99–103.
25. Robertson JL, Minhas BS, Palmer TV, et al. The absorption of ultraviolet light by the addition of para-amino benzoic acid to nutrient media used in vitro fertilization. Theriogenology. 1988;29:298.

Microbial Contamination of Culture Media

The IVF culture system provides a safe and stable environment for the survival and development of gametes and embryos in vitro. However, this stable, ideal environment is also hospitable to various microorganisms. The incidence of microbial contamination in IVF cycles has been reported in the literature to be approximately 0.1% to 1% [1]. Microbial contamination threatens the survival of gametes and embryos, causing degeneration, developmental arrest, and cross-infection in the culture system. The pathogens can even be transmitted to patients through embryo transfer. There have been previous incidents of patients being infected with hepatitis B virus (HBV) and human immunodeficiency virus (HIV) derived from IVF treatment [2, 3]. Although contamination of an IVF culture system can be detected in most cases, it is worth noting that insidious contamination may have even more severe consequences. Therefore, effective infection prevention is the foundation for ensuring the safe and stable operation of IVF laboratories. The asepsis principle should be strictly enforced in IVF laboratories to control infectious factors and inhibit the growth of pathogenic microorganisms.

7.1 Sources of Microbial Contamination

Microbial contamination in the IVF laboratory can originate from many sources, including the follicular fluid, semen, fresh or frozen gametes, embryos, laboratory staff, laboratory environment, air conditioning system, equipment, and consumables such as culture media, laboratory gases, and liquid nitrogen. This section will address microbial contamination from oocyte-derived contamination, semen-derived contamination, and manipulation-derived contamination.

7.1.1 Oocyte-Derived Contamination

Microorganisms often transiently colonize the female genital tract without causing symptoms of infection [4], and follicular fluid is not completely sterile. A study that included 263 follicular fluid specimens showed that microorganisms were detected in 100% of vaginal swabs collected after transvaginal oocyte retrieval, while bacteria were detected in 99% of follicular fluid speci-

D. Li, Y. Gao, *Quality Management in the Assisted Reproduction Laboratory*,
https://doi.org/10.1007/978-981-99-6659-2_7

mens [5]. In this case, 71% of the paired follicular fluid specimens and the vaginal swabs contained the same microorganism(s) ("contaminated" follicular fluid). The remaining 29% of the paired follicular fluid specimens and vaginal swabs contained different microorganisms ("colonized" follicular fluid). These results suggest that microbial contaminations in follicular fluid do not necessarily originate from the oocyte retrieval procedure but are most likely brought about by the follicular fluid itself. In this study, microorganisms identified in follicle fluid cultures were Lactobacillus, Actinomyces, Propionibacterium, Bifidobacterium, Staphylococcus, Streptococcus agalactiae, Peptostreptococcus, Escherichia coli, and Enterococcus faecalis, with Actinomyces being more prevalent in "colonized" follicle fluid specimens, and Peptostreptococcus being more prevalent in "contaminated" follicle fluid specimens. It was also found that follicles from the left and right ovaries had different microbiota, which may be related to their hematopoietic anatomy [6]. Furthermore, the study concluded that Actinomyces, Bifidobacterium, Propionibacterium, Streptococcus, and Staphylococcus were associated with poor pregnancy outcomes following in vitro fertilization. In contrast, the presence of Lactobacillus in follicular fluid of both ovaries seemed to be associated with a higher implantation rate, possibly due to the inhibition of other microbial growth by hydrogen peroxide and lactic acid produced by Lactobacillus. Other studies have suggested that certain bacteria in follicular fluid (e.g., Escherichia coli and Streptococcus) may inhibit follicle-stimulating hormone (FSH) from binding to receptors on granulosa cells. This inhibitory effect can impair the normal physiological function of FSH, destroy oocytes and cause an immune response during folliculogenesis or embryo implantation [7, 8]. Collectively, the above findings suggest that follicular fluid contains a variety of microorganisms and that different microbial species can affect IVF outcomes to varying degrees.

In another study, samples from the genital tract were collected and cultured from patients who underwent embryo transfer. The results showed that microorganisms were detected in 87.5% of the samples collected, and the presence of microbial contamination of the genital tract was associated with a significant decrease in the pregnancy rate. The authors suggest that this might be caused by microorganisms transferred from the lower genital tract into the uterine cavity during embryo transfer, which can change the biochemical or ultrastructural features of the endometrium and lead to a decrease in endometrial tolerance [9]. In summary, from oocyte retrieval to embryo implantation, microorganisms can contaminate oocytes and embryos at all stages of IVF and ultimately lead to poor IVF outcomes.

7.1.2 Semen-Derived Contamination

The most likely source of contamination in IVF laboratories is semen specimens, from which bacteria can be detected even when semen collection is performed under rigorous hygienic control. The literature has widely reported that 50% to 100% of cultured semen specimens are microorganism-positive. The most contaminating organisms are non-pathogenic, among which the most prevalent ones are Staphylococcus epidermidis, Streptococcus green, Escherichia coli, Staphylococcus aureus, Streptococcus faecalis, Streptococcus haemolyticus, and Enterobacter agglomerans [10]. Moreover, many of the bacteria in semen are also present in women's vagina, indicating that the bacteria may be transmitted between sexual partners [11]. Some studies have also demonstrated that the bacterial species present in semen do not differ significantly between sperm donors and infertile patients, and anaerobic bacteria may be biomarkers of low sperm quality.

In addition to bacteria, semen may also be infected by Chlamydia trachomatis [12] and mycoplasma. Clinical diagnosis of chlamydia and mycoplasma infections is routinely made by testing urine samples or urethral swabs. However, the infection cannot be completely ruled out even if the results are negative. Eley et al. analyzed 11 studies on Chlamydia trachomatis in urine and semen [13]. They found that Chlamydia trachomatis was detected in both semen and urine in 56% of patients who were positive for Chlamydia trachomatis. In contrast, Chlamydia trachomatis was only detected in urine in 20% of patients, and the percentage of patients with Chlamydia trachomatis detected only in semen was 23%. Mycoplasma in semen is difficult to detect, but its presence may adversely affect IVF outcomes in several ways, such as pH alteration, induction of oxidative stress, and secretion of harmful metabolites [14].

Microorganisms in semen mainly originate from the male urethra and skin. While non-pathogenic microorganisms such as aerobic bacteria, anaerobic bacteria, yeast, and mycoplasma genitalium are often detected in the male urethra, there may also be pathogenic microorganisms such as gonococci, Chlamydia trachomatis, and trichomonads. In addition, microorganisms from hands and vulvar skin may contaminate semen during sperm retrieval. Therefore, it is important to emphasize personal hygiene to the patients and make sure they wash their hands strictly before sperm collection.

7.1.3 Manipulation-Derived Contamination

Some studies have shown that besides semen, the most common source of contamination is inadequate aseptic manipulation. In humans, typical microorganisms found on the skin include staphylococci, coryne-like bacteria, Propionibacterium spp., Acinetobacter spp., and Malassezia furfur. Moreover, a smaller group of Micrococcaceae and Gram-negative bacteria are part of the resident flora, especially on the hands, such as Acinetobacter, Enterobacter, and Klebsiella spp. [15]. Each person sheds 30,000 to 40,000 skin cells per minute. These skin cells make up most of the dust in the laboratory and are the main reason for the increased airborne bacterial load inside the laboratory. Simple cleaning measures can reduce environmental microbial contamination by 80%, while disinfectants can reduce it by

95% [16]. The laboratory must therefore develop a strict hygiene management system to avoid as much possible contamination arising from human intervention.

7.2 Types of Microbial Contamination

Common microbial species in IVF laboratories include bacteria, fungi, mycoplasma, parasites, viruses, and prions.

7.2.1 Bacteria

The most common culprits of bacterial contamination in IVF laboratories are Escherichia coli, Pseudomonas, and Staphylococcus Albicans. Bacterial contamination is easier to detect once it occurs, mostly with manifestations such as cloudy or recolored culture media. Different bacterial contamination often occurs at different times, e.g., Escherichia coli contamination is often detected on day 1 [17]. All reported contamination events were derived from conventional IVF cycles during the literature search. It is probably because the ICSI is performed with a single sperm isolated from the PVP and an oocyte that has removed perivitelline granulosa cells. Both measures contribute to avoiding contamination. Also, given the ineffectiveness of prophylactic antibiotics, ICSI is recommended to patients with recurrent embryo contamination to reduce the risk of embryo contamination.

7.2.2 Fungi

Fungal contamination commonly occurs in IVF laboratories and can be attributed to the absence of anti-fungal agents in the culture media. It can originate from the follicle aspiration process and airborne contaminants or be brought in by staff. Aspergillus, for example, is one of the common fungal contaminants in the air, and sometimes its source can be traced to the heating or air conditioning system. Embryos exposed to fungal contamination should be removed from the contaminated culture medium immediately, as there is still a chance that they will survive and continue to develop [18]. Although fungi can be removed from cultures by repeated rinsing, fungal contamination may still compromise the embryo's development. Therefore, patients must be fully informed and sign informed consent before freezing or implanting embryos at risk.

7.2.3 Mycoplasma

Mycoplasma contamination has always been a more complex problem as its occurrence is often quite insidious. It is estimated that mycoplasma may contaminate up to 40% of tissue cultures. The numerous effects of mycoplasmas on cells include suppressing cell growth, altering pH, depleting cellular substrates, inducing oxidative stress, producing ammonia, and other harmful metabolites, and modifying DNA, RNA, and protein synthesis. In addition, mycoplasma is closely associated with infertility, stillbirth, preterm birth, and meningitis. Mycoplasma contamination in IVF laboratories may lead to many negative consequences [19], such as compromised embryo culture and pregnancy outcomes, embryo fragmentation and/or vacuolation, and poor quality or necrosis of embryos.

7.2.4 Viruses

Efforts to address viral contamination in IVF laboratories have primarily focused on a few viruses that can be transmitted during fertilization, such as HIV, HBV, and hepatitis C virus (HCV). When patients who carry these viruses seek help from assisted reproductive therapies, it is important to reduce the risk of transmitting the virus to their partners and/or the next generation. In the meantime, however, we must emphasize to patients that the risk of virus transmission cannot be eliminated with existing techniques. IVF laboratories are recommended to handle specimens originating from virus carriers individually, for example, by storing such embryos separately or

using fully enclosed carriers to cryopreserve these gametes and embryos to minimize the risk of cross-infection.

In conclusion, there are many types of microbial contamination in IVF laboratories and various sources. Most of the contamination cannot be eliminated upon occurrence, and it is, therefore, necessary for the laboratory to develop a strict hygiene management system and standardized management procedures to minimize microbial contamination.

7.3 Management of Microbial Contamination

The key to preventing microbial contamination lies in rigorous management: ensuring good aseptic operation, regularly cleaning and sterilizing the laboratory equipment, and preventing contaminated items from entering the operational area and culture system.

7.3.1 Culture Media

Gametes and embryos are cultured in vitro throughout the IVF process, so it is critical to ensure the sterility and stability of the culture medium. The stability of antibiotic supplements within culture media can be affected by temperature, pH, and light exposure. The establishment and strict implementation of principles related to culture media are mandatory in IVF laboratories:

1. Culture media should be stored at 4 °C, and repeated/frequent pickups should be avoided as much as possible.
2. Containers filled with culture media should be kept airtight. Culture media that have been left unsealed or heated should be discarded.
3. Moreover, appropriate specifications of the commercial culture medium should be selected based on the medium requirement decided by the mean number of IVF cycles per day, and ensure that it is used up as soon as possible after opening the bottle.

4. Before using the culture medium, its appearance should be checked/observed briefly, and the medium should be discarded once contamination is found.

5. The preparation of culture media and dishes should strictly follow the principle of asepsis. The prepared culture dishes or test tubes should be rechecked to ensure their cleanliness and sterility before placing them in the incubator. Moreover, all containers should be carefully checked for cracks.

6. Since most contamination incidents happen during the conventional IVF cycles, two medium microdroplets are always reserved for control when preparing insemination dishes (microdroplet insemination method) at our center: one is blank and the other microdroplet is with sperm (no oocyte). In this case, if contamination is detected on day 1 (contaminated microdroplets will show foggy turbidity, especially under the light of a stereoscopic microscope), a preliminary determination of the source can be made. For example, in the case of contaminated sperm-oocyte microdroplets—if neither the sperm microdroplet nor the blank microdroplet is contaminated, the contamination is most likely from oocytes; if the sperm microdroplet (with no oocyte) is also contaminated but not the blank control microdroplet, the contamination is more likely from the sperm; and if all microdroplets (sperm-oocyte, sperm, and blank microdroplets) are contaminated, the contamination is more likely from the culture medium. However, it is not always the case that we detect the contamination on day 1. For cases where no contamination is found on day 1, we would still preserve the processed semen for following three days, just in case to exclude the possibility of sperm-derived contamination.

7.3.2 Refrigerator

1. First, power off the refrigerator.
2. Clean the inside of the refrigerator entirely with purified water.

3. Splash the inside of the refrigerator with 75% ethanol and keep the refrigerator door closed for 24 h.
4. Wipe the inside of the refrigerator with pure water, and power up the refrigerator after the interior is completely dry.
5. Make a record in the refrigerator log book after the cleaning and sterilizing procedure.

7.3.3 Incubator

1. Clean the inside and outside surfaces of the incubator regularly with pure water or incubator-specific cleansers.
2. Internal components of some incubators can be removed for autoclaving, but UV sterilization is not recommended.
3. Change the water in the humidification tray or humidification bottle/tank weekly.

7.3.4 Consumables

Consumables commonly used in embryo laboratories include Pasteur glass pipettes, culture dishes, centrifuge tubes, microinjection pipettes, and oocyte denudation pipettes, among others. Endotoxin carried by consumables is a significant risk factor for embryo development. Therefore, IVF laboratories are advised to use specialized consumables that have passed the endotoxin and mouse embryo tests. Endotoxin is very heat resistant, and Pasteur glass pipettes made in-house should be sterilized by dry heat (250 °C/30 mins or 160 °C/2 h or more) to eliminate endotoxin.

7.3.5 Hygiene Management System of Embryo Laboratory

A disciplined hygiene management system is the foundation for the prevention and control of nosocomial infections:

1. Non-IVF laboratory personnel are prohibited from entering the laboratory without being authorized by the laboratory director.

2. The number of people entering the laboratory should be restricted, and even laboratory personnel should avoid entering if there is no operation need to be performed.

3. It is forbidden to bring non-work-related items into the laboratory, such as personal accessories, books or paper materials, and electronic products.

4. Before entering the laboratory, personnel should change into clean laboratory shoes and sterile barrier gowns, wear surgical masks and hats (with complete coverage of mouth, nose, and hair), and wash hands following the surgical seven-step handwashing procedure.

5. One must go through the air shower before entering the laboratory and change into laboratory shoes before entering the air shower.

6. Serological screening should be performed on patients to detect infections such as blood-borne viruses, mycoplasma, and chlamydia. All laboratory staff should wear gloves when handling virus carriers' specimens and change to new gloves promptly after accomplishing handling.

7. Wipe the workbench with sterilized injection water before and after each day's work. In case of any liquid contamination (e.g., follicular fluid, semen) on the bench during the manipulation, it can be cleaned and decontaminated with an IVF-specific disinfectant.

8. Laboratory reagents, consumables, and equipment should be removed from their outer packaging and wiped with IVF-specific disinfectant before entering the laboratory.

9. Waste should be sorted into medical and household waste, and sharp objects should be disposed of in special sharps containers. Medical waste from patients should be placed in medical waste bins, and no waste can be left in any sterile area. Medical waste should be cleared from the laboratory daily.

10. Cleaning staff should not enter the laboratory for cleaning until all work inside the laboratory has been finished and should also strictly comply with the requirements 1–5 mentioned above.

11. Airborne bacterial cultures should be performed regularly for each room and operating area of the IVF laboratory in cooperation with the nosocomial infection department.

7.3.6   Management of Embryo Contamination

1. For patients who have experienced embryo contamination in the previous cycle and are tentatively determined to be sperm-derived, ICSI and processing of semen by density gradient centrifugation associated with sperm upstream method may be recommended.

2. Normally, medium microdroplets with severe microbial contamination will appear cloudy to the naked eye. Once embryo contamination is detected, the culture medium droplets should be replaced immediately, and the embryos should be thoroughly rinsed with a clean culture medium. The contaminated embryos must then be placed in a separate incubator for further incubation and rinsed daily with a clean culture medium before being placed in new culture medium microdroplets. However, the bacteria attached to the zona pellucida cannot be removed entirely by simply rinsing the contaminated embryos, nor can rinsing prevent further contamination during embryo culture and implantation. In this case, one optional approach is to culture the embryos to the blastocyst stage and manually remove the zona pellucida (enzymatic digestion or laser method) before implantation or cryopreservation. However, given that the safety and reliability of this method have yet to be proven, it is essential to fully explain the procedure to the patients and sign informed consent before proceeding with implantation or cryopreservation.

References

1. Zhu GJ, Wei YL, Hu J, et al. Microorganism contamination in in vitro fertilization-embryo transfer system and their sources. Chin J Obstet Gynecol. 2004;39(6):382–4.

2. van Os HC, Drogendijk AC, Fetter WP, et al. The influence of contamination of culture medium with hepatitis B virus on the outcome of in vitro fertilization pregnancies. Am J Obstet Gynecol. 1991;165(1):152–9.

3. Matz B, Kupfer B, Ko Y, et al. HIV-1 infection by artificial insemination. Lancet. 1998;351(9104):728.

4. Viniker DA. Hypothesis on the role of sub-clinical bacteria of the endometrium (bacteria endometrialis) in gynaecological and obstetric enigmas. Hum Reprod Update. 1999;5(4):373–85.

5. Pelzer ES, Allan JA, Waterhouse MA, et al. Microorganisms within human follicular fluid: effects on IVF. PLoS One. 2013;8(3):e59062.

6. Misao F, Kiyomi F, Claus Y, et al. Right-sided ovulation favours pregnancy more then left-sided ovulation. Hum Reprod. 2000;15(9):1921–6.

7. Sluss PM, Lee K, Mattox JH, et al. Estradiol and progesterone production by cultured granulosa cells cryopreserved from in vitro fertilization patients. Eur J Endocrinol. 1994;130(3):259–64.

8. Sluss PM, Reichert LE Jr. Presence of bacteria in porcine follicular fluid and their ability to generate an inhibitor of follicle-stimulating hormone binding to receptor. Biol Reprod. 1983;29(2):335–41.

9. Selman H, Mariani M, Barnocchi N, et al. Examination of bacterial contamination at the time of embryo transfer, and its impact on the IVF/pregnancy outcome. J Assist Reprod Genet. 2007;24(9):395–9.

10. Huang GN, Sun HX. Laboratory techniques in in vitro fertilization and embryo transfer. Beijing: People's Medical Publishing House; 2012.

11. Hou D, Zhou X, Zhong X, et al. Microbiota of the seminal fluid from healthy and infertile men. Fertil Steril. 2013;100(5):1261–9.

12. Al-Mously N, Cross NA, Eley A, et al. Real-time polymerase chain reaction shows that density centrifugation does not always remove Chlamydia trachomatis from human semen. Fertil Steril. 2009;92(5):1606–15.

13. Eley A, Pacey AA. The value of testing semen for Chlamydia trachomatis in men of infertile couples. Int J Androl. 2011;34(5 Pt 1):391–401.

14. Macpherson. Mycoplasmas in tissue culture. J Cell Sci. 1996;1(2):145–68.

15. Lange-Asschenfeldt B, Marenbach D, Lang C, et al. Distribution of bacteria in the epidermal layers and hair follicles of the human skin. Skin Pharmacol Physiol. 2011;24(6):305–11.

16. Elder K, den Bergh MV, Woodward B. Troubleshooting and problem-solving in the IVF laboratory. Cambridge: Cambridge University Press; 2015.

17. Kastrop PM, de Graaf-Miltenburg LA, Gutknecht DR, et al. Microbial contamination of embryo cultures in an ART laboratory: sources and management. Hum Reprod. 2007;22(8):2243–8.

18. Ben-Chetrit A, Shen O, Haran E, et al. Transfer of embryos from yeast-colonized dishes. Fertil Steril. 1996;66(2):335–7.

19. Sylla L, Stradaioli G, Manuali E, et al. The effect of mycoplasma mycoides ssp. mycoides LC of bovine origin on in vitro fertilizing ability of bull spermatozoa and embryo development. Anim Reprod Sci. 2005;85(1–2):81–93.

Morphological Evaluation of Cleavage-Stage Embryos and Blastocysts

8

Over the last two decades, methodologies for assessing embryo implantation potential have emerged, including time-lapse imaging systems, various "-omics" techniques (genomics, metabolomics, etc.), and artificial intelligence. However, all the aforementioned methods are flawed or controversial in varying degrees [1–3]. Thus, conventional morphological indicators of embryos are still used as the main rating parameters or criteria.

8.1 The Main Reference Indicators and Criteria for Rating Cleavage-Stage Embryos

8.1.1 Morphological Indicators

The number of cells, fragmentation grade, cell size, and multinucleation profile of the embryo are the main morphological indicators for scoring cleavage-stage embryos [4].

8.1.1.1 Number of Cells
The cell number signifies the developmental rate of the embryo and is considered as the most important indicator of embryo scoring [5]. Generally, high-quality cleavage-stage embryos exhibit appropriate developmental kinetics and synchrony of division. In addition, the develop-

ment of an early zygote into an eight-cell embryo at 18–20 h/cell cycle is desirable [6], with proper shortening of the cell cycle in later stages.

8.1.1.2 Degree of Fragmentation
Embryo fragmentation is strongly associated with pregnancy outcomes [7]. The degree of fragmentation is usually expressed as the percentage of fragmented blastomeres in the total embryo volume, with <10% being preferable. When larger fragments are indistinguishable from blastomeres, an anucleate cytoplasm diameter of <45 μm on day 2 or < 40 μm on day 3 is the recommended definition of a fragment [8] (Fig. 8.1).

8.1.1.3 Symmetry
Theoretically, normal embryonic mitosis produces daughter cells of equal sizes. Embryos with symmetric cleavage have shown lower rates of multinucleation and aneuploidy, as well as a significantly elevated implantation rate. However, the equality and size of all blastomeres also depend on the developmental pattern and specific stage of the embryo, that is, the stage-specific cleavage pattern [6] (Table 8.1).

8.1.1.4 Multinucleation
An embryo is considered multinucleated if >1 nucleus is present in one or more blastomeres. However, the smaller size, larger number, and overlapping of embryonic blastomeres on day 3

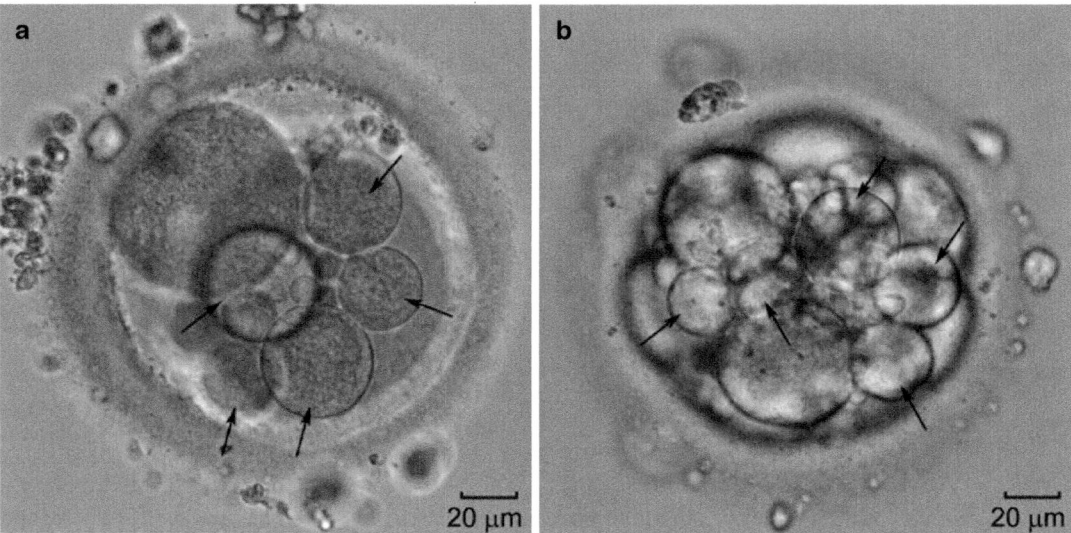

Fig. 8.1 Fragments of cleavage-stage embryos (200×). Note: Arrows indicate larger fragments. (**a**) Fragments in an embryo on day 2; (**b**) fragments in an embryo on day 3

would considerably increase the difficulty of observation. Therefore, for day-3 embryos, where multinucleation (MN) is difficult to observe, incorporating the observation results of multinucleation on day 2 for embryo scoring is possible.

8.1.2 Scoring Criteria for Cleavage-Stage Embryos

8.1.2.1 Scoring Criteria for Cleavage-Stage Embryos on Day 2

The scoring criteria for cleavage-stage embryos on day 2 are presented in Table 8.2. The superiority hierarchy of grade I, II-a, II-b, III, and IV embryos descends sequentially.

8.1.2.2 Scoring Criteria for Cleavage-Stage Embryos on Day 3

The scoring criteria for cleavage-stage embryos on day 3 is presented in Table 8.3 and Fig. 8.2. The following points should be noted:

(a) Grade I embryos should be 8-cell embryos (day 3) developing from 4-cell embryos (day 2), and these 4-cell embryos have no multinucleation phenomenon. In addition, grade I embryos should also be characterized by clear homogeneous cytoplasm (no pitting or vacuolation), tight intercellular junctions, and normal zona pellucida (no darkening, excessive thickness/thinness, abnormal shape, etc.). However, the impacts of several peculiar / abnormal morphological features on embryo development lack robust data support; therefore, these are not included as main scoring indicators (these peculiar /abnormal morphologies are shown in Fig. 8.3). (b) Relatively symmetric cells are represented by the following equation: (The largest cell diameter − the smallest cell diameter) / the largest cell diameter <20% [9]. (c) The superiority hierarchy of grade I, II-a, II-b, III-a, III-b, and IV embryos descends sequentially; however, no superiority difference exists within subgroups of grade II-a, II-b, or III-b embryos.

Table 8.1 Morphological diagram of embryos with stage-specific cleavage patterns

Embryos	Illustrations	Description
4-cell embryo		Four blastomeres of equal size
5-cell embryo		Two blastomeres are small and equally sized (purple), and three blastomeres are big and equally sized (blue)
6-cell embryo		Four blastomeres are small and equally sized (purple), and two blastomeres are big and equally sized (blue)
7-cell embryo		Six blastomeres are small and equally sized (purple), and one blastomere is big (blue)
8-cell embryo		Eight blastomeres of equal size

1. Division patterns other than these are considered as non-stage-specific cleavage patterns
2. For 4- to 7-cell embryos with the stage-specific cleavage patterns described above, this illustration simply shows that their cell division patterns are more plausible. However, they may still suffer from poor developmental rates or less synchronized cleavage. The specific or non-specific cleavage patterns indicates whether the embryo development conforms to the dynamic cleavage regularity, mainly based on cell size, without observation or judgment via a time-lapse imaging system

Table 8.2 Scoring criteria for cleavage-stage embryos (day 2)

Grade	No. of cells	Symmetry	Fragments	MN
I				
I	4	Good	<10%	No
II				
II-a	4	Good	10–25%	No
II-a	2/3/5	With a stage-specific cleavage pattern	<10%	No
II-b	2/3/5	With a stage-specific cleavage pattern	10–25%	No
III				
III	2–5	Without a stage-specific cleavage pattern or large difference in size between cells	<25%	/
III	2–5	/	26–50%	/
III	≥6	/	<50%	/
III	/	/	<50%	Yes
IV				
IV	/	/	>50%	/

The slash ("/") indicates that this item does not need to be considered. *MN* multinucleation

Table 8.3 Scoring criteria for cleavage-stage embryos (day 3)

Grade	No. of cells	Symmetry	Fragments	MN	Figure
I					
I	8	Good	<10%	No	8.2a
II					
II-a	8	Good	10–25%	No	8.2b
II-a	≥8	The blastomeres are relatively symmetric	<10%	No	8.2c
II-a	6–7	With a stage-specific cleavage pattern	<10%	No	8.2d
II-b	≥8	The blastomeres are relatively symmetric	10–25%	No	8.2e
II-b	6–7	With a stage-specific cleavage pattern	10–25%	No	8.2f
III					
III-a	4–5	With a stage-specific cleavage pattern	<25%	No	8.2g, h
III-b	≥4	Large difference in size between cells or without a stage-specific cleavage pattern	<25%	/	8.2i, j
III-b	≥4	/	26–50%	/	8.2k
III-b	/	/	<50%	Yes	8.2l, m
IV					
IV	<4	/	/	/	8.2n
IV	/	/	>50%	/	8.2o

The slash ("/") indicates that this item does not need to be considered. *MN* multinucleation

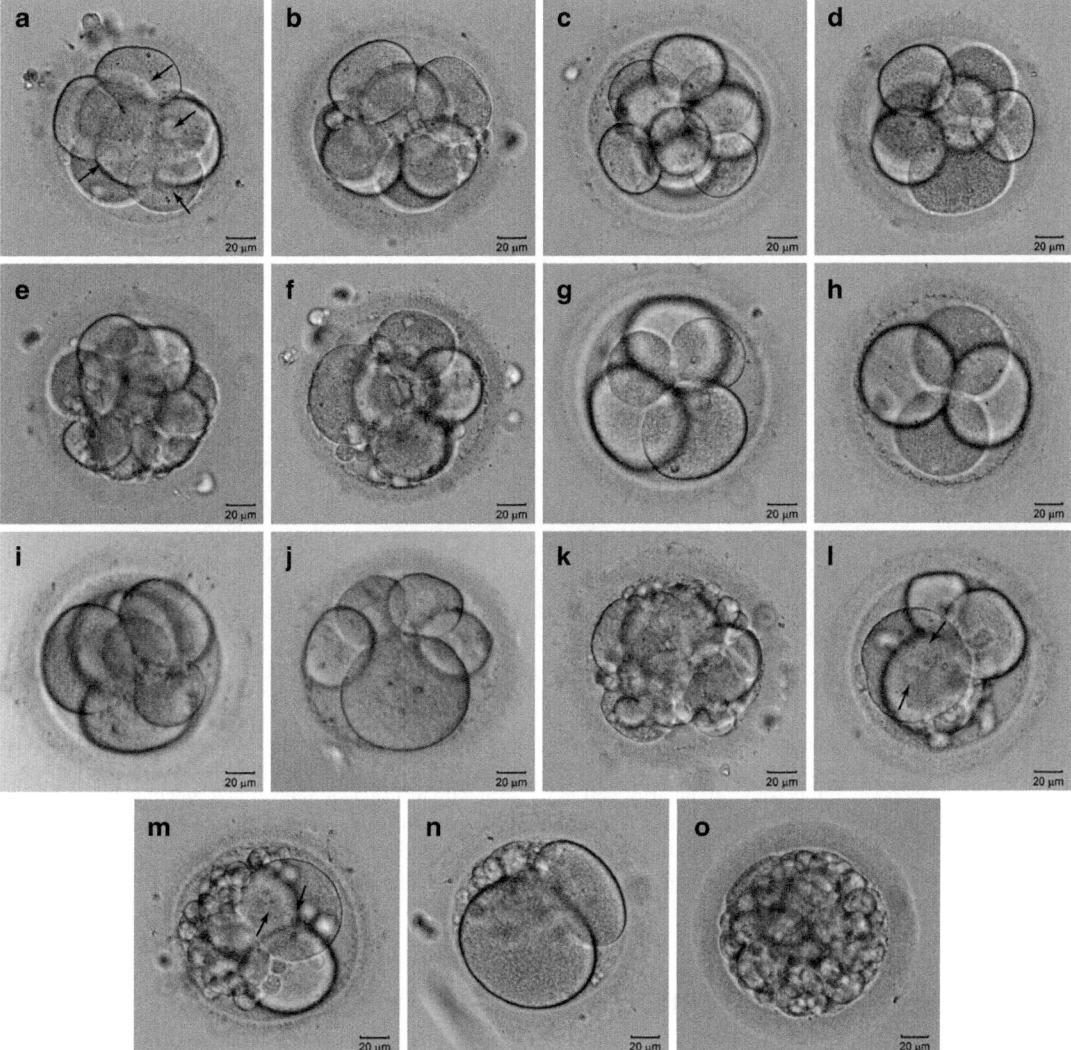

Fig. 8.2 Grade I–IV cleavage-stage embryos on day 3 (200×). (**a**) An 8-cell grade I embryo which has good symmetry and no fragment, and a visible mononucleated nucleus in most blastomeres (arrows indicate mononuclear blastomeres); (**b**) an 8-cell grade II-a embryo, with 10–15% fragments; (**c**) a 10-cell grade II-a embryo; (**d**) a 7-cell grade II-a embryo presenting a stage-specific cleavage pattern; (**e**) a 9-cell grade II-b embryo, with 15–25% fragments; (**f**) a 7-cell grade II-b embryo possessing a stage-specific cleavage pattern, with 15–20% fragments; (**g**) a 5-cell grade III-a embryo possessing a stage-specific cleavage pattern; (**h**) a 4-cell grade III-a embryo possessing a stage-specific cleavage pattern; (**i**–**j**) the embryos possess non-stage-specific cleavage patterns; (**i**) a 6-cell grade III-b embryo; (**j**) a 5-cell grade III-b embryo; (**k**) an 8-cell grade III-b embryo, with relatively equal blastomeres and fragments >25%; (**l**) a 4-cell grade III-b embryo (arrows indicate multinucleated nuclei of blastomeres); (**m**) a 4-cell grade III-b embryo, with fragments >25% (arrows indicate multinucleated nuclei of blastomeres); (**n**) a developmental arrested embryo graded IV; (**o**) a grade IV embryo with fragments >50%

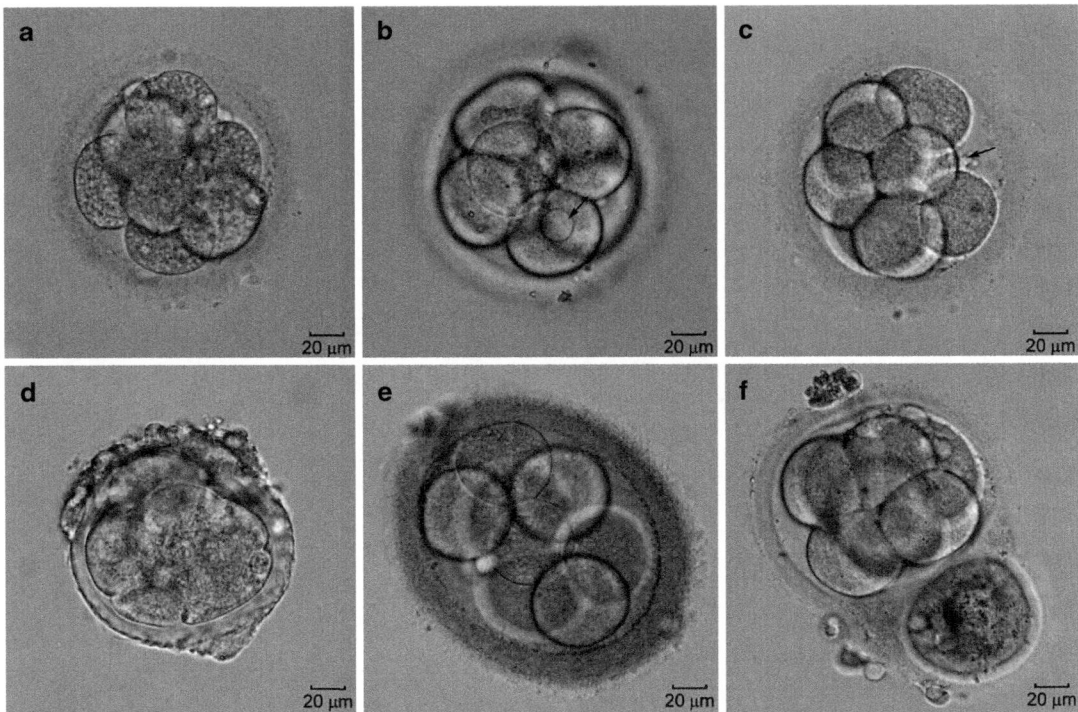

Fig. 8.3 Peculiar/abnormal embryo morphologies on day 3 (200×). (**a**) Cytoplasmic pitting phenomenon: blastomeres exhibit increased cytoplasmic granularity and are covered with numerous small pits of approximately 1.5 μm in diameter; (**b**) a vacuole >10 μm in diameter is evident in the blastomere indicated by the arrow; (**c**) the arrow indicates a distinct gap between two blastomeres; (**d**) the zona pellucida looks condensed, bright and agar-like; (**e**) the zona pellucida is darkened, and the embryo is oval with insufficient intercellular junctions; (**f**) conjoined embryos. Embryos with any of the above peculiar /abnormal morphological features cannot be assessed as grade I or considered the preferred choice

8.2   Blastocyst Scoring Criteria

Blastocyst culture is an effective method of enabling embryo preference and selective single embryo transfer. This blastocyst scoring criterion is based on the Gardner and Schoolcraft blastocyst scoring system [10] combined with the *Consensus on Human IVF-ET Laboratory Manipulation (2016)* developed by Chinese experts [11]. It divides embryonic grading into six stages based on the expansion and hatching status of the blastocyst (Table 8.4, Fig. 8.4). Herein, grade D is added for evaluating inner cell mass (ICM) (Table 8.5, Fig. 8.4), the generic grading scale is provided for trophectoderm (TE) (Table 8.6, Fig. 8.4), and the specialized grading scale of TE cells is provided for stage-6 blastocysts (Table 8.7, Fig. 8.5).

Table 8.4 Staging criteria for blastocysts (day 5/6/7)

Stage	Name	Morphological description	Figure
1	Early blastocyst I	Blastocoel <1/2 of total embryo volume	8.4a
2	Early blastocyst II	Blastocoel ≥1/2 of total embryo volume	8.4b
3	Expansion-stage blastocyst	Fully expanded blastocoel filling the entire embryo	8.4c
4	Fully expanded blastocyst	Significant increase in embryo size and a thinner[a] zona pellucida	8.4d
5	Hatching blastocyst	Trophectoderm cells begin to hatch from the zona pellucida	8.4e, f
6	Hatched blastocyst	Complete hatching of the blastocyst from the zona pellucida	8.4g

[a]Typically, when the zona pellucida thickness is <5 μm, the blastocyst is almost maximally expanded

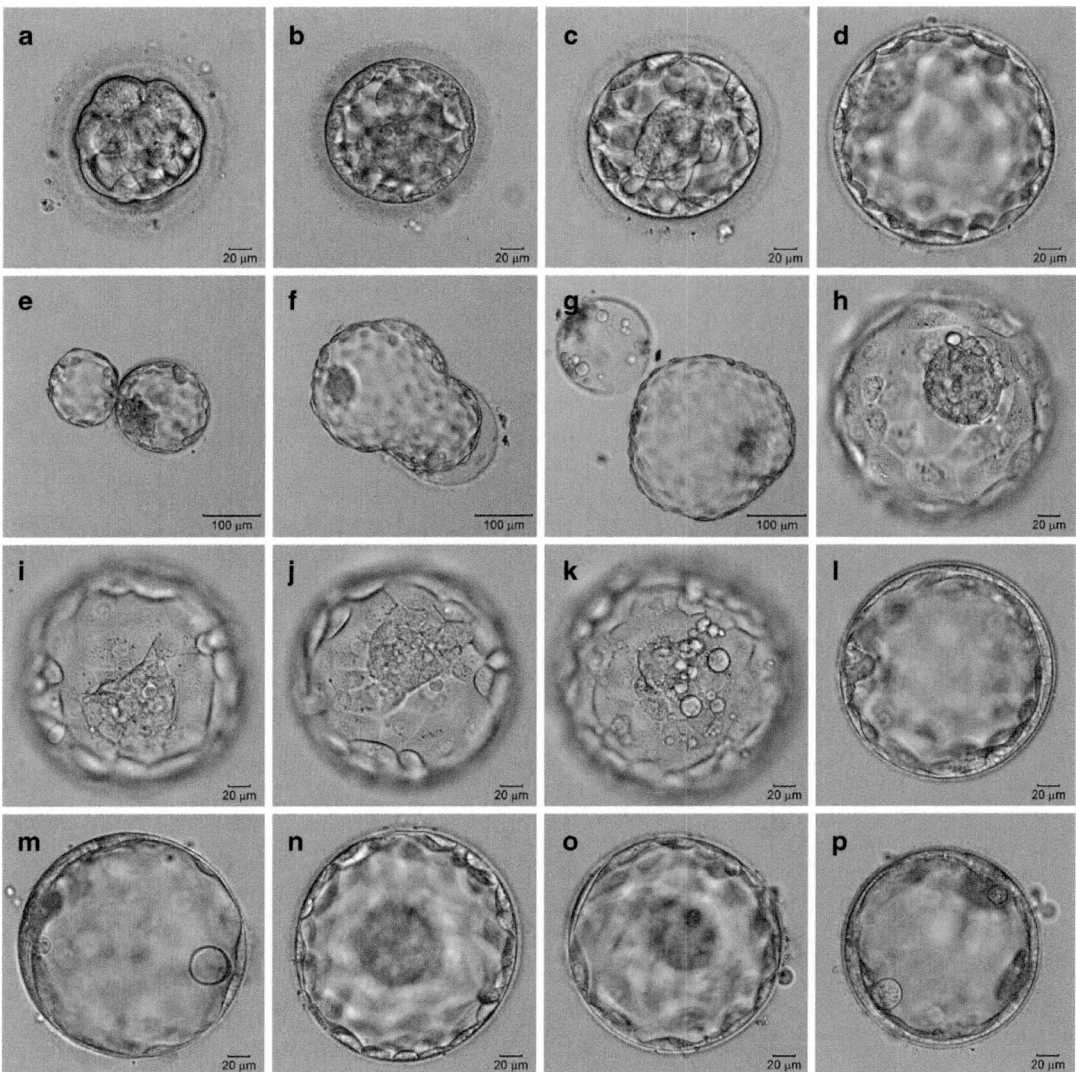

Fig. 8.4 Blastocysts at different developmental stages and with different grades (**a–d** 200×, **e–g** 100×, **h–p** 200×). *ICM* inner cell mass, *TE* trophectoderm. (**a**) A stage-1 blastocyst; (**b**) a stage-2 blastocyst; (**c**) a stage-3 blastocyst; (**d**) a stage 4 blastocyst; (**e**) an 8-shaped stage-5 blastocyst; (**f**) a peanut-shaped stage-5 blastocyst; (**g**) a stage-6 blastocyst; (**h**) a stage-4 blastocyst with grade A ICM; (**i** and **j**) two stage-4 blastocyst with grade B ICM; (**k** and **l**) a stage-4 blastocyst with grade C ICM; (**m**) a stage-4 blastocyst with grade D ICM; (**n**) a stage-4 blastocyst with grade A TE; (**o**) a stage-4 blastocyst with grade B TE; (**p**) a stage-4 blastocyst with grade C TE

Table 8.5 Grading scale for the ICM of stage 3–6 blastocysts

Grade	Morphological description	Figure
A	Many cells, tightly packed and fused with regular morphology (stage 4–6 blastocyst, diameter > 60 μm)	8.4h
B	A few cells, but more loosely grouped with irregular morphology (stage 4–6 blastocysts, diameter > 60 μm)	8.4i, j
C	Very low cell count, small or inconspicuous cell mass, degeneration or apoptosis in some cells	8.4k, l
D	No ICM-like cell mass or completely degenerated	8.4m

Table 8.6 Generic grading scale for TE of stage 3–6 blastocysts

Grade	Morphological description	Figure
A	Many cells present along the "equatorial plane" of the blastocyst, tightly packed, uniform in size, with clear morphology on the bottom surface of the blastocyst, and mostly with clearly visible nuclei (number of cells along the equatorial plane of a stage-4 blastocyst >15)	8.4n
B	Adequate number of cells present along the "equatorial plane" of the blastocyst, relatively loosely arranged, and not uniform in size. Some of the cells on the bottom surface of the blastocyst are well-defined and some of them have visible nuclei (8–15 cells along the equatorial plane of a stage-4 blastocyst)	8.4o
C	Very few cells present along the "equatorial plane" of the blastocyst, with significant heterogeneity in size, obvious fragmentation between the trophoblast and zona pellucida, and indistinct cells on the bottom surface of the blastocyst (<8 cells along the equatorial plane of a stage-4 blastocyst)	8.4p

TE cells of a high-quality fully expanded blastocyst have been stretched sufficiently during development, which facilitates the observation of TE nuclei located at the bottom of the blastocyst

Table 8.7 Specialized grading scale for TE of stage 6 blastocysts

Grade	Morphological description	Figure
A	The diameter of the blastocyst is approximately more than twice the diameter of the residual zona pellucida	8.5a
B	The diameter of the blastocyst is approximately 1.5–2 times that of the residual zona pellucida	8.5b
C	The diameter of the blastocyst is less than 1.5 times that of the residual zona pellucida	8.5c

Not applicable to stage-6 blastocysts with collapsed blastocoel and stage-6 blastocysts formed after assisted hatching performed on day 3/4

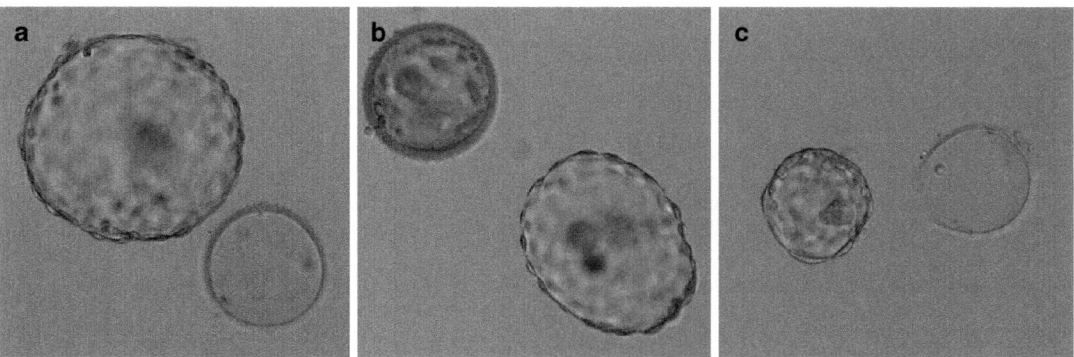

Fig. 8.5 The Stage-6 blastocyst TE cells of different grades (100×). (**a**) The stage-6 blastocyst is graded as A; (**b**) the stage-6 blastocyst is graded as B; (**c**) the stage-6 blastocyst is graded as C

8.3 Setting Time Points for Embryo Observation

Referring to the *Istanbul Consensus* [12], time points for embryo observation include 44 ± 1 h (day 2) and 68 ± 1 h (day 3) after insemination for cleavage-stage embryos; 116 ± 2 h (day 5), 140 ± 2 h (day 6), and 164 ± 2 h (day 7) after insemination for blastocysts. Furthermore, each center may refine the timetable for embryo observation according to the characteristics of embryo development and working schedule in their own laboratories; however, they should ensure consistency in the observation time.

8.4 Recording Methods of Embryo Grading

(i). Writing format for cleavage-stage embryo grading: Cell number and grade (e.g., I/8 or 8I). Given that the cell number is the most important indicator for embryo scoring, cell number is reflected in the writing format.

(ii). Writing format for blastomere nuclei: Not all embryos have visible blastomere nuclei (either mono- or multinucleated) on day 3 of observation. The clear presence of mononucleated blastomeres in the embryo and the proportion of mononucleated blastomeres to total blastomeres may be positively correlated with the developmental potential of the embryo and live birth [13, 14]; therefore, this phenomenon can be recorded specifically. To report this, N indicates mononucleated blastomeres, MN indicates multinucleated blastomeres, and a number indicates the number of mono- or multinucleated blastomeres observed. Furthermore, blastomeres without nuclei are not recorded. For example, an 8-cell class I embryo with six blastomeres observed as mononucleated is recorded as $I/8^{6N}$. Moreover, a 6-cell grade III embryo with one blastomere observed as multinucleated is recorded as $III/6^{1MN}$. This labeling approach may help improve the preferential selection of embryos. However, the pres-

ence and number of visible mononucleated blastomeres are not the main reference indicators for embryo assessment.

(iii). Writing format for blastocyst: The writing format for blastocyst grading is relatively consistent, and the scoring system can be further refined by adding a "+" or "−" to the blastocyst TE and ICM grades, e.g., $4B^+A$ and $4BB^-$. This annotation approach may facilitate the preferential selection of embryos at additional levels.

8.5 Definition of High-Quality and Usable Embryos

8.5.1 Cleavage-Stage Embryos

Based on the *Vienna Consensus* [15] and combined with the practical experience of multiple centers, the definitions of high-quality and usable cleavage-stage embryos are showed in Table 8.8.

All usable embryos (including high-quality embryos) can be used for embryo transfer, cryopreservation, or blastocyst culture. The grade I/8 (day 3) embryos, developed from I/4 (day 2) embryos (without fragments), are defined as optimal embryos and are preferred for transfer. Early compaction on day 3 is commonly observed during embryonic development (Fig. 8.6). Embryos with ≥7 cells and <10% fragments may be associated with increased implantation potential [16, 17]. With reference to relevant research and the experience of many centers, it is recommended that early compaction embryos with ≥7 cells and fragments <10% are classified as high-quality embryos. Blastocyst culture is recommended for grade III-b embryos (day 3). Grade IV embryos

Table 8.8 Definitions of high-quality and usable cleavage-stage embryos

Cleavage-stage embryos	Day 2	Day 3
High-quality embryos	I/4 II-a/2–5	I/8 II-a/7–14 Early compaction (≥7 cells)
Usable embryos	Grade I–III	Grade I–III

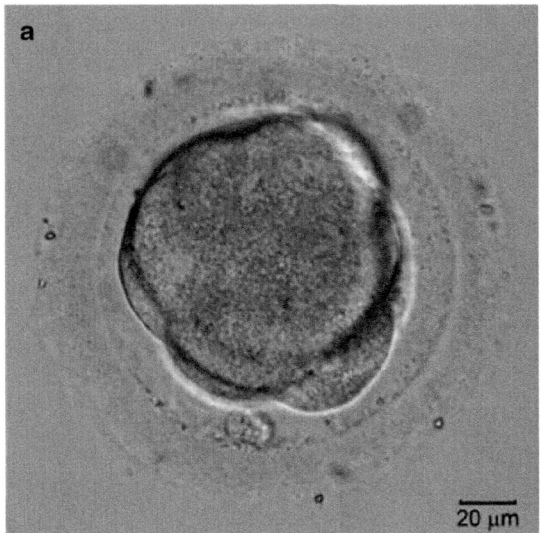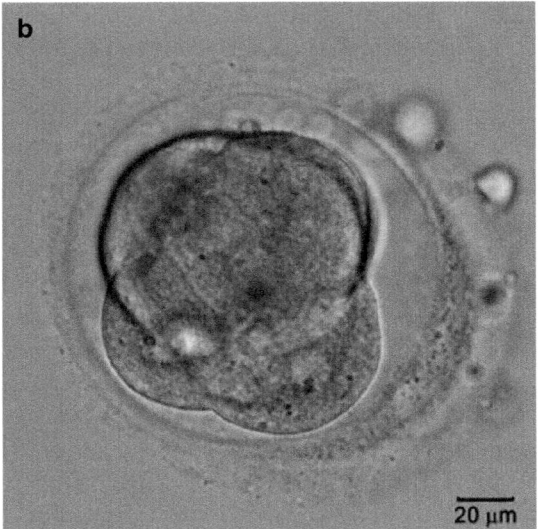

Fig. 8.6 Day 3 embryos exhibiting early compaction (100×). (**a**) The embryo with approximately 10 cells, which developed into a high-quality blastocyst; (**b**) the embryo with approximately 6 cells, which failed to develop into a blastocyst

Table 8.9 Definitions of high-quality and usable blastocysts

Blastocytes	Day 5	Day 6	Day 7
High-quality blastocysts	Stage 3 and higher blastocysts graded as AA, AB, BA, or BB	Stage 4 and higher blastocysts graded as AA, AB, BA, or BB	/
Usable blastocysts	High-quality blastocysts, stage 3 and higher blastocysts graded as AC, CA, BC, or CB.		Stage 4 and higher blastocysts graded as AA, AB, BA, or BB

The slash ("/") indicates that this item does not need to be considered

should be discarded, and are not recommended for embryo transfer or cryopreservation.

8.5.2 Blastocysts

Based on *the Gardner and Schoolcraft blastocyst scoring system* [10] and combined with the practical experience of multiple centers, the definitions of high-quality and usable blastocysts are given in Table 8.9.

A grade D for ICM is added to the conventional Gardner blastocyst scoring system with the aim of refining the conventional grade C for ICM. For blastocysts with an ICM grade of C based on the conventional scoring system, the clinical outcomes reported by different centers vary considerably [18], and the primary probable explanation is that grade C level ICM cells assessed based on the conventional Gardner scoring system include both low ICM cell counts and complete absence of ICM. Stage-3 and higher blastocysts graded as CC on day 5/6 could be implanted, cryopreserved, or discarded depending on the patient's condition and the low-quality blastocyst management strategy of each center. Early blastocysts that are still at stage 1 or 2 on day 6 are recommended to be cultured until day 7. By this time, if the blastocysts can reach stage 4 and above with a grade of AA, AB, BA, or BB, without large degenerative foci, they can be used for embryo transfer or cryopreservation. Blastocysts with an ICM grade D is recommended to be discarded to reduce the unnecessary financial burden on patients and the workload of laboratory personnel.

8.6   Notes of the Evaluation Criteria

8.6.1   Abnormal or Peculiar Morphological Features of Embryos

Based on these evaluation criteria, reference to some of the abnormal or peculiar morphological features of embryos for further screening is recommended, such as cytoplasmic features of the blastomere (pitting, presence of vacuoles, etc.), spatial arrangement of the blastomeres (four-leaf clover-shaped arrangement or excessive blastomere gap), abnormal zona pellucida (darkened or condensed), early compaction of cleavage-stage embryos, conjoined embryos, blastocysts with residual cells or fragments under the zona pellucida, and the hatching pattern of stage 5 blastocysts. However, because the predictive value of the above abnormal or peculiar morphological features for embryo quality or implantation potential is unclear, they are not presented as the main reference indicators for embryo assessment.

8.6.2   Specialized TE Grading Criteria for Stage 6 Blastocysts

All stage 6 blastocysts that hatch naturally have a certain number of TE cells (usually >15 cells dis-tributed along the equatorial plane of the blasto-cyst); however, the number of TE cells varies greatly and is difficult to count. The generic grad-ing scale for TE of stage 3–6 blastocysts is not fully applicable to stage 6 blastocysts. Therefore, a more objective assessment is facilitated by combining the generic with the specialized TE grading criteria for stage 6 blastocysts. However, stage 6 blastocysts that are in a temporary col-lapse state can only be graded after waiting for complete expansion. Additionally, the special-ized criteria cannot be applied to stage 6 blasto-cysts which have undergone assisted hatching on day 3/4 in preimplantation genetic testing cycle, because the zona pellucida is not sufficiently expanded and thinned.

8.6.3   Definition of Stage 5 Blastocysts

For stage 5 blastocysts, the exact number of "par-tially hatched" TE cells is controversial. We sug-gest that a blastocyst can be defined as a stage 5 blastocyst, as long as the TE cells start to hatch. However, it is controversial whether blastocysts hatching with a small number of TE cells can be defined as stage 5 blastocysts. Some blastocysts may appear one or more TE cells projection site (or sites), which are not the final sites of blasto-cyst hatching [19] (Fig. 8.7a). Such small TE cells projections without evident lumen forma-

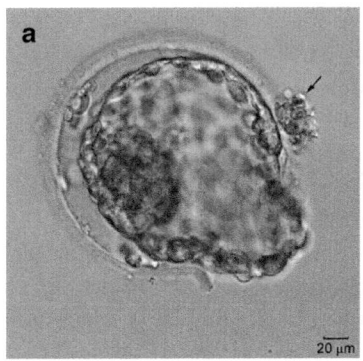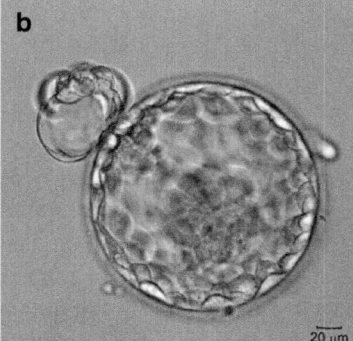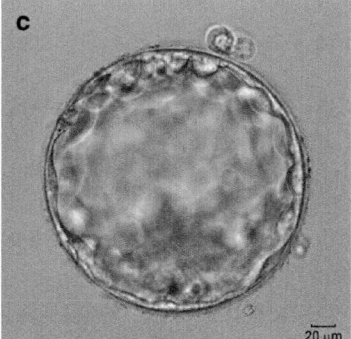

Fig. 8.7 Different hatching types of 5-stage blastocysts (200×). (**a**) A peanut-shaped stage-5 blastocyst, with a penetration of the ZP by small trophectoderm projections; (**b**) an 8-shaped stage-5 blastocyst with an evident lumen formed by the hatched TE cells; and (**c**) a stage-5 blasto-cyst without evident lumen formation

tion cannot exactly predict blastocyst hatching ability. Therefore, different types of stage 5 blastocysts, such as peanut-shaped hatching (large opening of zona pellucida), 8-shaped hatching (hatching with lumen formation), and hatching of a small number of TE cells (hatching without lumen formation), should be specially marked on the basis of the scoring of stage 5, which is helpful for the distinction and optimization of embryos (Fig. 8.7).

8.6.4 Grading for Delayed-Fertilization, Late Rescue ICSI, and Nonpronuclear (0PN) / Monopronuclear (1PN) -Derived Embryos

Delayed-fertilization, late-rescue ICSI, and 0PN/1PN-derived embryos can all be graded using the grading criteria described above.

8.6.4.1 Grading for Delayed-Fertilization and Late-Rescue ICSI Embryos

Delayed-fertilization and late-rescue ICSI embryos should be marked accordingly and should not be selected as the preferred embryos for transfer. Late-rescue ICSI embryos refer to those embryos that undergo rescue ICSI after overnight fertilization failure of conventional IVF, or those embryos that undergo artificial oocytes activation after fertilization failure of ICSI.

8.6.4.2 Grading for 0PN-Derived Embryos

0PN-derived embryos (without pronuclear on day 1 but with normal cleavage) should not be selected as the preferred embryos for transfer, regardless of their grades. High-quality 0PN-derived embryos have similar incidences of chromosomal normalities and proportions of biparental diploid and pregnancy outcomes as 2PN-derived embryos [20], it is recommended to perform blastocyst culture for high-quality 0PN-derived embryos, provide patients with genetic counseling, and ensure that they are fully

informed of the potential risks before 0PN-derived embryo transfer or cryopreservation.

8.6.4.3 Grading for 1PN-Derived Embryos

Similarly, 1PN-derived embryos should not be selected as the preferred embryos for transfer. As for 1PN-derived embryos which were fertilized via conventional IVF and has good quality, it is therefore also recommended to extend to culture them to the blastocyst stage. If usable blastocysts have formed, patients should be provided with the necessary genetic counseling, and embryo transfer or cryopreservation should be conducted after obtaining full informed consent [20, 21].

The above source embryos can be separately calculated when performing key performance indicator (KPI)-related statistics.

8.6.5 Grading of Embryos on Day 4 (Morulae)

The morula stage is usually considered to be a short and uninformative developmental stage; however, day-4 embryo implantation has recently gained attention [22]. The *Istanbul Consensus* classifies day-4 embryos into the following three grades [12]: Grade 1, the fourth round of cleavage occurs and the whole embryo is compacted; Grade 2, the fourth round of cleavage occurs, and the majority of the embryonic volume is compacted; and Grade 3, less than half of the embryo is compacted and is accompanied by 2–3 free discrete blastomeres. However, time-lapse observations have revealed that embryonic compaction is a dynamic process, and the grade of the same embryo may differ at different time points. Therefore, the combination of time-lapse observations may enable a more objective and accurate evaluation of day 4 embryos.

Although we attempted to maximally objectify the indicators, the evaluation of some indicators remains influenced by objective conditions and subjective factors as follows: (a) Fragmentation ratio: fragments usually demonstrate the features of varying size, uneven distribution, dynamic changes in cell division, and a wide variation in subjective evaluations; (b) Stage-specific cleavage pattern: time-lapse reveals that some of the cleavage-stage embryos with good developmental potential may not precisely follow the theoretical stage-specific cleavage pattern, possibly because their cells do not divide in a completely symmetric manner; (c) ICM grading: although ICM grading is partially quantified, even grade A ICM is only required to be relatively regular in morphology and not absolutely round or oval in shape.

References

1. Armstrong S, Bhide P, Jordan V, et al. Time-lapse systems for embryo incubation and assessment in assisted reproduction. Cochrane Database Syst Rev. 2019;5(5):Cd011320.
2. Brouillet S, Martinez G, Coutton C, et al. Is cell-free DNA in spent embryo culture medium an alternative to embryo biopsy for preimplantation genetic testing? A systematic review. Reprod Biomed Online. 2020;40(6):779–96.
3. Zaninovic N, Rosenwaks Z. Artificial intelligence in human in vitro fertilization and embryology. Fertil Steril. 2020;114(5):914–20.
4. Lundin K, Ahlström A. Quality control and standardization of embryo morphology scoring and viability markers. Reprod Biomed Online. 2015;31(4):459–71.
5. Machtinger R, Racowsky C. Morphological systems of human embryo assessment and clinical evidence. Reprod Biomed Online. 2013;26(3):210–21.
6. Prados FJ, Debrock S, Lemmen JG, et al. The cleavage stage embryo. Hum Reprod. 2012;27(Suppl_1):i50–71.
7. Ebner T, Yaman C, Moser M, et al. Embryo fragmentation in vitro and its impact on treatment and pregnancy outcome. Fertil Steril. 2001;76(2):281–5.
8. Johansson M, Hardarson T, Lundin K. There is a cutoff limit in diameter between a blastomere and a small anucleate fragment. J Assist Reprod Genet. 2003;20(8):309–13.
9. Hardarson T, Hanson C, Sjögren A, et al. Human embryos with unevenly sized blastomeres have lower pregnancy and implantation rates: indications for aneuploidy and multinucleation. Hum Reprod. 2001;16(2):313–8.
10. Schoolcraft WB, Gardner DK, Lane M, et al. Blastocyst culture and transfer: analysis of results and parameters affecting outcome in two in vitro fertilization programs. Fertil Steril. 1999;72(4):604–9.
11. Chinese Medical Association, Reproductive Medicine Branch. Expert consensus on human in vitro fertilization-embryo transfer laboratory operations (2016). J Reprod Med. 2017;26(1):1–8.
12. Alpha Scientists in Reproductive Medicine and ESHRE Special Interest Group of Embryology. The Istanbul consensus workshop on embryo assessment: proceedings of an expert meeting. Hum Reprod. 2011;26(6):1270–83.
13. Rhenman A, Berglund L, Brodin T, et al. Which set of embryo variables is most predictive for live birth? A prospective study in 6252 single embryo transfers to construct an embryo score for the ranking and selection of embryos. Hum Reprod. 2015;30(1):28–36.
14. Setti AS, Figueira RCS, Braga D, et al. Blastomere nucleation: predictive factors and influence of blastomere with no apparent nuclei on blastocyst development and implantation. JBRA Assist Reprod. 2018;22(2):102–7.
15. ESHRE Special Interest Group of Embryology and Alpha Scientists in Reproductive Medicine. The Vienna consensus: report of an expert meeting on the development of ART laboratory performance indicators. Reprod Biomed Online. 2017;35(5):494–510.
16. Skiadas CC, Jackson KV, Racowsky C. Early compaction on day 3 may be associated with increased implantation potential. Fertil Steril. 2006;86(5):1386–91.
17. Iwata K, Yumoto K, Sugishima M, et al. Analysis of compaction initiation in human embryos by using time-lapse cinematography. J Assist Reprod Genet. 2014;31(4):421–6.
18. Kemper JM, Liu Y, Afnan M, et al. Should we look for a low-grade threshold for blastocyst transfer? A scoping review. Reprod Biomed Online. 2021;42(4):709–16.
19. Kirkegaard K, Hindkjaer JJ, Ingerslev HJ. Hatching of in vitro fertilized human embryos is influenced by fertilization method. Fertil Steril. 2013;100(5):1277–82.
20. Li M, Huang J, Zhuang X, et al. Obstetric and neonatal outcomes after the transfer of vitrified-warmed blastocysts developing from nonpronuclear and monopronuclear zygotes: a retrospective cohort study. Fertil Steril. 2021;115(1):110–7.
21. Si J, Zhu X, Lyu Q, et al. Obstetrical and neonatal outcomes after transfer of cleavage-stage and blastocyst-stage embryos derived from monopronuclear zygotes: a retrospective cohort study. Fertil Steril. 2019;112(3):527–33.
22. Simopoulou M, Sfakianoudis K, Tsioulou P, et al. Should the flexibility enabled by performing a day-4 embryo transfer remain as a valid option in the IVF laboratory? A systematic review and network meta-analysis. J Assist Reprod Genet. 2019;36(6):1049–61.

Quality Management of Gamete and Embryo Cryopreservation

The cryopreservation of gametes and embryos is one of the routine practices within the IVF laboratory. The increasingly sophisticated gamete and embryo cryopreservation technology secure the safety and effectiveness of assisted reproduction treatment. With the widespread use of the whole embryo freezing strategy, single blastocyst implantation strategy, and the development of preimplantation genetic testing technology, embryo cryopreservation has become a crucial part of assisted reproduction treatment. In this chapter, we will have a comprehensive overview of the various aspects of cryopreservation involved in the IVF laboratory: we will introduce the basics involved in cryopreservation, i.e., the forms of damage to gametes and embryos during cryopreservation, as well as the principles of cryoprotectants; we will outline the steps and principles of slow freezing and thawing; we will explain in detail the principles and steps of vitrification and postvitrification thawing of eggs and embryos; we will describe the steps and clinical outcomes of sperm cryopreservation; we will list and compare open versus closed cryopreservation carriers; we will explain specifically the artificial shrinkage and assisted hatching techniques involved in embryo cryopreservation; and finally, we will discuss matters related to the management of cryostorage room.

9.1 Risks During Freezing and Thawing of Gametes and Embryos

The risks during freezing and thawing of gametes and embryos refer to their vulnerability to a series of damages during the handling process, including three major aspects: ice crystal formation; solution effects; and osmotic shock.

9.1.1 Ice Crystal Formation

Cell damage caused by ice crystal formation is the most common and important form of cell damage during cryopreservation. The water inside the cell forms ice crystals when the temperature drops below the freezing point and causes damage to the cell membrane, organelles, and cytoskeleton by mechanical effects. Intracellular water molecules can be divided into bound water and free water. Bound water is water molecules that can bind to intracellular membranous structures, organelles, and proteins. During the icing process, these bound water molecules are abstracted, changing the stability of the structure of their original bound objects, and thereby causing cellular damage. Therefore, most cryoprotection protocols utilize permeating and nonpermeating cryoprotectants to reduce the intracellular water content, which can replace water molecules to bind to intracellular membranous structures, organelles, and proteins, thereby reducing the damage caused by icing.

Solutions: (1). Reduce the cooling rate where appropriate to allow sufficient dehydration of the embryos before freezing (e.g., slow freezing). (2). Increase the cooling rate so that intracellular water is vitrified rapidly and does not form ice crystals during the freezing process (e.g., vitrification).

However, it should be noted that: (a) When the freezing is too slow, although the intracellular water can be fully excreted to reduce the damage caused by ice crystals, it may also cause structural abnormalities and impaired functions of macromolecules (such as proteins and nucleic acids) due to severe dehydration; (b) when the cooling rate is relatively fast, but not yet fast enough to allow sufficient dehydration of the cells, then there will be ice crystals formed and physical damage to the cells during the freezing process; (c) when the cooling rate is very fast, the intracellular water can appear as irregularly arranged vitrification. In this case, although many small ice crystals are formed, the formation of large ice crystals is avoided, and the cells can still survive when a rapid rewarming approach is adopted for thawing. However, if the rewarming is too slow during thawing, a phenomenon of re-freezing, where small intracellular ice crystals re-freeze and become large ice crystals, can still result in fatal damage to the embryo.

9.1.2   Solution Effects

During cell cooling, the water in the extracellular fluid freezes first, causing the extracellular fluid to concentrate and the osmolality to rise (i.e., the solute concentration to increase), which can damage the cells. Suppose the cooling rate is too slow or the cell is exposed to high osmolality for a long time. In that case, a significant outflow of intracellular water molecules and an extreme increase in intracellular solute concentration can damage the cells by denaturing the cell mem-

brane lipoprotein complexes and some other functional proteins in the cytoplasm.

Solution: The duration of the intra-embryonic hyperosmotic state can be shortened by rapid freezing to attenuate the damage caused by the solution effects on the embryo.

9.1.3   Osmotic Shock

When cells are placed in a solution with osmolality much lower than the intracellular fluid, extracellular water molecules will rapidly enter the cells, causing them to swell and rupture, i.e., resulting in osmotic shock. During cell cryopreservation, due to the very high concentration of cryoprotectants, a large amount of permeating cryoprotectants will accumulate inside the cells, resulting in a high intracellular osmolality. When thawing embryos, if they are placed directly in a comparatively hypotonic culture medium, a massive number of water molecules will enter the embryonic cells, causing a dramatic increase in cell volume or even rupture, leading to the osmotic shock of the embryos.

Solution: During embryo thawing, sugar solutions (e.g., sucrose solutions) or polymer solutions with decreasing concentration gradients can be added to the thawing medium as osmotic buffers to slow the flow of water molecules into the cells and avoid osmotic shock.

9.2   Cryoprotectants

Cryoprotectants are a class of chemicals that can reduce cellular damage caused by low or ultra-low temperatures, thereby improving cellular freeze–thaw outcomes. In 1949, Polge's team discovered by chance that glycerol could be used as a cryoprotectant to freeze poultry sperm with favorable results [1]. In the decades since then, cryoprotectants have been developed, and biologists have discovered many kinds of substances that provide cryoprotection. The commonly used cryoprotectants fall into three main categories (Table 9.1):

Table 9.1 Category of cryoprotectants

Permeating cryoprotectants	Non-permeating cryoprotectants	Other types of cryoprotectants
Glycerin	Sucrose	Blood serum albumin (BSA)
Dimethyl sulfoxide (DMSO)	Trehalose	Fetal calf serum (FCS)
Ethylene glycol (EG)	Cottonseed sugar	Ficoll
Propylene glycol (PG)	Fructose	Polyvinylpyrrolidone (PVP)
	Lactose	Polyethylene glycol (PEG)

9.2.1 Permeating Cryoprotectants

Permeating cryoprotectants (e.g., glycerol, dimethyl sulfoxide (DMSO), ethylene glycol (EG), and propylene glycol (PG)) are a class of compounds with small relative molecular masses that can enter the cell by permeation. The function principles of permeating cryoprotectants are as follows: (a) Extracellular cryoprotectants at high concentrations can promote cell dehydration and increase intracellular viscosity, which in turn increases the critical temperature for vitrification, making it easier for cells to become vitrified. (b) Permeating cryoprotectants can alter the interaction between water molecules and the interaction between water molecules and other solutes inside the cell by affecting the formation of hydrogen bonds. (c) Permeating cryoprotectants can change the nucleation process in the crystallization of water molecules so that when water molecules are combined with cryoprotectants they are less likely to form ice. (d) Permeating cryoprotectants can replace water molecules to bind to biological macromolecules such as DNA, RNA, and proteins inside cells and maintain their structural stability.

Because oocytes and embryonic cells at each developmental stage differ in terms of the structure and function of their cell membranes, they also have different transmembrane transport modes for permeating cryoprotectants [2] (Table 9.2). Oocytes and early embryos are generally less permeable to cryoprotectants, while blastocysts are highly permeable. Although it is impossible to quantitatively assess the motility of cryoprotectants passing through the plasma membrane, reasonable estimates regarding their motility patterns can be made based on permeability and Arrhenius activation energy (E_a value). A cryoprotectant with low permeability and a high E_a value indicates that its motility mode is mainly simple diffusion. A cryoprotectant with high permeability and a low E_a value indicates that its motility mode is mainly facilitated diffusion. The permeation of cryoprotectants into the cell is accompanied by the efflux of water. The transmembrane transport of water is primarily accomplished by simple diffusion in oocytes and cleavage-stage embryos and by facilitated diffusion in morulas and blastocysts (Fig. 9.1).

Glycerol: Glycerol was the first cryoprotectant discovered. Glycerol has a small relative molecular mass (92.09) and is featured by low toxicity, good solubility in water, and slow permeation rate. It can reduce the intracellular electrolyte concentration, promote the efflux of intracellular water molecules during freezing, and stabilize the cell membrane conformation. Oocytes and embryos at early stage exhibit low glycerol permeability and high E_a values. Thus, glycerol moves through oocytes and embryos at early stage mainly by simple diffusion. In contrast, morulas have a higher and lower E_a value, indicating that glycerol passes through morulas mainly by facilitated diffusion (mediated by aquaporin-3).

DMSO: It has a smaller relative molecular mass (78.12) than glycerol, which provides higher cell permeability and faster permeation. At lower concentrations, DMSO can decrease membrane conformational disorder [3]. However, it can also be cytotoxic under certain circumstances, e.g., DMSO can reduce the protein denaturation temperature when heated. DMSO enters oocytes mainly by simple diffusion and morulas by facilitated diffusion. The facilitated diffusion of DMSO in morulas is not dependent on aquaporin 3, but on other channel proteins.

EG: With a relative molecular mass of only 67.02, it is smaller than both glycerol and

Table 9.2 Transmembrane transport modes of cryoprotectants

Cryoprotectant	Oocytes and cleavage-stage embryos			Morulas and blastocysts		
	Permeability[a]	E_a^b	Transport mode	Permeability[a]	E_a^b	Transport mode
Glycerin	$0.01–0.02 \times 10^{-3}$	42	Simple diffusion	$4–5 \times 10^{-3}$	10	Facilitated diffusion
DMSO	1.0×10^{-3}	18	Simple diffusion	3.0×10^{-3}	12	Facilitated diffusion
EG	0.6×10^{-3}	17	Simple diffusion	10×10^{-3}	9	Facilitated diffusion
PG	1.7×10^{-3}	20	Simple diffusion	3.8×10^{-3}	20	Simple diffusion

E_a Arrhenius activation energy
[a]Unit of permeability: cm/min
[b]Unit of E_a: kcal/mol

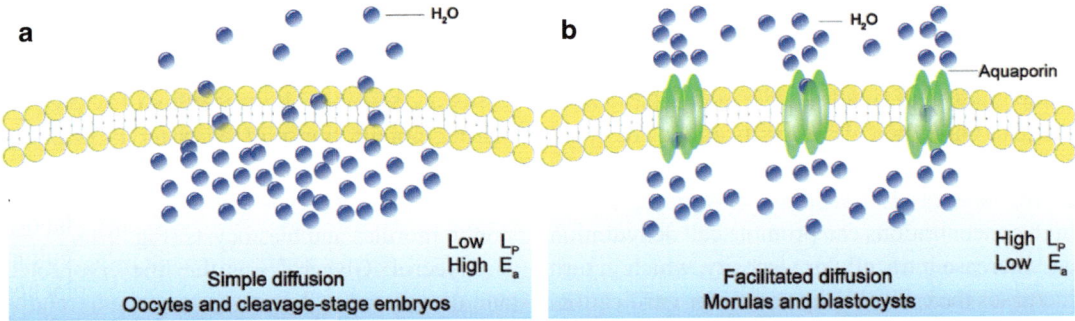

Fig. 9.1 Transmembrane transport of water. (**a**) simple diffusion, (**b**) facilitated diffusion. L_p permeability of water; E_a Arrhenius activation energy

DMSO and therefore has a faster permeation rate. The permeability of oocytes to EG (P_{EG}) is low, and the E_a value is high. As a result, EG passes through oocytes mainly by simple diffusion. In contrast, morulas exhibit a high P_{EG} value and a low E_a value, which is why EG passes through morulas mainly by facilitated diffusion.

PG: The relative molecular mass of PG is 76.07. The permeability of oocytes to PG (P_{PG}) is relatively low, while the E_a value is high. Therefore, PG passes through oocytes mainly by simple diffusion. However, the permeability of oocytes to PG is higher than to other cryoprotectants, which is probably related to the fact that PG is more hydrophobic than other cryoprotectants. The P_{PG} value of morulas is more than twice as high as that of oocytes, but the E_a value of PG is also quite high in morulas, with the result that PG also passes through morulas mainly by simple diffusion.

9.2.2 Non-permeating Cryoprotectants

Non-permeating cryoprotectants, such as sucrose, trehalose, cottonseed sugar, fructose, and lactose, have large molecular masses and cannot penetrate the cells by permeation. They all contain hydrophilic and lipophilic groups (i.e., they are amphiphilic compounds). They can increase the osmolality of the extracellular fluid and induce cell dehydration, thereby reducing intracellular ice crystal formation. Dehydration can alter the structure and function of cell membranes. Sugars can bind to polar residues on the cell membrane surface in place of water molecules, preserving their structural integrity. Although both monosaccharides and disaccharides can be used as cryoprotectants, sucrose and trehalose, which are disaccharides, are more effective in this regard. Sucrose, for example, can be used as an active ingredient in osmotic buffers to stabilize the cell membrane structure and prevent cell swelling by binding to lipid bilayers.

9.2.3   Other Types of Cryoprotectants

Some other macromolecules are also often added to the vitrification and thawing medium. They can nourish the cells, reduce or avoid cell damage by various physical and chemical stresses, and ultimately improve the vitrification and thawing processes. However, these macromolecules possess huge relative molecular masses and low molar concentrations and thus have little effect on osmolality and should not be grouped with non-permeating cryoprotectants.

Such macromolecules mainly include blood serum albumin (BSA), fetal calf serum (FCS), Ficoll, polyvinylpyrrolidone (PVP), and polyethylene glycol (PEG), among others.

9.2.4   Toxicity of Cryoprotectants

The toxicity of cryoprotectants is cell-specific and highly correlated with exposure time, concentration and temperature. Because different exposure modes can generate different outcomes, the toxicity magnitude of a particular cryoprotectant should be addressed based on its specific mode of action. It has long been established that the toxicity of cryoprotectants is related to the temperature at which the exposure happens [4]. For example, ethylene glycol decreases protein homeostasis at temperatures above 0 °C and increases protein homeostasis at temperatures below 0 °C. Furthermore, the decrease in exposure temperature can mitigate the toxicity of cryoprotectants. On the other hand, prolonged exposure to cryoprotectants can cause damage to cells. For example, prolonged (24 h) exposure of astrocytes to DMSO at room temperature can cause damaging alterations in mitochondrial membrane potential [5].

9.2.5   How to Control the Toxicity of Cryoprotectants

The toxicity of cryoprotectants can be attenuated by combining multiple cryoprotectants. For example, the dilution effect of formamide can attenuate the toxicity of DMSO [6]; the combination of ethylene glycol, glycerol, and DMSO can attenuate their toxicity in general [7]; Propylene glycol alone is not effective in cryopreservation of mouse oocytes, whereas the combination of low concentration propylene glycol with DMSO can significantly improve the freezing effect [8].

Researchers are also constantly identifying new cryoprotectants. For example, hyaluronic acid [9], a natural, non-toxic, non-sulfated glycosaminoglycan, can be used as an alternative non-permeating cryoprotectant and features good cryoprotective effects.

In summary, the toxicity of cryoprotectants can be controlled by optimizing various conditions, such as: adjusting the exposure time of cells in cryoprotectants and the operating temperature; limiting the concentration of cryoprotectants below the toxicity threshold; using multiple cryoprotectants in combination to attenuate their toxicity. When embryos are thawed, they are transferred into a highly concentrated non-permeating thawing solution and gradually replaced with thawing solutions of decreasing concentrations. This procedure helps remove residual permeating cryoprotectants from the cells and allows the cells to recover their physiological state progressively. Therefore, although cryoprotectants are of certain toxicity, it is still possible to achieve successful cell thawing and recovery without impairing cell function as long as effective methods are taken.

9.3   Overview of the Principles of Slow Freezing and Thawing

Whittingham first reported successful cryopreservation of mouse cleavage embryos by a slow freezing method in 1972 [10]. Slow freezing, also known as slow programmable freezing (SPF), utilizes a programmable freezer with a controlled cool-down rate to fully dehydrate the cells and reduce the formation of intracellular ice crystals, achieving a better freezing effect. The process, principles, and key points of slow freezing and thawing are outlined as follows.

9.3.1 Osmotic Equilibrium and Dehydration of Embryos

The embryos are first fully osmotically equilibrated in a solution containing permeating cryoprotectants and then further dehydrated in a solution containing both permeating and nonpermeating cryoprotectants. The concentration of cryoprotectants used in slow freezing is lower compared to vitrification.

9.3.2 Programmable Cooling Process of Slow Freezing

1. Phase I: The starting temperature is 20 °C, and the cooling rate is controlled at 2–3 °C/min until the temperature drops to −7 °C.
2. Phase II: When the temperature falls to −7 °C, the so-called seeding procedure is carried out, with a soaking time of 5–10 min. "Seeding": When the temperature is down to −7 °C, ice crystal formation is induced by "seeding" in the extracellular area. "Seeding" is performed using a knife, forceps, or cotton balls previously immersed in liquid nitrogen. The "seeding" process is a key step in determining the success or failure of slow freezing and is an effort to prevent undercooling. Undercooling is a phenomenon defined as when the temperature of an aqueous solution has fallen below the freezing point corresponding to the current pressure of the liquid, but then it is still not solidified. And the purer the solution, the more pronounced the undercooling phenomenon. This is because when the solution is very clean, it will lack the "crystallization nuclei" required for solidification. This "unsolidified state" is thermodynamically unstable.

If a small amount of solid material is thrown into this aqueous solution, or if the aqueous solution is shaken, it will solidify rapidly. Undercooling can damage embryos: on the one hand, when supercooled solution freezes, a large amount of latent heat is released, resulting in drastic changes in the temperature around the cells and causing damage to them; and on the other hand, the freezing process of an undercooled solution is rapid and erratic, leading to insufficient cell dehydration, and making it easy for intracellular ice crystals to emerge. Therefore, artificial "seeding" to trigger icing is a key step in slow freezing to prevent supercooling.

It is important to note that the specimens must be kept at icing temperatures close to −7 °C for 5–10 min. As the temperature drops, extracellular ice crystals will evolve aggressively. The icing process releases heat outward from the solution, and this latent heat release causes a slight increase in the surrounding temperature. Therefore, by maintaining the temperature for 5–10 min, the latent heat can be fully released before further freezing.

3. Phase III: The subsequent cooling rate is controlled at 0.3 °C/min until the temperature drops to −30 °C. As the water in the extracellular fluid crystallizes, the amount of water that dissolves extracellular salt ions and cryoprotectants decreases, and the extracellular fluid concentration and osmolality subsequently increase. Meanwhile, the embryo is further dehydrated to compensate for the elevated extracellular osmolality. As the concentration of intracellular fluid increases, the cells gradually shrink. Ideally, the cell can be dehydrated to an extreme level when the cooling rate is extremely slow and balanced with the rate of cell dehydration, allowing sufficient time for the intracellular water molecules to exit the cell. In this case, as the slow freezing proceeds, the intracellular concentration is high enough when the temperature is lowered to −30 to −40 °C. Since a dilute salt solution's freezing point decreases as the solution's concentration increases, the solu-

Fig. 9.2 Phase change process of the solution

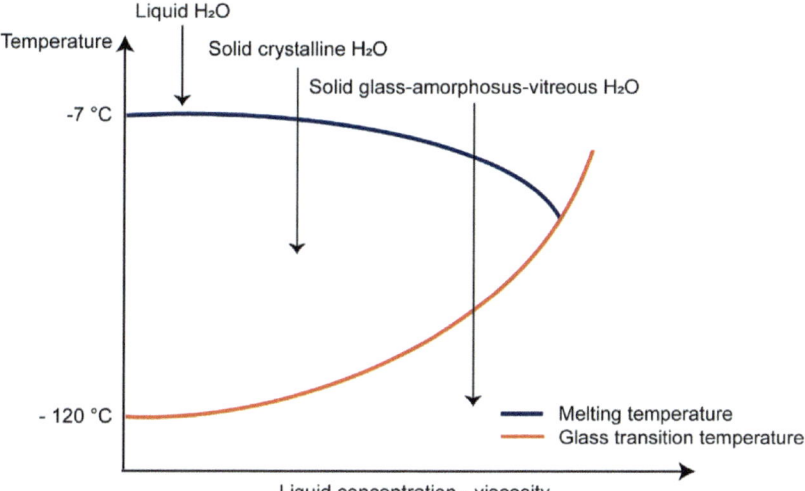

tion's glass transition temperature increases as the solution's concentration increases (Fig. 9.2). When the embryonic intracellular concentration is sufficiently high, and the extracellular temperature reaches the glass transition temperature, there will be no ice formation inside the cell even if the embryo is placed in liquid nitrogen. This state of an indefinite increase in intracellular concentration and cellular solidification is called vitrified ("vitrification"). However, during actual slow freezing, the process of cell dehydration is often accompanied by repeated formation and dissolution of intracellular ice crystals, which cause irreversible damage to cell organelles.

4. Phase IV: When the temperature drops to −30 °C, the cooling rate is controlled at −30 °C/min until the temperature drops to −150 °C, at which point the embryos are put into liquid nitrogen.

9.3.3   Thawing

The thawing process of slow-frozen cells should, on the one hand, bring the cells back to normal physiological temperature while avoiding the re-formation of ice crystals that can damage the cells. On the other hand, it should allow water molecules to get into the cells and displace the intracellular permeating cryoprotectants so that the cells can restore their physiological functions.

Rapid thawing is usually applied for slow-frozen cells. During the gradual rewarming of the cells as they are taken out of the liquid nitrogen, their temperature will pass through the temperature range where ice crystals are formed, risking re-icing and causing damage to the cells, so it is important to move quickly through this temperature range. Rapid thawing is performed by holding the oocyte or embryo in the air for 30 s after removing it from liquid nitrogen, then placing it in warm water at around 30 °C.

When the cells are just thawed, a significant amount of permeating cryoprotectants remain in the cytoplasm, leaving the cytoplasm in a hyperosmotic state. By using a thawing solution with an osmolality slightly lower than that of the cytoplasm, water molecules are facilitated to enter the cells. At the same time, the permeating cryoprotectants are driven out of the cells. To prevent cellular osmotic shock, the concentration of the thawing solution should not differ too much from the physiological cytoplasmic concentration. The thawing solutions are usually including three gradually decreasing concentrations. The thawing solution with the lowest concentration is physiologically isotonic. The components of the thawing solution are usually non-permeating cryoprotectants, with sucrose being the most commonly used.

9.4   Overview of the Principles of Vitrification and Thawing

9.4.1   What Is Vitrification?

Vitrification (derived from the Latin word vitrum) of a liquid is a complex physical process that can be described in simplified terms as the solidification of a liquid at low temperatures yielding an extremely high viscosity in the absence of ice crystal formation. It is sometimes referred to as "amorphous ice" or "glass-water." But it is not "ice" in the strict sense because there is no crystal structure. Water or dilute salt solutions must be cooled down extremely rapidly to the critical temperature for the glass transition of water molecules before they can be vitrified.

9.4.2   The Process of Vitrification

The basic principle of vitrification technology is to use a highly concentrated solution of cryoprotectants to displace the water molecules inside the cells and to transform the liquid component of the cells directly into a glassy state by rapid cooling. During the entire vitrification process, no ice crystals are formed inside or outside the cells. The steps of vitrification are (1) Place the embryos in an equilibration solution for perme-

ation until osmotic equilibrium is reached; (2) Place the embryos in a more concentrated vitrification solution for further dehydration; (3) Load the embryos and quickly plunge the carrier into liquid nitrogen. Detailed functions and principles of each step of vitrification are as follows:

9.4.2.1   The First Step of Vitrification: Osmotic Equilibration

The first step of vitrification is to place the gametes or embryos in an equilibration solution composed of permeating cryoprotectants at a lower concentration. In this step, embryos can be observed under the microscope as first shrinking and then recovering (Fig. 9.3). This cellular response is because: when an embryo is first placed into the equilibration solution, the higher osmolality of the extracellular fluid causes the intracellular water molecules to be rapidly expelled; as the water molecules permeate faster than cryoprotectants, the embryo will initially shrink in shape; then as the cryoprotectants gradually enter the cell, the cell will asymptotically expand until it returns to its initial volume, which marks the osmotic equilibrium between water molecules and cryoprotectants inside and outside the cell.

Two to three permeating cryoprotectants are usually used in combination in the equilibration solution with the aim of reducing cryoprotectant-induced cytotoxicity. The effects of permeating cryoprotectants upon entry into the cell include increasing intracellular viscosity, decreasing intracellular water content, and reducing ice crystal formation. The increased intracellular viscos-

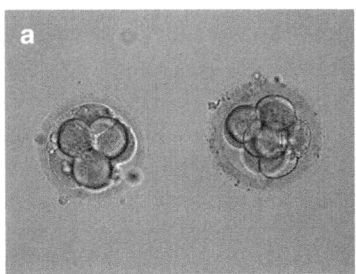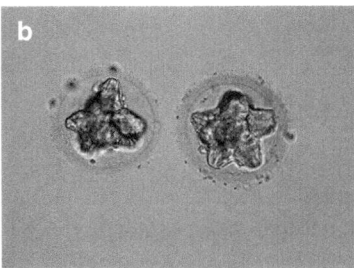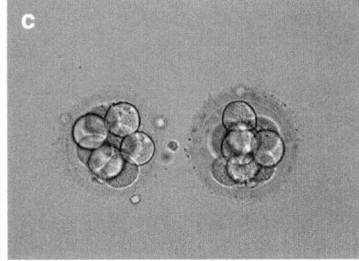

Fig. 9.3 Morphological changes of embryos in equilibration solution at different times. (**a**) Embryonic morphology in culture medium. The embryo will initially shrink in shape (**b**) when entering equilibration solution, and then recovering (**c**)

ity reduces the critical temperature of intracellular fluid crystallization and increases the critical temperature of glass transition. When water molecules bind to cryoprotectants, the crystallization nucleation process of water molecules will be altered, making them less likely to form ice. Moreover, the cryoprotectants that enter the cells can replace the water molecules originally bound to biomolecules such as proteins and prevent the conformational changes of these biomolecules.

9.4.2.2 The Second Step of Vitrification: Further Dehydration

The second step of vitrification is to place the embryos in a vitrification solution consisting of permeating and non-permeating cryoprotectants at higher concentrations. The more concentrated vitrification solution induces further dehydration of the cells and increases intracellular viscosity, facilitating cell vitrification. The non-permeating cryoprotectants in the solution can protect the cell membrane structure and maintain its stability by wrapping closely around the cell membrane surface. The embryos are then loaded onto the carriers. The types of vitrification carriers and the details of loading operation are described in Sect. 9.6 and 9.10 of this chapter.

The components and concentration of cryoprotectants vary among different commercial vitrification kits, but sucrose is usually chosen as a non-permeating cryoprotectant in the vitrification solution. Depending on the concentrations and types of cryoprotectants and the temperature (room temperature or 37 °C), the exposure time of embryos in the equilibration solution varies from 3 min to 15 min; and the exposure time of embryos in the vitrification solution plus the loading time varies from 30 s to 60 s.

9.4.2.3 The Third Step of Vitrification: Plunging Loaded Carriers in Liquid Nitrogen

The third step of vitrification is rapidly plunging the already loaded vitrification carrier into liquid nitrogen. The cooling rate during this process can be up to 23,000 °C/min. Ideally, no ice crystals are formed inside or outside the cells during the whole vitrification process of the embryo, and the

intracellular water molecules do not have enough time to form ice but are directly transformed into the vitrified state, avoiding cell damage induced by icing.

9.4.3 Thawing

The principle of post-vitrification thawing is similar to that after slow freezing. It consists of two elements: rewarming the cells and replacing the intracellular permeating cryoprotectants, as described in Sect. 9.8 of this chapter.

9.5 Comparison of Slow Freezing and Vitrification

9.5.1 Principles of Slow Freezing and Vitrification

Slow freezing utilizes a low concentration solution of cryoprotectants and a slow cooling rate to achieve a balance between cellular osmotic dehydration and temperature reduction, which would theoretically prevent the formation of ice crystals within the cells. Vitrification employs a high concentration solution of cryoprotectants and an extremely rapid cooling rate to transform the cells directly from the physiological state to the vitrified state, avoiding the formation of intracellular ice crystals.

9.5.2 Operating Procedures for Slow Freezing and Vitrification

Slow freezing requires large equipment (a programmable freezer), consumes more liquid nitrogen, takes several hours, and has more complex operating procedures. Vitrification, by contrast, mostly employs commercial kits, consumes less liquid nitrogen, takes a very short time (about 15 min), and has simple procedures. However, the operator has to be trained repeatedly before he/she can actually perform either slow freezing or vitrification.

9.5.3 Clinical Outcomes of Slow Freezing and Vitrification

Vitrification is more advantageous in clinical outcomes [11], showing higher post-thaw survival and embryonic developmental potential in cleavage-stage embryos and blastocysts. Vitrified-thawed embryos have demonstrated higher clinical pregnancy and birth rates, lower premature birth rates, and lower risk of preterm delivery and low birth weight babies than fresh cycles. Vitrification has also proven more effective in oocyte cryopreservation, with a higher post-thaw survival rate and more intact meiotic spindles [12]. The time has, therefore, come for the slow freezing technique to be gradually replaced by vitrification in embryo cryopreservation.

9.6 Procedures of Embryo Vitrification

Before the actual operation begins, the relevant reagents, consumables, and embryos should be made ready (Fig. 9.4). When performing vitrification, the standardized laboratory operation protocol and the commercial kit instructions should be strictly adhered to, and proper registration and archiving (electronic and paper files) should be done after the vitrification operation is completed. In this section, the procedure and practical tips for vitrification are explained in detail based on the case of using a commercial vitrification kit.

9.6.1 Pre-work Preparation

1. Embryo transfer pipette: Pasteur glass pipettes pulled on a flame of an alcohol lamp are used in our center for transferring embryos.
2. A thermal box specifically for liquid nitrogen: Prepare a polystyrene thermal box specifically for liquid nitrogen and place it on a flat operating bench, preferably adjacent to the microscope, to ensure that the loaded embryos can be immediately placed into the liquid

nitrogen. If the vitrification operation continues for a long time, the volume of liquid nitrogen in the box should be monitored and refilled in a timely manner. And this box should be inspected for rupture and defects ordinarily.
3. Timer: Each operation step should strictly adhere to the timing specified in the operating protocol provided by the (vitrification) reagent kit manufacturer.
4. Equilibrate the vitrification solution to room temperature: Equilibrate all solutions used in operation to room temperature in advance and mix the reagents well before use.
5. Preparation of operating dishes
   (a) Operating dish for equilibration solution: The first step of vitrification is to place the embryos in the equilibration solution. The equilibration solution dishes are prepared in our center using the microdroplet method (approximately 30 μL per drop), and the microdroplets are covered with tissue culture oil (approximately 3 mL). Depending on how many embryos need to be processed that day, all the required equilibration solution dishes can be prepared at one time and left at room temperature before starting vitrification.
   (b) Operating dish for vitrification solution: One vitrification solution dish should be prepared per time right before use to avoid prolonged exposure to air (Fig. 9.5).
6. Carrier and carrier label: Label the carrier appropriately before loading embryos (Fig. 9.6).
7. Define the storage place of the carriers: Make sure of the storage place of the embryos before putting the loaded carriers into the dewars.

9.6.2 Embryo Preparation

Prior to freezing, identify the embryos to be frozen. Cleavage-stage embryos can be frozen directly; blastocysts undergo artificial shrinkage before freezing (see Sect. 9.11 of this chapter).

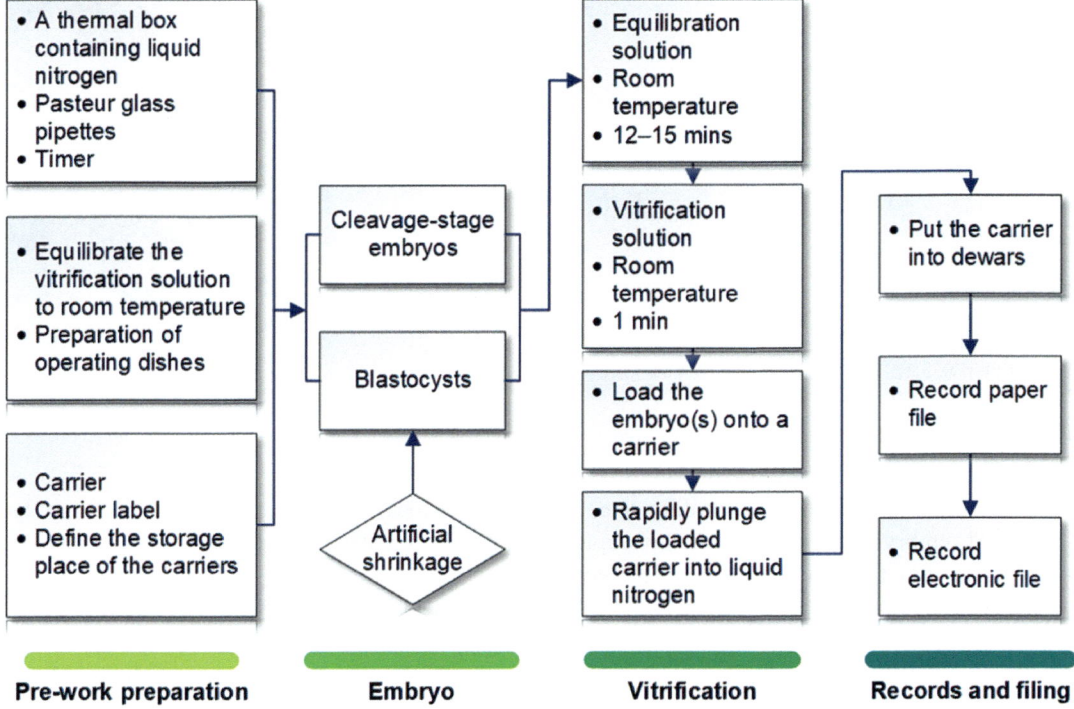

Fig. 9.4 Flow chart of embryo vitrification operation

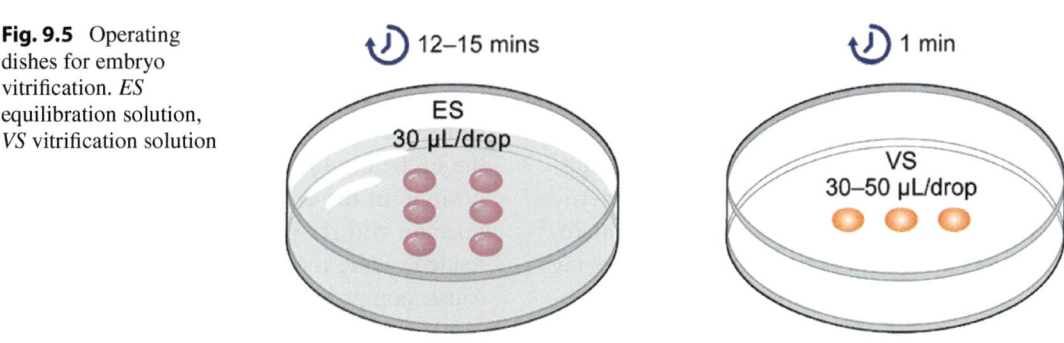

Fig. 9.5 Operating dishes for embryo vitrification. *ES* equilibration solution, *VS* vitrification solution

9.6.3 Vitrification Procedures

1. The vitrification procedures usually start with placing the embryos in an equilibration solution (12–15 min) to make them osmotically equilibrated, followed by placing them in a more concentrated vitrification solution (1 min) for further dehydration (Figs. 9.4 and 9.5), and finally loading the embryo(s) onto a carrier and rapidly plunging the loaded carrier into liquid nitrogen.

2. The operator should remain focused while performing the vitrification operation.

3. Double-checking should always be performed when freezing embryos, verifying that the patient's name labeled on the culture dish matches the information labeled on the carrier.

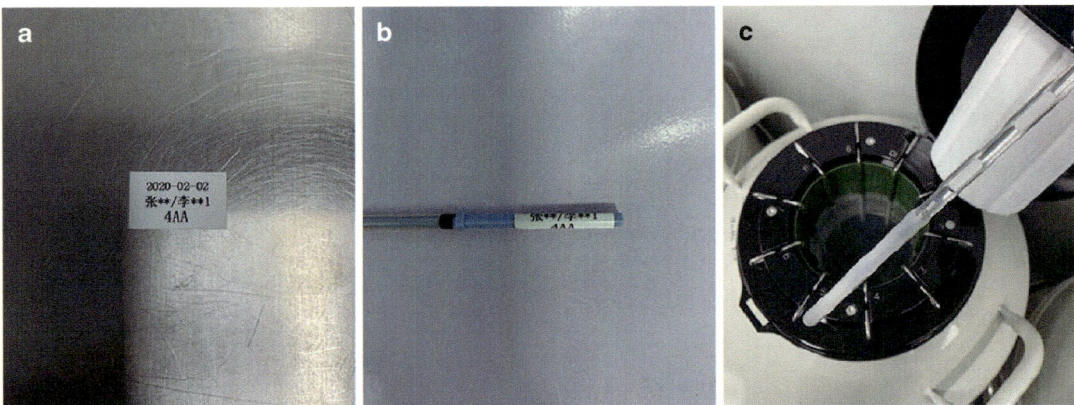

Fig. 9.6 (**a**) Label; (**b**) carrier, and (**c**) carrier holder

4. To ensure a sufficiently fast cooling rate, the loaded embryo carrier should be rapidly plunged into the liquid nitrogen and never pause in the liquid nitrogen vapor.

9.6.4   Records and Filing

Records should be made in both electronic and paper files, including the patient's name (both spouses), age, medical record number, cycle type (IVF/ICSI/preimplantation genetic testing), oocyte type (fresh oocyte/frozen-thawed oocyte), sperm type (husband sperm (fresh sperm)/husband sperm (frozen-thawed sperm)/donor sperm/epididymal puncture/testicular puncture/microdissection testicular sperm extraction), freezing date, freezing tube number, embryo quality, number of embryos, freezing carrier storage location and freezing operator.

9.6.5   Quality Management of Embryo Loading

The amount of liquid (vitrification solution) loaded onto the carrier will directly affect the cooling rate of the embryos during freezing. Therefore, the operator should strictly control the amount of liquid loaded with the embryo and minimize the volume of cryoprotectants loaded. Our center uses manually pulled fine caliber Pasteur glass pipettes and open-type carriers for

embryo loading. Some practical tips on embryo loading are listed below:

1. Appropriate liquid volume: The volume of liquid loaded with the embryo should be as small as possible, as too much liquid will affect the cooling rate. The volume of vitrification solution loaded should be just enough to wrap the embryo (Fig. 9.7).
2. Caliber of the embryo transfer pipette: The caliber of the embryo transfer pipette is very important for embryo loading. The embryo should be kept inside the pipette and close to the tip before loading (Fig. 9.8). A backward position of the embryo or too thick a pipette opening will result in too much liquid being loaded, while too thin a pipette opening will cause compression damage to the embryo. Usually, oocytes and cleavage-stage embryos require pipettes of the same caliber (approximately 150 μm), and stage-4 and stage-5 blastocysts require thicker caliber pipettes (150–200 μm). In comparison, finer caliber pipettes should be applied to stage-6 blastocysts after sufficient shrinkage. Commercial oocyte denudation pipettes or hand-pulled Pasteur glass pipettes can be employed for embryo loading. Commercial oocyte denudation pipettes are available in defined sizes, so the appropriate size can be selected as needed. In contrast, hand-pulled Pasteur glass pipettes are less costly but require repeated training to master the handcrafting skills.

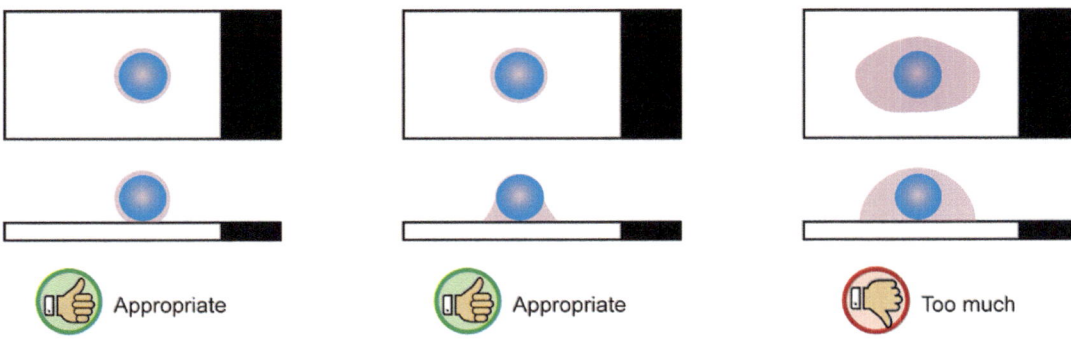

Fig. 9.7   Volume of liquid loaded with the embryo

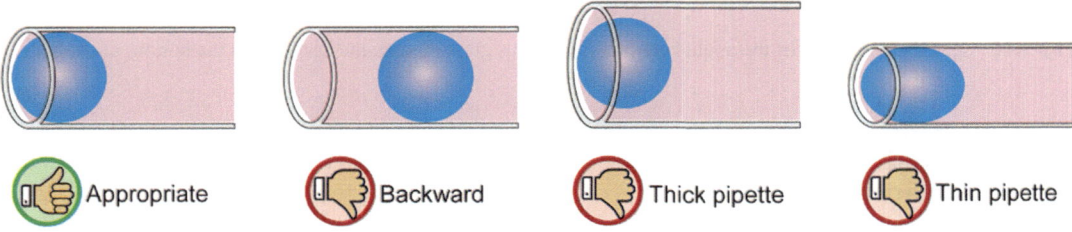

Fig. 9.8   Embryo position and pipettes with different calibers

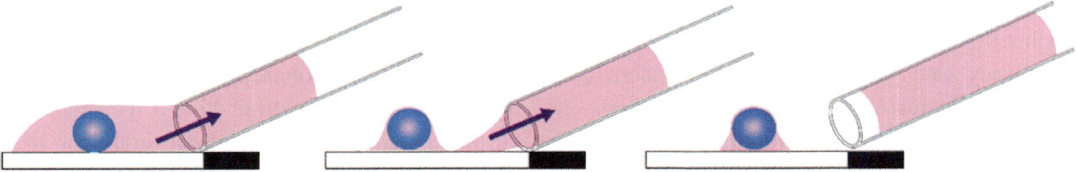

Fig. 9.9   Aspiration of excess liquid

3. Aspiration of excess liquid: The ideal state for embryo loading before freezing is to have the pipette tip gently touch the carrier and have the embryo been gently dripping on the carrier with only a small volume of liquid coating the embryo. If an excess liquid is accidentally brought in, it must be aspirated away. When aspirating the liquid, the pipette tip should be directed away from the embryo (Fig. 9.9).

4. Position of the carrier sheet and the pipette tip: If a commercial oocyte denudation pipette with a flat opening is used for embryo load-ing, the operator may hold the carrier in the left hand during the loading process and tilt the carrier slightly so that the carrier sheet is parallel to the opening of the oocyte denuda-tion pipette, which facilitates a smooth spit-ting out of the embryo. In the case of using a hand-pulled Pasteur glass pipette with a slop-ing opening, the orientation of the sloping opening should be adjusted. The front end of the carrier should be gently pressed against the bottom of the culture dish so that the slop-ing opening of the pipette is parallel to the front end of the carrier sheet (Fig. 9.10).

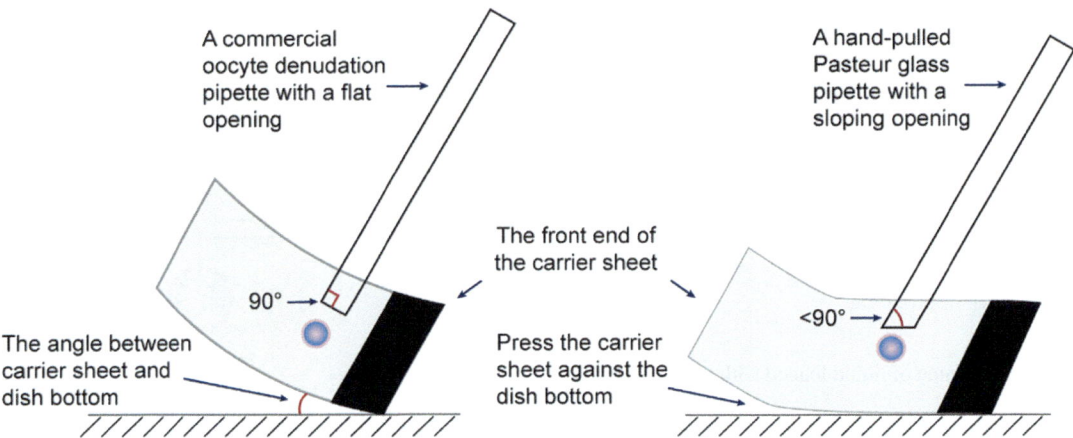

Fig. 9.10 Schematic diagram of the angle between the Pasteur glass pipette, the carrier, and the bottom of the dish

9.7 Procedures of Oocyte Vitrification

Oocyte freezing technology came into the limelight in 1986 with the birth of the first baby conceived from a frozen oocyte. With the increasingly sophisticated freezing technology and the rising pregnancy rate with frozen oocytes, there is a growing interest in the cryopreservation of oocytes. Oocyte cryopreservation will serve as an effective approach for females to preserve their fertility, and the demand for oocyte cryopreservation is bound to become increasingly stronger. There are various clinical reasons for oocyte cryopreservation, and examples include: the male partner being unable to retrieve sperm on the day of oocyte collection; some of the oocytes are to be frozen as too many oocytes are retrieved from the female partner; and in case of oocyte donation.

9.7.1 Changes in Oocyte Ultrastructure by Cryopreservation

Under the light microscope, slowly frozen oocytes have no change in appearance, the zona pellucida structure is normally intact, and vacuoles can sometimes be found in some frozen-thawed oocytes. Under transmission electron microscopy, on the other hand, changes in the

ultrastructure can be observed in oocytes that have been slowly frozen and thawed [13]. Many vesicles, multivesicular bodies, secondary lysosomes, and dysplastic mitochondrial-smooth endoplasmic reticulum aggregates may be present in these oocytes [14]. Delamination of the zona pellucida could be observed in some oocytes, which is probably related to the increased density of the zona pellucida and the release of cortical granules. The cortical granules of a mature oocyte are distributed uniformly and in strips under its membrane. As a result of oocyte freezing, the cortical granules under the oocyte membrane are reduced and the cortical granules are released into the perivitelline space. In contrast, freezing and thawing have no significant impacts on the distribution and number of mitochondria in oocytes [15].

9.7.2 Vitrification Procedure for Oocytes

The oocytes usually need to be digested with hyaluronidase to remove the granulosa cells before freezing. There are now commercial kits available specifically for oocyte freezing. Meanwhile, it should be noted that oocytes take longer to equilibrate in cryoprotectant solutions than embryos because they have a lower surface area/volume ratio (Fig. 9.11), which affects the

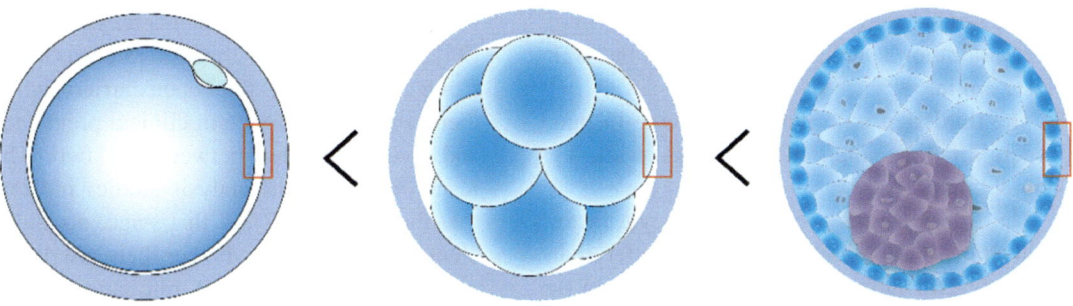

Fig. 9.11 Ratio of surface area to volume of oocytes and embryos

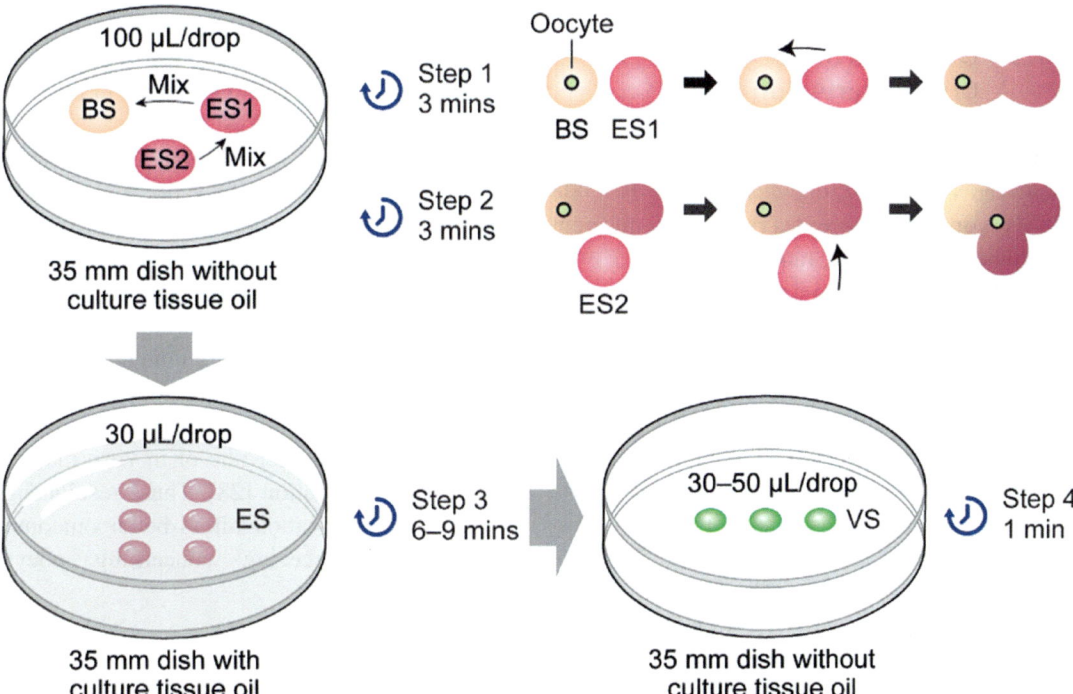

Fig. 9.12 Schematic diagram of oocyte freezing steps. *BS* basal solution, *ES* equilibration solution, *VS* vitrification solution

efficiency of transmembrane movement of water molecules, resulting in less efficient expulsion of water from the oocytes and less efficient permeation of cryoprotectants into them. Moreover, the oocytes themselves are more inclined to preserve water and are more susceptible to damage by intracellular ice crystals. Therefore, it is important to allow sufficient time for the oocytes to dehydrate and "load" with cryoprotectants during the freezing process to prepare for vitrification.

The laboratory materials to be prepared for oocyte vitrification are the same as for embryo vitrification (see Sect. 9.6 of this chapter). The steps of oocyte vitrification are described here with the example of using a commercial kit (Fig. 9.12).

1. The first step is to place the oocyte in the basal solution (BS), followed immediately by mixing the equilibration solution (ES1) with it and waiting for 3 min.

2. The second step is to mix the second drop of equilibration solution (ES2) with it and wait for 3 min.
3. The third step is to place the oocyte in pure equilibration solution (ES) and wait for 6–9 min.
4. The fourth step is to place the oocyte in the vitrification solution (VS) and transfer it in VS several times within 1 min, followed by loading it onto a carrier and plunging it into liquid nitrogen.

9.7.3 Outcomes of Oocyte Cryopreservation

1. Comparison of clinical outcomes of cryopreserved versus fresh oocytes: The survival rate of cryopreserved oocytes reported in different studies varies and ranges from 74.5% to 96.9% [16]. A meta-analysis including five randomized controlled trial (RCT) studies and six non-RCT studies showed no difference in fertilization rate between cryopreserved oocytes (77.8%) and fresh oocytes (80.8%) [17]. According to the results of several RCT studies, there is no difference in cleavage rate or good quality embryo rate between cryopreserved versus fresh oocytes [18, 19]. The results also showed that: the live birth rate of slowly frozen oocytes is lower than that of fresh oocytes [20]; whereas the live birth rate of vitrified oocytes does not differ from that of fresh oocytes [11]; and there are no significant differences in the incidence of adverse obstetric outcomes (including diabetes, gestational hypertension, premature birth, anemia, and neonatal pathological jaundice), gestational week, birth weight, Apgar score, and incidence of neonatal congenital anomalies in frozen oocytes compared with fresh oocytes [21–24].
2. Comparison of clinical outcomes of cryopreserving oocytes with open versus closed carriers: Results of a prospective cohort study on clinical outcomes of cryopreserved oocytes showed that the survival rate of oocytes frozen and preserved using closed carriers (94.5%)

was higher than that of open carriers (88.9%) [25]. However, the fertilization rate was lower using closed carriers than open carriers, while there was no difference in clinical pregnancy and live birth rates between the two. The results of two meta-analysis studies indicate that there is [26, 27], at this stage, not sufficient evidence about whether there are differences in oocyte survival rate and clinical outcomes between open and closed carriers. Therefore, there is no definitive conclusion about the advantages and disadvantages of open and closed carriers. Further studies are needed to determine if there are differences between the two types of carriers in terms of oocyte cryopreservation.

3. Comparison of clinical outcomes between slow-frozen and vitrified oocytes. Similar results have been reported in several studies: higher survival rate, pregnancy rate, and live birth rate were obtained with vitrification compared to slow freezing of the oocytes [11]. In addition, a study on the developmental potential of frozen-thawed immature oocytes showed that vitrified immature oocytes had a higher rate of in vitro maturation and fertilization [28]. These results suggest that vitrification offers better outcomes than slow freezing concerning oocyte cryopreservation.

9.8 Procedures of Oocyte and Embryo Thawing

The thawing process of vitrified oocytes and embryos is to place them in a thawing solution containing a certain concentration of nonpermeating cryoprotectants. This allows water molecules to progressively enter the cells and replace the permeating cryoprotectants within the cells so that the oocytes and embryos are gradually restored to their physiological state. The thawing solution usually contains only nonpermeating cryoprotectants (e.g., sucrose). Since water molecules enter the cells faster than the permeating cryoprotectants move out, multiple thawing solutions with decreasing sucrose con-

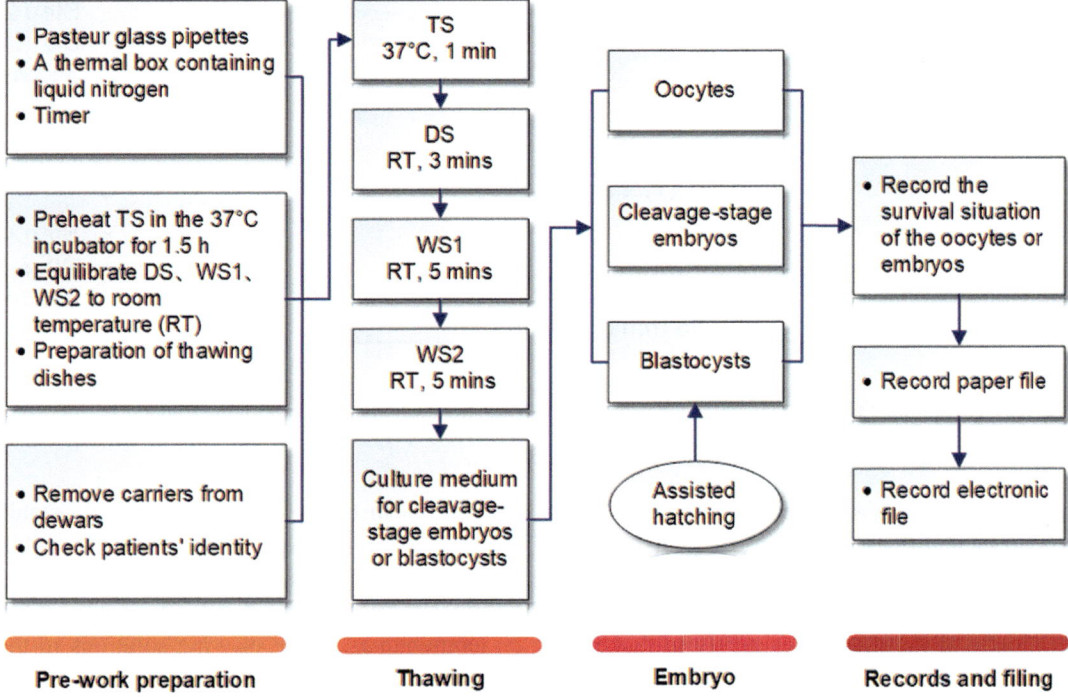

Fig. 9.13 Flow chart of oocyte and embryo thawing. *TS* thawing solution, *DS* diluent solution, *WS* washing solution, *RT* room temperature

centrations are used to prevent osmotic shock caused by too many water molecules entering the cells. This section explains the operating procedure and practical tips for thawing in detail, with an example of using a commercial thawing kit (Fig. 9.13).

9.8.1   Pre-work Preparation

1. Embryo transfer pipettes, polystyrene thermal box for liquid nitrogen, and a timer, as described in Sect. 9.6 of this chapter.
2. The thawing solution and dishes for the first step of thawing need to be preheated at 37 °C for more than 1.5 h.
3. The diluent solution required for the second step of thawing, the washing solution 1 required for the third step, and the washing solution 2 required for the fourth step must be equilibrated to room temperature in advance.
4. Preparation of thawing dishes.

(a) Preparation of thawing solution dishes in our center: drop 200 μL of thawing solution into the culture dish and cover it with tissue culture oil (4–5 mL) (Fig. 9.14), followed by preheating at 37 °C for more than 1.5 h.
(b) Preparation of the operating dish for the diluent solution, washing solution 1, and washing solution 2: make diluent solution, washing solution 1, and washing solution 2 microdroplets (30 μL/droplet) and cover them with tissue culture oil in the same culture dish at room temperature (Fig. 9.14).

9.8.2   Steps for Thawing

1. Step 1 (thawing solution): Place the thawing solution dish on a clean bench with the temperature set to 37 °C. After the carrier is removed from the liquid nitrogen, rapidly plunge it into the thawing solution and wait

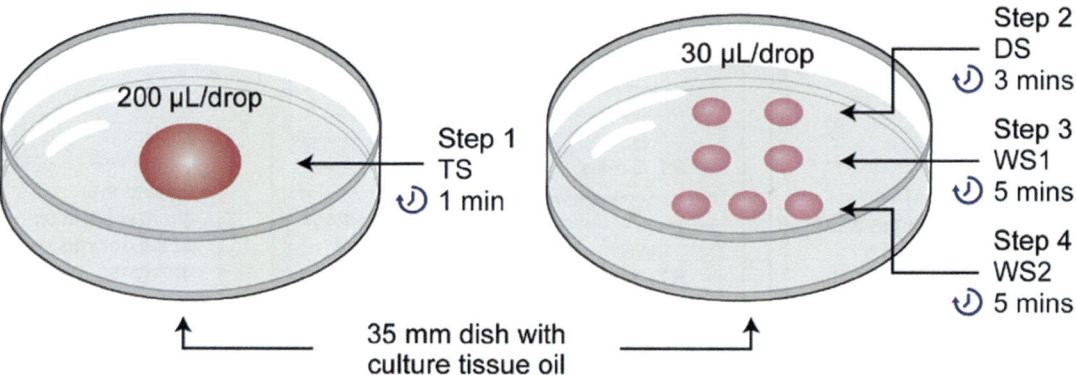

Fig. 9.14 Operating dishes for thawing. *TS* thawing solution, *DS* diluent solution, *WS1* washing solution 1, *WS2* washing solution 2

for 1 min. Suppose the embryo attaches to the carrier and does not come off easily. In that case, one can either pipette thawing solution toward the embryo repeatedly with a Pasteur pipette or tap the carrier gently to make the embryo come off. Then gently aspirate the embryo with a Pasteur pipette and transfer it to the diluent solution.

To investigate the effect of covering tissue culture oil on the temperature of the thawing solution, we divided thawing solution dishes into oil-covered and uncovered groups and monitored the temperature changes in both groups. The thawing solution volume was set to increase by 50 µL each time. A total of 23 dishes were set in each group, including 20 dishes with total thawing solution volumes ranging from 50 µL to 1000 µL and 3 dishes with thawing solution volumes of 2, 3, and 4 mL, respectively. After the two groups of thawing solution dishes were preheated at 37 °C for 1.5 h, they were placed on the clean bench at 37 °C with the ventilator turned on (room temperature was about 25 °C). A precision thermometer was used to measure the temperature changes in two groups within 1 min with a value read every two seconds, and a temperature change curve was plotted accordingly. The carrier was removed from the liquid nitrogen at the 0th second, quickly plunged into the thawing solution, and taken out at the 10th second. The results are shown in Fig. 9.15. The temperature of the thawing

solution in the oil-covered group was stable and was maintained at about 37 °C within 1 min, while the solution volume had no significant effect on the temperature. The initial temperatures of the thawing solutions in the uncovered group were all lower than 36 °C, which gradually decreased with time. Moreover, the smaller the volume of the thawing solution in the uncovered group, the lower its temperature. The initial temperatures of the small volume thawing solutions (50 µL, 100 µL, 150 µL) in the uncovered group were much lower than 37 °C (32.4 °C, 33.4 °C, 34.3 °C). Furthermore, the insertion and take-out of the carrier did not affect the temperature of thawing solutions in both groups. The above experiments can be concluded as follows: the temperature of thawing solutions in the oil-covered group can be effectively always maintained at 37 ± 0.2 °C; for thawing solutions without oil coverage, even when the volume is as large as 4 mL, the temperature of the solution decreased significantly within 1 min (temperature reduction range was about 1.5–2 °C).

Therefore, given that the required operating temperature for the thawing solution in the first step of thawing is 37 °C, the presence of covering oil has a major contribution to maintaining the temperature of the thawing solution. Figure 9.16 shows the morphology of the thawed oocytes in thawing solution without versus with oil coverage. It is evident

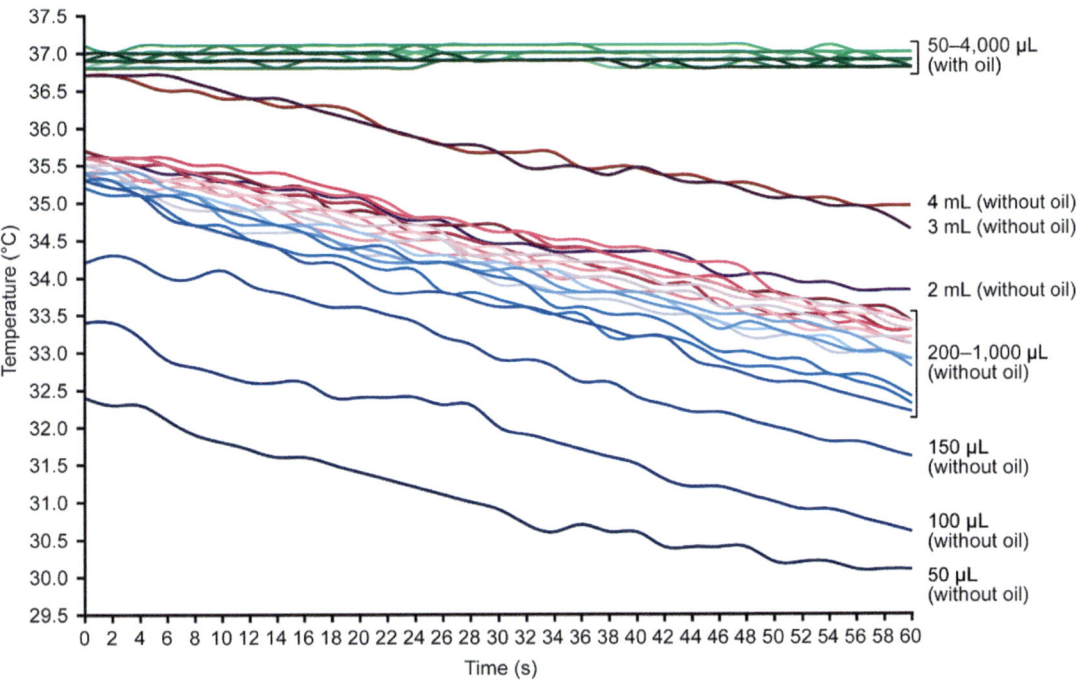

Fig. 9.15 Temperature variations of thawing solution in different volumes with and without tissue culture oil coverage

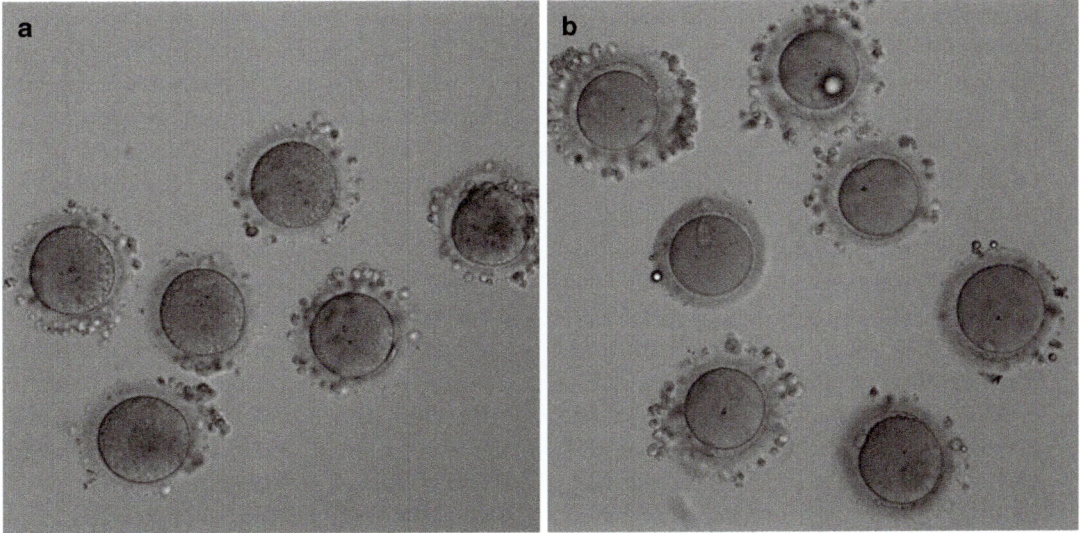

Fig. 9.16 Morphological comparison of thawed oocytes in the thawing solution without (**a**) versus with (**b**) oil coverage

that the cytoplasm of the thawed oocytes without oil coverage is coarse and with a significant number of vacuoles (Fig. 9.16a). In contrast, the cytoplasm of the thawed oocytes with oil coverage is homogeneous (Fig. 9.16b).

2. Steps 2–4 (diluent solution, washing solution 1, washing solution 2): The second step of thawing is to transfer the embryos into diluent solution and leave them for 3 min at room temperature. The third step is to transfer the

embryos into washing solution 1 and leave them for 5 min at room temperature. The fourth step is to transfer the embryos into washing solution 2 and leave them for 5 min at room temperature. It is important to note that a small amount of fluid is always carried with the embryos when transferring them from thawing solution to diluent solution and from diluent solution to washing solution 1. Finally, the embryos are transferred to a blastocyst culture medium to await implantation. After thawing and recovery, cleavage-stage embryos can be implanted immediately, while blastocysts require assisted hatching (see Sect. 9.12 of this chapter) before implantation.

9.8.3 Recording and Filing

1. Record the thawing profile of the embryos: (a) Morphology: After thawing, the oocytes and cleavage-stage embryos should first be evaluated for their morphological condition in terms of cell membrane and cytoplasm. The criteria for cell survival are as follows: clear cell membrane; normal cytoplasmic refractivity; no cracked zona pellucida; and no cytoplasmic leakage, expansion, or solidification of the cell [29]. Similarly, the post-thawing conditions of blastocysts should also be assessed by the cell membrane and cytoplasm states. The survival of a cleavage-stage embryo after thawing is defined as $\geq 50\%$ of the blastomeres being intact after thawing; the complete survival of a cleavage-stage embryo is defined as all blastomeres being intact after thawing; the survival of a blastocyst after thawing is defined as $\geq 75\%$ of all cells being intact after thawing. Post-thawing survival rate = the number of survival cleavage-stage embryos or blastocysts/total number of cleavage-stage embryos or blastocysts thawed × 100%; complete survival rate = the number of completely survival cleavage-stage embryos/total number of thawed cleavage-stage embryos × 100%. (b) Developmental status: ICSI is usually performed after the oocytes are thawed. The fertilization rate, embryo formation rate, and blastocyst formation rate are valid indicators to assess the thaw-recovery outcome of the cryopreserved oocytes. If the frozen-thawed cleavage-stage embryos need further culture before embryo transfer, good survival can be determined by observing whether the number of blastomeres increases and whether the embryos are compact. Blastocysts usually expand again within a few hours after thawing, which is a sign of good survival.

The frozen-thawed blastocysts usually need to be incubated in vitro for a while before being transferred. To investigate the relationship between different post-thaw incubation times of blastocysts and pregnancy outcomes, we followed up on the pregnancy outcomes of 232 patients who underwent frozen-thawed blastocyst(s) transfer in our unit. The subjects of this study included: 22 patients who received embryo transfer within 1 h after blastocyst thawing, 77 patients who received embryo transfer between 1 and 2 h after blastocyst thawing, 86 patients who received embryo transfer between 2 and 3 h after blastocyst thawing, and 47 patients who received embryo transfer more than or equal to 3 h after blastocyst thawing. The results of this study revealed no statistical difference in clinical pregnancy and implantation rates among the four groups of patients (Table 9.3), thus tentatively indicating that the time of in vitro incubation after blastocyst thawing does not affect pregnancy outcomes. With this finding, embryo laboratory operators are given the flexibility to schedule blastocyst thawing and embryo transfer according to the actual circumstances of each case.

2. Register electronic files and paper files

Both electronic and paper files are required to contain the following information: embryo score after thawing, embryo transfer date and time, whether the embryo transfer process was smooth, whether the transfer catheter was with blood during the process, and the distance of the transfer catheter opening from the uterine fundus.

Table 9.3 Clinical outcomes of different in vitro incubation times after blastocyst thawing

Key indicators	<1 h (N = 22)	1–2 h (N = 77)	2–3 h (N = 86)	≥3 h (N = 47)	P-Value
Clinical pregnancy rate	72.7%	67.5%	64.0%	63.8%	>0.05
Implantation rate	56.1%	56.8%	51.7%	49.4%	>0.05

9.9 Sperm Cryopreservation and Thawing

Sperm cryopreservation is a well-established technology that safeguards the success of IVF treatment cycles. Sperm freezing can be implemented in the following situations: the male partner has difficulty in sperm retrieval, and sperm freezing in advance would facilitate a normal embryo culture cycle; the male partner has severe oligoasthenoteratozoospermia, making it unfeasible to fertilize the oocytes with fresh sperm; surgical sperm retrieval cannot be performed simultaneously with oocyte retrieval; the male partner cannot be present on the day of oocyte retrieval; in cases of sperm and oocyte donations.

9.9.1 Treatment Outcomes of Sperm Cryopreservation

For azoospermia patients requiring surgical sperm retrieval, frozen-thawed sperm have shown more reliable treatment outcomes than fresh sperm retrieved surgically. A meta-analysis of testicular sperm retrieval surgery in patients with nonobstructive azoospermia showed that cryopreserved testicular-derived sperm had a similar ICSI fertilization rate, high-quality embryo rate, and clinical pregnancy rate as fresh testicular-derived sperm [30]. However, other studies have also demonstrated that fresh testicular biopsy samples are associated with a higher good quality embryo rate, a higher clinical pregnancy rate, and a higher implantation rate [31, 32]. Meanwhile, a study by Kalsi et al. indicates no statistical difference in fertilization rate, pregnancy rate, and live birth rate between fresh and cryopreserved epididymal spermatozoa [33]. Therefore, for patients who have undergone surgical sperm retrieval, the sperm obtained can be frozen and preserved in advance to facilitate the subsequent treatment and avoid additional surgical retrieval.

9.9.2 Changes in Physicochemical Properties of Cryopreserved Sperm

The resistance of spermatozoa to freezing is related to their basal state. It has been observed under light microscopy that cryopreservation can impair sperm morphology, viability, and motility to a certain extent [34]. However, in most cases, frozen-thawed sperm are adequate for ART treatment owing to the large basal sperm count and the application of intracytoplasmic sperm injection technology. Under scanning electron microscopy, swelling of the acrosome of the sperm head and peeling of the acrosomal inner membrane from the cell nuclear membrane can be observed in cryopreserved sperm [35]. Some sperm cryopreservation solutions have added cholesterol to stabilize the sperm cell membrane. The literature has also reported that sperm cryopreservation can lead to DNA damage and increased sperm DNA fragmentation accompanied by elevated expression of oxidative stress-related factors [36, 37].

9.9.3 Sperm Cryopreservation Procedure

Different commercial sperm cryopreservation kits are available in the market. Sperm cryopreservation approaches can be divided into three categories based on the principle of freezing. (a) Slow freezing: This method of freezing involves a gradient cooling of the sperm in 2–3 steps with the help of a programmed freezer before placing the sperm in liquid nitrogen, taking a total of 2 to 4 h to complete the freezing of the sperm. In the interval from 20 °C to 5 °C, the temperature is cooled down by 0.5–1 °C per minute; in the interval from 5 °C to −80 °C, the temperature is cooled down by 1–10 °C per minute before putting the sperm into liquid nitrogen. (b) Rapid freezing: After adding an equal amount of freezing medium drop by drop, the sperm are loaded into the freezing tubes. Let the loaded freezing tubes stand at room temperature for 10 min, then place them horizontally in the vapor phase for 30 min, and submerge them into liquid nitrogen. (c) Vitrification: Mix the sperm with the freezing medium at room temperature, drop the suspension mixture directly into the liquid nitrogen, and retrieve the frozen droplets into the cryovial using a metal strainer previously submerged in liquid nitrogen. This method is fast and inexpensive, but the semen specimen will directly contact liquid nitrogen in this process. The rapid freezing method is a comparatively mature technique, which is largely adequate for clinical needs. A systematic review has concluded that vitrification yields a higher motile sperm rate and forward-moving sperm rate when comparing these three freezing methods [38]. However, the effectiveness of vitrification is influenced by semen quality and correlates with whether cryoprotectants are applied, so more studies are needed to confirm this conclusion.

9.9.4 Sperm Thawing

Compared to sperm cryopreservation methods, fewer studies have been conducted on sperm thawing methods. Cryopreserved sperm are usually thawed by rapid warming, i.e., by using a 37 °C water bath (or incubator) to warm them for 10–15 min, while some centers thaw sperm at room temperature.

9.10 Open Vs. Closed Carriers

The carriers used for vitrification principally include open and closed carriers. The difference between the two is whether the gametes or embryos are in contact with liquid nitrogen during the cryopreservation process. There are at least thirty different carriers, at least fifteen fully commercialized. Nevertheless, most carriers feature only minor improvements based on the earlier ones, and many closed carriers are only slightly modified from the earlier open carriers. This section presents examples of some commercial open and closed carriers (Fig. 9.17) and compares the two in terms of the risk of pathogen transmission and cooling rate.

9.10.1 Open Carriers

When using open carriers, the specimens are exposed to liquid nitrogen during the freezing process. The sleeve used to protect the carrier is also open-ended so that the specimens remain in direct contact with liquid nitrogen during cryopreservation, resulting in the potential risk of cross-contamination. Open carriers also feature fast cooling rates. Two common open-type carriers are listed as follows:

1. Cryotop: It is a completely open carrier. When using a Cryotop carrier, the specimens are loaded on a transparent, flat, and slim-shaped plastic sheet with the observation spot clearly visible. The operating procedure is as follows: load the specimens onto the carrier with the recommended medium volume in the instructions, then rapidly plunge the carrier into liquid nitrogen, followed by covering it with the outer straw.
2. VitriFit: It is also a completely open carrier. However, unlike Cryotop, the loading area of VitriFit is curved, which is designed to protect the embryo and facilitate the operation of aspirating excess medium.

9.10.2 Closed Carriers

Specimens are not directly exposed to liquid nitrogen during cryopreservation using closed carriers. Once the specimens are loaded onto the carrier, a closed straw is placed to block contact between the specimens and the liquid nitrogen, preventing cross-contamination, and nosocomial

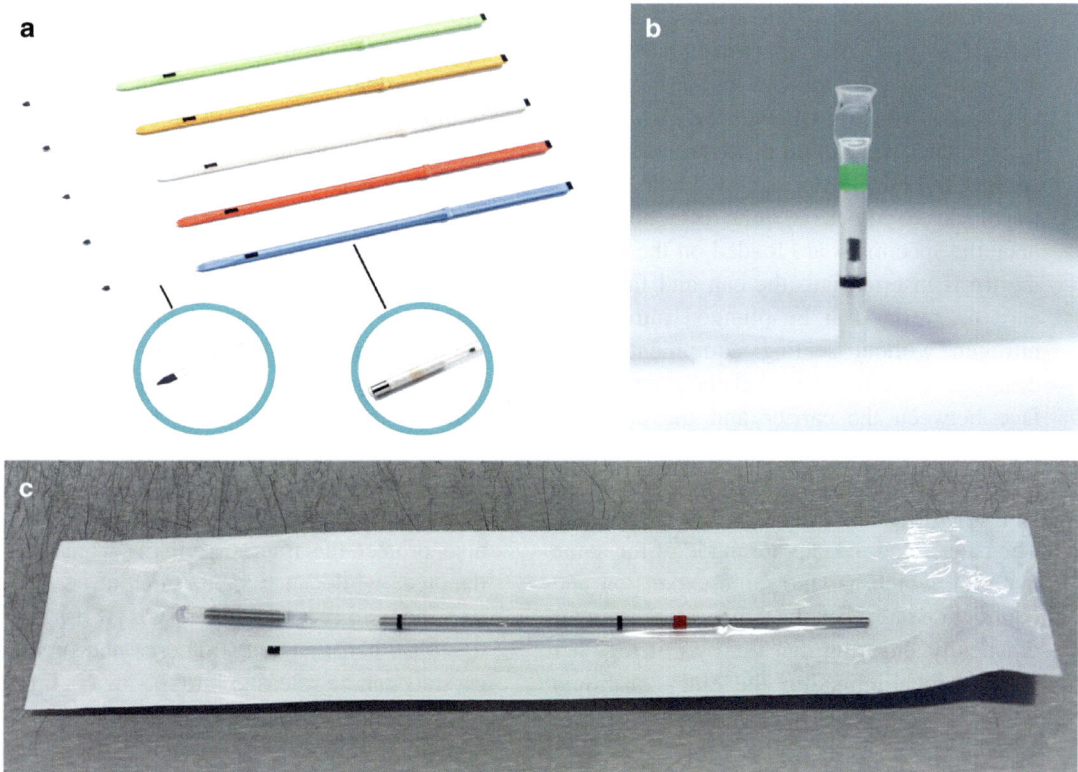

Fig. 9.17 Open vs. closed cryopreservation carriers. (Image **a** kindly supplied by KITAZATO CORPORATION, Japan. www.kitazato.co.jp. Images **b** and **c** supplied by CooperSurgical, Inc., Australia. www.coopersurgical.com)

infections yet also slowing down the cooling rate. There are many kinds of closed carriers, and depending on their design principles, the cooling rate during freezing and rewarming rate during thawing can also be different. Four common types of closed carriers are listed as follows:

1. HSV: After the specimens are loaded onto the carrier, the carrier is packed into a thin-walled plastic capillary straw, which is then sealed with a sealer and subsequently plunged into liquid nitrogen. When thawing, the plastic straw is cut open with a matching cutter, and the carrier is taken out for thawing and recovery of the specimens. This carrier has the highest hermeticity and isolates the specimens from the liquid nitrogen throughout the freezing and thawing process. However, the cool-ing rate during freezing and the rewarming rate during thawing are also reduced.

2. Rapid-i: This product comes with a specially designed liquid nitrogen box. A small hole is reserved on the lid of the liquid nitrogen box for RapidStraw. The RapidStraw is pre-cooled by prior insertion into the hole. The loaded Rapid-i is inserted into the RapidStraw sitting in liquid nitrogen, and the straw is then sealed with the matching sealer. The unique design of the lid of the liquid nitrogen box greatly reduces the evaporation of liquid nitrogen.

3. CVM: A unique design is adopted to utilize a metal block pre-cooled to a temperature equivalent to that of liquid nitrogen. The carrier loaded with specimens is then brought into contact with the metal surface for cool-ing. This design not only ensures the cooling

rate of the specimens but also avoids direct contact between the specimens and liquid nitrogen. However, this product does not provide instructions on whether the metal block is in contact with liquid nitrogen during precooling and how to sterilize the block.

4. Cryolock: Cryolock is quite easy to use—once the specimens are loaded on the carrier, the tip is inserted into the cap and fastened, and the carrier can be plunged into liquid nitrogen without sealing equipment. It is designed in such a way that the contact surface between the carrier and the cap is a unique conical interface. The carrier is completely sealed and isolated from liquid nitrogen when the cap is snapped and fastened. The carrier and the cap are made of the same material, which has the same expansion and contraction rate when the temperature changes drastically, ensuring that the two fit together tightly and eliminating the entry of liquid nitrogen.

9.10.3 Comparison of Open Vs. Closed Cryopreservation Carriers

The comparison of open and closed carriers has been the subject of extensive "debates" in recent years, mostly concerning pathogen transmission and the cooling rate. From time to time, we hear not only objective evaluations of these two technical approaches but also biased opinions. These biases may stem from experimental conclusions based on uncritical scientific design, distractions caused by commercial interests, or even overthinking of ethical and legal issues.

1. Risk of pathogen transmission: The safety of cryopreservation has received increasing attention since Tedder first reported a case of cross-contamination of hepatitis B virus due to leakage of blood specimens stored in liquid nitrogen in 1995 [39]. Results on microbial contamination have also been reported in studies in animal reproductive medicine

[40]. In one study, a total of 32 bacterial species and one fungus were identified by examining animal embryos and semen stored in liquid nitrogen for 6–35 years. The most common contaminant was Stenotrophomonas maltophilia [41], which can significantly inhibit gamete fertilization and embryo development.

It is indisputable that some pathogens can survive in liquid nitrogen and that particles in the atmosphere or on the surface of the container will gradually mix into the liquid nitrogen over time [42]. These particles may carry pathogenic microorganisms, most of which can survive in liquid nitrogen [43]. The cryoprotectants applied to protect the embryos can also protect the microorganisms from cryodamage, while such contamination will, in turn, poses a risk to the embryos. It has been demonstrated that fungal spores and organic crystals can be released into the air via liquid nitrogen, indicating that there is still a risk of contamination of the specimens or facility by the gas phase above the liquid nitrogen.

Cryopreservation carriers harbor human lives, and their biosafety concerns human offspring's health and has been a topic of great interest. Since specimens loaded on open carriers are exposed to liquid nitrogen during freezing and storage, some have argued that pathogens carried by infertile couples may cause cross-contamination during assisted reproductive treatment. However, studies have shown that no viral sequences were detected in waste culture media and vitrification solutions collected from oocyte/embryo culture processes in patients who were seropositive for human immunodeficiency virus, hepatitis C virus, and hepatitis B virus, and that there is no risk of cross-contamination in seropositive patients, even when open vitrification device is used [44]. It is estimated that at least one million patients annually have their embryos or oocyte frozen with open carriers. However, no cases of pathogen cross-contamination have been reported to date [45]. There is no direct evidence showing that pathogens can be transmitted between vitri-fied/frozen embryos via liquid nitrogen [46], and there have been no cases of bacterial or fungal contamination when using either open or closed carriers in oocyte and embryo banks [47]. The most likely explanation is that the pathogen level in liquid nitrogen in which the gametes or embryos are stored is well below the infection threshold and that the pathogen level is negligible after multiple dilutions and rinses throughout the IVF process. It is esti-mated by available data that >500,000 implan-tations of frozen embryos using fully open carriers do not seem to result in a single detectable infection, i.e., the probability of infection is less than 0.0002% [45].

Biological contamination via liquid nitro-gen can be disinfected by ultraviolet irradiation or filtration. Ultraviolet light can effectively destroy bacteria (*Stenotrophomonas malto-philia*, *Pseudomonas aeruginosa*, *Escherichia coli*) and fungi (*Aspergillus niger*) in liquid nitrogen [48]. If embryos are cryopreserved using closed carriers, these closed carriers need to be cut open in liquid nitrogen when the embryos are going to be thawed. There is a theoretical possibility that the carriers could get contaminated as the liquid nitrogen evaporates. To guarantee the biosafety of the specimens during the cryopreservation-thawing process and to prevent any potential contamination, the outer surface of the straw/sleeve/casing and the cutter should be disinfected before cutting. Another effective way to remove contamina-tion from the surface of the carrier is to rinse it with ultraviolet-sterilized liquid nitrogen [49].

2. Cooling rate: Embryos cryopreserved using open carriers are left exposed and are cooled at a rate of up to 23,000 °C/min when immersed directly into liquid nitrogen from a room temperature environment. Embryos cryopreserved with closed carriers are sleeved in straws. Although these straws have been made to be as thin-walled and slim as possible to transfer heat at maximum speed, the cooling rate of these embryos is <1500 °C/min when they are plunged into

liquid nitrogen from a room temperature environment. Based on the solution-crystal-vitrification phase transition process (Fig. 9.2), the solution has to go through a crystal phase before getting vitrified, and the intracellular ice formation can only be mini-mized when the solution passes through the crystal phase fast enough. It can be deduced that closed carriers could increase the prob-ability of intracellular ice crystal formation. However, recent studies have almost lopsid-edly suggested that the vitrification effect of closed carriers does not seem to affect mor-phological characteristics, developmental potential, or even reproductive outcomes of oocytes and embryos compared to open car-riers [50–54]. In contrast, the opposite con-clusion has not been reported as much [55, 56]. But we cannot ignore that most of the previous experimental data were not derived from prospective randomized controlled tri-als and multicenter studies, so the evidence level is not very high.

In summary, we still need higher-level evi-dence to fully understand the advantages and disadvantages of open and closed carriers and to make a scientific choice of carrier type weighing the benefits and risks.

9.11   Artificial Shrinkage of Blastocysts

Artificial shrinkage aims to release fluid from the blastocyst cavity and reduce the extracellular ice formation during vitrification. After the blasto-cyst develops to the expansion stage, a large amount of fluid is present in the blastocyst cavity, which can form ice during freezing, causing cell damage. It has been well established that artifi-cial shrinkage of blastocysts prior to freezing can improve their post-thaw recovery rate, increase the hatching rate of stage-4 blastocysts, and improve treatment outcomes [57, 58]. There are various methods of artificial shrinkage, which can be classified into laser and mechanical meth-ods according to their principles.

9.11.1 Laser Method

The laser method is widely used because it is less expensive, simple, and fast, reduces the exposure time of the embryo to the environment, and has been shown to result in good pregnancy outcomes [59]. When performing artificial shrinkage by laser method, the following precautions should be taken:

1. Laser intensity: The laser intensity should be set according to the specific conditions of each device. For example, the laser pulse duration applied in our center is 400–500 μs, and the ablation aperture is about 5–7 μm. The principle is to use the lowest possible laser intensity while effectively releasing the fluid in the blastocoel to reduce the cell damage.
2. Perforation location: Laser perforation should be sited away from the inner cell mass, where the trophectoderm cells are loosely connected, and two cells are joined (Fig. 9.18).

9.11.2 Mechanical Method

The mechanical method can be performed by repeatedly pipetting the blastocyst with a pulled fine-tip Pasteur glass pipette, which promotes blastocyst shrinkage via mechanical compres-

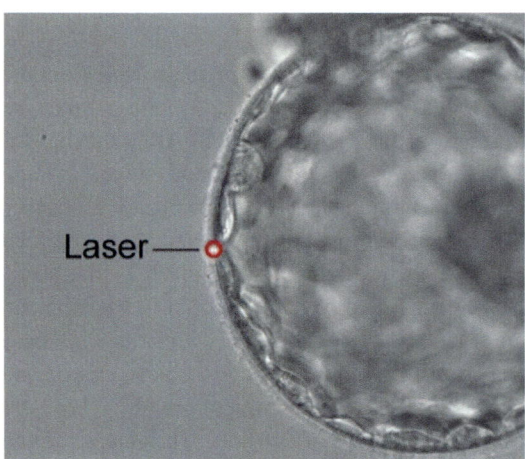

Fig. 9.18 Laser perforation position

sion; or by puncturing an ICSI pipette into the blastocoel and aspirating the fluid from the cavity with the help of a microscopic manipulation system. However, regardless of the approach taken, care should be taken to avoid damaging the inner cell mass during the manipulation.

9.12   Assisted Hatching

Assisted hatching is a technique to improve the hatching rate of blastocysts by manually removing or thinning the zona pellucida to reduce the resistance encountered during hatching. Studies concluded that in vitro culture and freezing/thawing would alter the physical and chemical properties of the zona pellucida and increase its hardness, thus requiring assisted hatching after thawing the embryos [60].

9.12.1 Zona Pellucida

The zona pellucida has a multilayered structure, and its three-layer structure can be observed by polarized light microscopy [61]. The zona pellucida is composed of four glycoproteins (ZP1, ZP2, ZP3, and ZPB) and plays different roles in each stage of embryonic development: before fertilization, the sperm binds to the zona pellucida to induce the acrosome reaction; after fertilization, the cortical granules released by the oocyte change the structure of the zona pellucida and can prevent polyspermous fertilization; during the cleavage stage, the zona pellucida maintains the integrity of the blastomeres as they are poorly attached to each other; and when the development proceeds to the blastocyst stage, the blastocyst will break through the zona pellucida and attach itself to the endometrium. Under physiological conditions, blastocyst hatching is the result of embryo-maternal interaction. When cultured in vitro, the hatching of blastocysts relies on the tension generated by their repeated contraction and expansion and the digestion of the zona pellucida by proteases released from trophoblast cells [62].

9.12.2 Assisted Hatching Methods

1. Laser method: The laser emitter is normally mounted on an inverted microscope and does not need to touch the embryo to perform assisted hatching (Fig. 9.19). Laser-assisted hatching is widely used because of its low cost and easy operation. The laser-assisted hatching method include the creation of an opening in the zona pellucida by drilling with laser photoablation. The opening should be well away from the inner cell mass and at a spot where there is a large gap between the trophectoderm cells and the zona pellucida, and the laser intensity should be carefully adjusted to avoid accidental cell injury.

2. Chemical method: Acidic Tyrode's solution and pronase can be used for perforation [63]. When using acidic Tyrode's solution: Hold the embryo in place with an oocyte-holding pipette at 9 o'clock with the assistance of a micro-manipulation system, and use a micro-pipette to expel acidic Tylenol's solution at 3 o'clock against the embryo, which will dissolve the zona pellucida. Pronase digestion method: Immerse the embryos in pronase

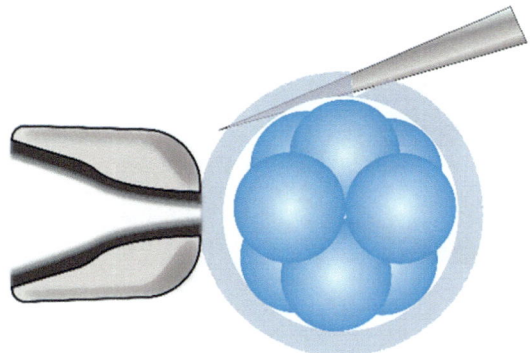

Fig. 9.20 Schematic diagram of mechanical method

dilution for 60–120 s to thin the zona pellucida by digestion (but not completely remove the zona pellucida).

3. Mechanical method: The mechanical method involves using a holding pipette and a microneedle to incise the zona pellucida. This method partially eliminates the zona pellucida by mechanical dissection [64] (Fig. 9.20).

4. Piezo method: The embryo is fixed with a holding pipette, and an opening in the zona pellucida is created using a piezo-micromanipulator. After applying a piezo-electric pulse, the zona pellucida is peeled off by the vibration of a micro-manipulation needle [65] (Fig. 9.21).

9.12.3 Treatment Outcomes of Assisted Hatching

The results of several systematic reviews and meta-analyses have shown that assisted hatching can improve clinical pregnancy and implantation rates [66, 67]. However, it has also been proposed that assisted hatching can increase the risk of twin pregnancy while not affecting the live birth or miscarriage rate.

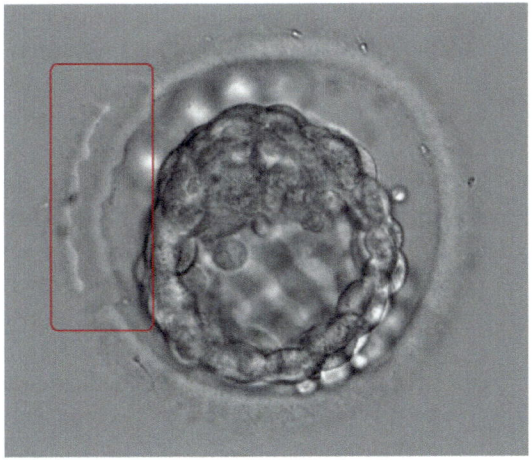

Fig. 9.19 Schematic diagram of laser method

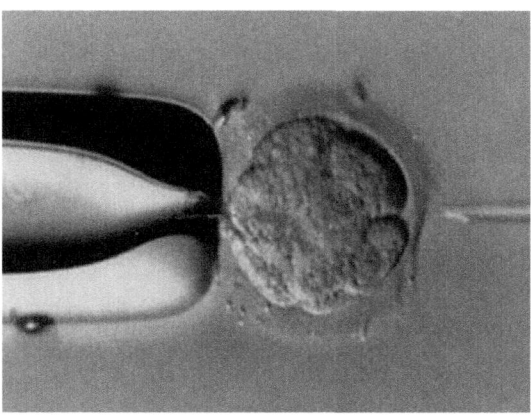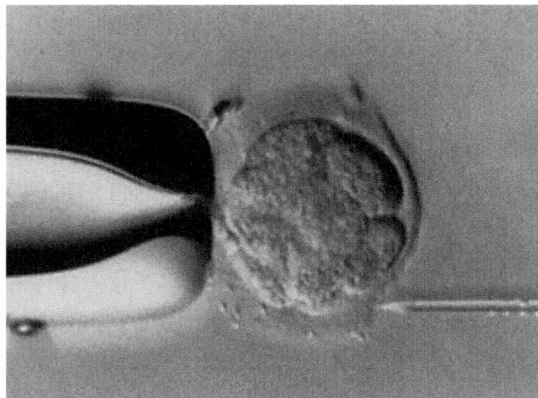

Fig. 9.21 Schematic diagram of the piezo method

9.13 Quality Management of Cryostorage Room

With the increase in the number of ART treatment cycles, coupled with the widespread use of the whole embryo freezing strategy, the number of specimens to be stored in IVF laboratories is also increasing, making the quality management of the cryostorage room increasingly important.

9.13.1 Use of Dewars and Risk Control

1. Dewars: Specimens are usually stored in dewars, where sperm, oocytes, and embryos are stored directly in liquid nitrogen for thermal stability. Take the dewar shown in Fig. 9.22 as an example, it has a sturdy and durable lid that can be locked, which is tamper-resistant. Its neck is constructed with glass fiber, reducing liquid nitrogen loss, and providing maximum liquid nitrogen storage efficiency. The surface of the dewar is made of high-strength, lightweight insulating aluminum, and the interior features an advanced chemical vacuum retention system. Depending on the size of the dewar, the number of internal specimen containers can vary from 6 to 10. The dewar in the figure also features a spider-shaped platform

for easy removal and return of the specimen containers.

2. Precautions when using a dewar: It is strictly forbidden to hit the dewar violently during use, which may damage the neck tube or cause vacuum failure. The container and packaging should be inspected for damage during shipping when purchasing a new dewar. After the first filling with liquid nitrogen, observe whether there is frost or "sweating" on the outer surface of the dewar, which would indicate a possible break in the vacuum mechanism inside the dewar (note: some frost near the top is normal after the first filling with liquid nitrogen). Each IVF laboratory should keep 1–2 empty dewars filled with liquid nitrogen for emergency use. When the dewar is filled with liquid nitrogen for the first time, the following should be noted:
   (a) Use a funnel or delivery tube to slowly inject a small amount of liquid nitrogen into the new dewar.
   (b) Let the liquid nitrogen settle in the dewar for 2 h so that the interior is completely cooled.
   (c) After cooling, fill the dewar with liquid nitrogen to the desired level.
   (d) When filling the dewar from a pressurized source, make sure that the pressure inside the liquid nitrogen source tank is below 22 psi.

Fig. 9.22 Exterior and interior structure of the dewar

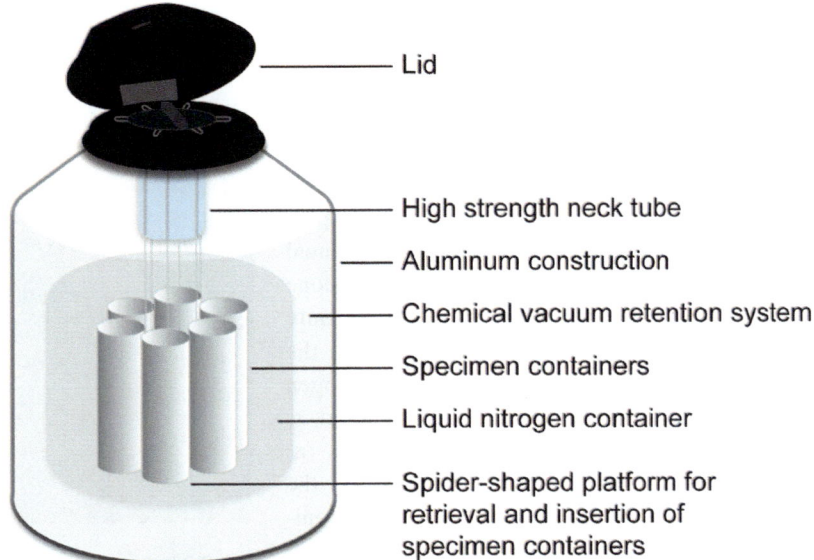

Lid

High strength neck tube

Aluminum construction

Chemical vacuum retention system

Specimen containers

Liquid nitrogen container

Spider-shaped platform for retrieval and insertion of specimen containers

(e) If a conveying hose is used to extract liquid nitrogen from a pressurized source, always use a phase separator on the end of the hose.

(f) Never overfill the dewar with liquid nitrogen. Overfilling the tank may cause pumpout components to leak leading to immediate or premature vacuum failure to occur.

3. Staff protection: Due to the Leidenfrost effect, the liquid nitrogen will instantly vaporize when in brief contact with the skin, and the air film and air on the surface of the skin are poor conductors of heat, so there will be no frostbite to the skin in this case. However, prolonged exposure to liquid nitrogen can cause frostbite, so that the laboratory may have an ointment for frostbite just in case. However, in the case of extensive frostbite, medical attention should be sought as soon as possible. To avoid frostbite, staff should be extra careful when handling liquid nitrogen and should pay attention to the following matters:

(a) Do not leave the skin exposed.

(b) Always wear protective clothing: face mask, cryogenic gloves, cryogenic apron.

(c) Do not overfill the liquid nitrogen container.

(d) Keep the liquid nitrogen container upright at all times.

(e) Do not completely seal the liquid nitrogen container.

(f) Take extra care to prevent spillage and splashing of liquid nitrogen during transfer.

(g) The evaporation of liquid nitrogen will substantially reduce the oxygen content in the air, which may lead to asphyxiation or even death. Dewars with liquid nitrogen should be stored and operated in a well-ventilated area.

9.13.2 Management and Risk Control of the Cryostorage Room

1. Management of the cryostorage room: First, the cryostorage room must be equipped with good ventilation and preferably located at the periphery of the laboratory with direct access to the outside. If the cryostorage room is located in the interior area of the laboratory, it must be equipped with appropriate ventilation ducts. In addition, the door of the cryostorage room should be equipped with a viewing window, and the floor should be made of frost-resistant materials such as steel plates.

2. Liquid nitrogen level detection system: Liquid nitrogen level detection systems can be divided into manual and automatic measurement systems. The purpose of either system is to monitor the liquid nitrogen balance during daily use to prevent the liquid nitrogen balance from getting too low and thus compromising the safety of embryo storage. Manual measurement of liquid nitrogen level is done using a wooden or plastic dipstick to measure and record the liquid nitrogen level in the dewar daily. The automatic liquid nitrogen level detection system, on the other hand, is available in various types, such as: (a) Tempurity system can indirectly monitor the level of liquid nitrogen in the dewar by monitoring the weight of the dewar in real-time and display the reading on a monitor. Its measurement data can be transmitted to the staff's computer via the internet. When the weight drops to a critical level, the system will notify the staff via SMS and phone. (b) MVE TEC 3000 system is designed based on the principle of differential pressure. It also monitors the temperature and liquid level in the dewar in real-time and is equipped with an alarm and communication system.

3. Inspection of dewars: All dewars in the laboratory should be checked regularly for damage to ensure that the vacuum is functioning properly. The main observations are as follows: (a) Whether there is a "cold spot" on the outer surface of the dewar, which may indicate a vacuum failure. In this case, a significant temperature change can be detected by placing a hand on the outer surface of the dewar. (b) Detect any damage to the foam in the neck, which can jeopardize the effectiveness of the dewar.

4. Filling of liquid nitrogen
   (a) Adding liquid nitrogen manually: Liquid nitrogen is mostly supplied by liquid nitrogen cylinders. The liquid nitrogen cylinders commonly used in IVF laboratories feature a low gravity center and a polished stainless steel housing. They normally have stainless steel casters that allow free movement within the embryo room. The

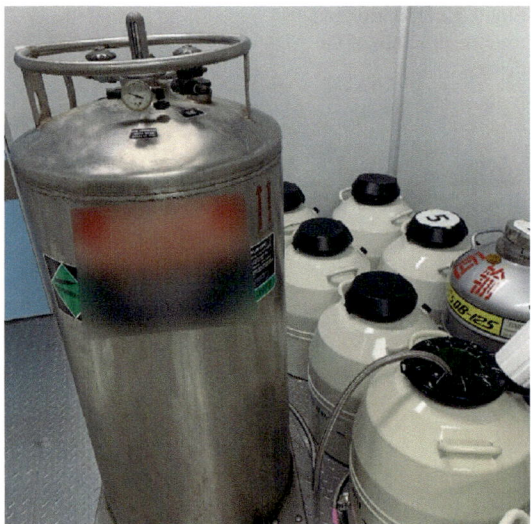

Fig. 9.23 Liquid nitrogen cylinder

liquid nitrogen cylinder used in our laboratory has a capacity of 270 L and is connected to a metal hose approximately 2 m in length (Fig. 9.23). The staff should determine the interval between each refill of liquid nitrogen according to the actual conditions of each laboratory. For example, they may choose to refill all dewars every 7 days. Also, the amount of liquid nitrogen refilled in each dewar should be monitored and recorded to calculate each dewar's liquid nitrogen loss rate. These records will indicate which dewars are less efficient at holding liquid nitrogen and whether they should be replaced.

   (b) Liquid nitrogen piping system
       Due to their high maintenance costs, piping systems for liquid nitrogen are often only employed by very large-scale reproduction centers. Such piping systems are usually equipped with a main dewar bottle that is connected through a piping system to the embryo cryostorage room, where a terminal switch is installed that allows the liquid nitrogen to be discharged like tap water.

   (c) Automatic liquid nitrogen filling system
       The automatic liquid nitrogen filling system is installed on each dewar, which

can automatically open the solenoid valve, refill liquid nitrogen according to the liquid nitrogen level measured by the detector, and close the valve when the liquid nitrogen level approaches the upper limit. The liquid nitrogen filling system and the liquid nitrogen level monitoring system are completely independent, ensuring that the monitoring system's measurements are not interfered with while the liquid nitrogen is being filled [68, 69].

5. Removal and return of embryos

When the embryos are frozen and put into the dewar, the storage location should be recorded, and two copies, electronic and paper, must be kept and filed. Double-checking is always required when placing embryos. When embryos need to be thawed and removed from the dewar, the procedure should also be done under double-checking, verifying the patient's name, the date of freezing, and the grade of the embryos to be thawed.

6. Personnel training

All staff working with liquid nitrogen or who may be involved in liquid nitrogen emergencies must receive adequate training. This training is conducted on-site at the cryogenic storage facility by an instructor with comprehensive health and safety expertise. Written records should be kept to document the training completed, and no one is allowed to handle liquid nitrogen without adequate training.

References

1. Polge C, Smith AU, Parkes AS. Revival of spermatozoa after vitrification and dehydration at low temperatures. Nature. 1949;164(4172):666.
2. Edashige K. Permeability of the plasma membrane to water and cryoprotectants in mammalian oocytes and embryos: its relevance to vitrification. Reprod Med Biol. 2016;16(1):36–9.
3. Spindler R, Wolkers WF, Glasmacher B. Effect of Me(2)SO on membrane phase behavior and protein denaturation of human pulmonary endothelial cells studied by in situ FTIR spectroscopy. J Biomech Eng. 2009;131(7):074517.
4. Elmoazzen HY, Poovadan A, Law GK. Dimethyl sulfoxide toxicity kinetics in intact articular cartilage. Cell Tissue Bank. 2007;8(2):125–33.
5. Yuan C, Gao J, Guo J, et al. Dimethyl sulfoxide damages mitochondrial integrity and membrane potential in cultured astrocytes. PLoS One. 2014;9(9):e107447.
6. Fahy GM, Lilley TH, Linsdell H, et al. Cryoprotectant toxicity and cryoprotectant toxicity reduction: in search of molecular mechanisms. Cryobiology. 1990;27(3):247–68.
7. Jomha NM, Weiss AD, Fraser Forbes J, et al. Cryoprotectant agent toxicity in porcine articular chondrocytes. Cryobiology. 2010;61(3):297–302.
8. Szurek EA, Eroglu A. Comparison and avoidance of toxicity of penetrating cryoprotectants. PLoS One. 2011;6(11):e27604.
9. Gurruchaga H, Saenz Del Burgo L, Orive G, et al. Low molecular-weight hyaluronan as a cryoprotectant for the storage of microencapsulated cells. Int J Pharm. 2018;548(1):206–16.
10. Whittingham DG, Leibo SP, Mazur P. Survival of mouse embryos frozen to -196 degrees and -269 degrees C. Science. 1972;178(4059):411–4.
11. Rienzi L, Gracia C, Maggiulli R, et al. Oocyte, embryo and blastocyst cryopreservation in ART: systematic review and meta-analysis comparing slow-freezing versus vitrification to produce evidence for the development of global guidance. Hum Reprod Update. 2017;23(2):139–55.
12. Martínez-Burgos M, Herrero L, Megías D, et al. Vitrification versus slow freezing of oocytes: effects on morphologic appearance, meiotic spindle configuration, and DNA damage. Fertil Steril. 2011;95(1):374–7.
13. Nottola SA, Macchiarelli G, Coticchio G, et al. Ultrastructure of human mature oocytes after slow cooling cryopreservation using different sucrose concentrations. Hum Reprod. 2007;22(4):1123–33.
14. Nottola SA, Coticchio G, De Santis L, et al. Ultrastructure of human mature oocytes after slow cooling cryopreservation with ethylene glycol. Reprod Biomed Online. 2008;17(3):368–77.
15. Stimpfel M, Vrtacnik-Bokal E, Virant-Klun I. No difference in mitochondrial distribution is observed in human oocytes after cryopreservation. Arch Gynecol Obstet. 2017;296(2):373–81.
16. Cobo A, Diaz C. Clinical application of oocyte vitrification: a systematic review and meta-analysis of randomized controlled trials. Fertil Steril. 2011;96(2):277–85.
17. Potdar N, Gelbaya TA, Nardo LG. Oocyte vitrification in the 21st century and post-warming fertility outcomes: a systematic review and meta-analysis. Reprod Biomed Online. 2014;29(2):159–76.
18. Cobo A, Meseguer M, Remohí J, et al. Use of cryobanked oocytes in an ovum donation programme: a prospective, randomized, controlled, clinical trial. Hum Reprod. 2010;25(9):2239–46.
19. Rienzi L, Romano S, Albricci L, et al. Embryo development of fresh 'versus' vitrified metaphase II

oocytes after ICSI: a prospective randomized sibling-oocyte study. Hum Reprod. 2010;25(1):66–73.

20. Kushnir VA, Barad DH, Albertini DF, et al. Outcomes of fresh and cryopreserved oocyte donation. JAMA. 2015;314(6):623–4.

21. Seshadri S, Saab W, Exeter H, et al. Clinical outcomes of a vitrified donor oocyte programme: a single UK centre experience. Eur J Obstet Gynecol Reprod Biol. 2018;225:136–40.

22. Noyes N, Porcu E, Borini A. Over 900 oocyte cryopreservation babies born with no apparent increase in congenital anomalies. Reprod Biomed Online. 2009;18(6):769–76.

23. Chian RC, Huang JY, Tan SL, et al. Obstetric and perinatal outcome in 200 infants conceived from vitrified oocytes. Reprod Biomed Online. 2008;16(5):608–10.

24. Cobo A, Serra V, Garrido N, et al. Obstetric and perinatal outcome of babies born from vitrified oocytes. Fertil Steril. 2014;102(4):1006–15.

25. Pujol A, Zamora MJ, Obradors A, et al. Comparison of two different oocyte vitrification methods: a prospective, paired study on the same genetic background and stimulation protocol. Hum Reprod. 2019;34(6):989–97.

26. Youm HS, Choi JR, Oh D, et al. Survival rates in closed and open vitrification for human mature oocyte cryopreservation: a meta-analysis. Gynecol Obstet Investig. 2018;83(3):268–74.

27. Cai H, Niringiyumukiza JD, Li Y, et al. Open versus closed vitrification system of human oocytes and embryos: a systematic review and meta-analysis of embryologic and clinical outcomes. Reprod Biol Endocrinol. 2018;16(1):123.

28. Zhang Z, Liu Y, Xing Q, et al. Cryopreservation of human failed-matured oocytes followed by in vitro maturation: vitrification is superior to the slow freezing method. Reprod Biol Endocrinol. 2011;9:156.

29. Alpha Scientists in Reproductive Medicine. The Alpha consensus meeting on cryopreservation key performance indicators and benchmarks: proceedings of an expert meeting. Reprod Biomed Online. 2012;25(2):146–67.

30. Yu Z, Wei Z, Yang J, et al. Comparison of intracytoplasmic sperm injection outcome with fresh versus frozen-thawed testicular sperm in men with nonobstructive azoospermia: a systematic review and meta-analysis. J Assist Reprod Genet. 2018;35(7):1247–57.

31. Aoki VW, Wilcox AL, Thorp C, et al. Improved in vitro fertilization embryo quality and pregnancy rates with intracytoplasmic sperm injection of sperm from fresh testicular biopsy samples vs. frozen biopsy samples. Fertil Steril. 2004;82(6):1532–5.

32. Wu B, Wong D, Lu S, et al. Optimal use of fresh and frozen-thawed testicular sperm for intracytoplasmic sperm injection in azoospermic patients. J Assist Reprod Genet. 2005;22(11–12):389–94.

33. Kalsi J, Thum MY, Muneer A, et al. Analysis of the outcome of intracytoplasmic sperm injection using fresh or frozen sperm. BJU Int. 2011;107(7):1124–8.

34. Ozkavukcu S, Erdemli E, Isik A, et al. Effects of cryopreservation on sperm parameters and ultrastructural morphology of human spermatozoa. J Assist Reprod Genet. 2008;25(8):403–11.

35. Pedersen H, Lebech PE. Ultrastructural changes in the human spermatozoon after freezing for artificial insemination. Fertil Steril. 1971;22(2):125–33.

36. de Paula TS, Bertolla RP, Spaine DM, et al. Effect of cryopreservation on sperm apoptotic deoxyribonucleic acid fragmentation in patients with oligozoospermia. Fertil Steril. 2006;86(3):597–600.

37. Thomson LK, Fleming SD, Aitken RJ, et al. Cryopreservation-induced human sperm DNA damage is predominantly mediated by oxidative stress rather than apoptosis. Hum Reprod. 2009;24(9):2061–70.

38. Li YX, Zhou L, Lv MQ, et al. Vitrification and conventional freezing methods in sperm cryopreservation: a systematic review and meta-analysis. Eur J Obstet Gynecol Reprod Biol. 2019;233:84–92.

39. Tedder RS, Zuckerman MA, Goldstone AH, et al. Hepatitis B transmission from contaminated cryopreservation tank. Lancet. 1995;346(8968):137–40.

40. Bielanski A, Bergeron H, Lau PC, et al. Microbial contamination of embryos and semen during long term banking in liquid nitrogen. Cryobiology. 2003;46(2):146–52.

41. An SQ, Berg G. Stenotrophomonas maltophilia. Trends Microbiol. 2018;26(7):637–8.

42. Bielanski A, Vajta G. Risk of contamination of germplasm during cryopreservation and cryobanking in IVF units. Hum Reprod. 2009;24(10):2457–67.

43. Grout BW, Morris GJ. Contaminated liquid nitrogen vapour as a risk factor in pathogen transfer. Theriogenology. 2009;71(7):1079–82.

44. Cobo A, Bellver J, de los Santos MJ, et al. Viral screening of spent culture media and liquid nitrogen samples of oocytes and embryos from hepatitis B, hepatitis C, and human immunodeficiency virus chronically infected women undergoing in vitro fertilization cycles. Fertil Steril. 2012;97(1):74–8.

45. Vajta G, Rienzi L, Ubaldi FM. Open versus closed systems for vitrification of human oocytes and embryos. Reprod Biomed Online. 2015;30(4):325–33.

46. Castello D, Cobo A, Mestres E, et al. Pre-clinical validation of a closed surface system (Cryotop SC) for the vitrification of oocytes and embryos in the mouse model. Cryobiology. 2018;81:107–16.

47. Molina I, Mari M, Martinez JV, et al. Bacterial and fungal contamination risks in human oocyte and embryo cryopreservation: open versus closed vitrification systems. Fertil Steril. 2016;106(1):127–32.

48. Parmegiani L, Accorsi A, Cognigni GE, et al. Sterilization of liquid nitrogen with ultraviolet irradiation for safe vitrification of human oocytes or embryos. Fertil Steril. 2010;94(4):1525–8.

49. Parmegiani L, Accorsi A, Bernardi S, et al. A reliable procedure for decontamination before thawing of human specimens cryostored in liquid nitrogen: three washes with sterile liquid nitrogen (SLN2). Fertil Steril. 2012;98(4):870–5.

50. De Munck N, Belva F, Van de Velde H, et al. Closed oocyte vitrification and storage in an oocyte donation programme: obstetric and neonatal outcome. Hum Reprod. 2016;31(5):1024–33.

51. De Munck N, Santos-Ribeiro S, Stoop D, et al. Open versus closed oocyte vitrification in an oocyte donation programme: a prospective randomized sibling oocyte study. Hum Reprod. 2016;31(2):377–84.

52. Gook DA, Choo B, Bourne H, et al. Closed vitrification of human oocytes and blastocysts: outcomes from a series of clinical cases. J Assist Reprod Genet. 2016;33(9):1247–52.

53. Papatheodorou A, Vanderzwalmen P, Panagiotidis Y, et al. How does closed system vitrification of human oocytes affect the clinical outcome? A prospective, observational, cohort, noninferiority trial in an oocyte donation program. Fertil Steril. 2016;106(6):1348–55.

54. Papatheodorou A, Vanderzwalmen P, Panagiotidis Y, et al. Open versus closed oocyte vitrification system: a prospective randomized sibling-oocyte study. Reprod Biomed Online. 2013;26(6):595–602.

55. Bonetti A, Cervi M, Tomei F, et al. Ultrastructural evaluation of human metaphase II oocytes after vitrification: closed versus open devices. Fertil Steril. 2011;95(3):928–35.

56. Youm HS, Choi JR, Oh D, et al. Closed versus open vitrification for human blastocyst cryopreservation: a meta-analysis. Cryobiology. 2017;77:64–70.

57. Van Landuyt L, Polyzos NP, De Munck N, et al. A prospective randomized controlled trial investigating the effect of artificial shrinkage (collapse) on the implantation potential of vitrified blastocysts. Hum Reprod. 2015;30(11):2509–18.

58. Darwish E, Magdi Y. Artificial shrinkage of blastocoel using a laser pulse prior to vitrification improves clinical outcome. J Assist Reprod Genet. 2016;33(4):467–71.

59. Cao S, Zhao C, Zhang J, et al. Retrospective clinical analysis of two artificial shrinkage methods applied prior to blastocyst vitrification on the outcome of frozen embryo transfer. J Assist Reprod Genet. 2014;31(5):577–81.

60. Schiewe MC, Araujo E Jr, Asch RH, et al. Enzymatic characterization of zona pellucida hardening in human eggs and embryos. J Assist Reprod Genet. 1995;12(1):2–7.

61. Montag M, Schimming T, Köster M, et al. Oocyte zona birefringence intensity is associated with embryonic implantation potential in ICSI cycles. Reprod Biomed Online. 2008;16(2):239–44.

62. Gonzales DS, Bavister BD, Mese SA. In utero and in vitro proteinase activity during the Mesocricetus auratus embryo zona escape time window. Biol Reprod. 2001;64(1):222–30.

63. Balaban B, Urman B, Alatas C, et al. A comparison of four different techniques of assisted hatching. Hum Reprod. 2002;17(5):1239–43.

64. Cieslak J, Ivakhnenko V, Wolf G, et al. Three-dimensional partial zona dissection for preimplantation genetic diagnosis and assisted hatching. Fertil Steril. 1999;71(2):308–13.

65. Nakayama T, Fujiwara H, Yamada S, et al. Clinical application of a new assisted hatching method using a piezo-micromanipulator for morphologically low-quality embryos in poor-prognosis infertile patients. Fertil Steril. 1999;71(6):1014–8.

66. Li D, Yang DL, An J, et al. Effect of assisted hatching on pregnancy outcomes: a systematic review and meta-analysis of randomized controlled trials. Sci Rep. 2016;6:31228.

67. Practice Committee of the American Society for Reproductive Medicine; Practice Committee of the Society for Assisted Reproductive Technology. Role of assisted hatching in in vitro fertilization: a guideline. Fertil Steril. 2014;102(2):348–51.

68. Deniz E, Eberl KB, Bredenbeck J. Note: An automatic liquid nitrogen refilling system for small (detector) Dewar vessels. Rev Sci Instrum. 2018;89(11):116101.

69. Koizumi M, Oshima M, Toh Y, et al. An automatic liquid-nitrogen filling system for multiple Ge detectors. Rev Sci Instrum. 2009;80(1):016102.

Quality Management of Intracytoplasmic Sperm Injection

Intracytoplasmic sperm injection (ICSI) is assisted reproduction laboratories' most routine microscopic procedure. It includes a set of equipment and a technique and solves most infertility caused by male factors, such as severe oligospermia, malformed sperm, and sometimes azoospermia. This chapter will provide a comprehensive overview of the ICSI technique and its risks and management during manipulation.

10.1 Development and Indications of Intracytoplasmic Sperm Injection

10.1.1 Development of ICSI

The conventional in vitro fertilization technique applied at the early stage of ART development mainly addressed female and male infertility caused by mild oligozoospermia. However, it failed to provide a more effective solution for severe male infertility. This deficiency has led researchers to try to increase the chance of sperm-oocyte binding, thereby improving the fertilization rate through measures including concentrating the sperm and reducing culture medium volume during insemination. Nevertheless, these efforts ended with little success in patients with severe oligospermia. In the 1980s, zona pellucida drilling [1] or mechanical

partial zona dissection [2] was used to facilitate sperm entry. However, these methods did not improve fertilization outcomes but resulted in a greater probability of polyspermic fertilization. Even when the sperm was injected directly into the perivitelline space using an injection pipette bypassing the zona pellucida, i.e., subzonal insemination (SUZI), the benefits of this treatment for severe male infertility were still very limited. Later, Lanzendorf et al. demonstrated successful fertilization by directly injecting sperm into the cytoplasm, but no successful pregnancy was obtained [3]. It was not until 1992 that the Palermo et al. reported the first live birth of an ICSI baby. His assistant recalled that during a SUZI procedure for 12 oocytes, the cytoplasm of one oocyte was inadvertently punctured, and the sperm was injected into the cytoplasm. Instead of degenerating, this oocyte formed the only embryo, leading to humans' first successful ICSI pregnancy [4]. Subsequently, numerous studies have confirmed the advantages of ICSI technology in improving fertilization, which led to the rapid promotion of this technology in assisted reproduction.

10.1.2 Indications for ICSI

ICSI technology has been widely used worldwide, with a higher application proportion. With the advances in ICSI technology, it is now implemented not only for the treatment of male infertility but also for many non-male conditions [5, 6], such as (a) thawed oocytes or immature oocytes cultured in vitro—as the zona pellucida may harden due to cryopreservation or prolonged in vitro culture, preventing sperm from penetrating the zona pellucida; (b) preimplantation genetic testing (PGT)—to avoid paternal or maternal contamination; (c) complete lack of fertilization or low fertilization (usually <30%) in the previous conventional IVF cycle; (d) certain oocyte abnormalities, such as oocytes without perivitelline gaps combined with heterogeneous zona pellucida (oocytes presenting indented zona

pellucida). However, it is still controversial whether ICSI should be performed in patients of advanced age or with a poor ovarian response (only a few oocytes were obtained). And there is a lack of high-level evidence to support the claim that ICSI improves pregnancy outcomes in this patient population [7–10]. Although ICSI has some advantages in treating male infertility and in improving the fertilization rate, it is, after all, an invasive technique that still involves unpredictable biological risks to the offspring. Therefore, the indications for ICSI should be strictly defined (Fig. 10.1) and implemented with caution [11, 12].

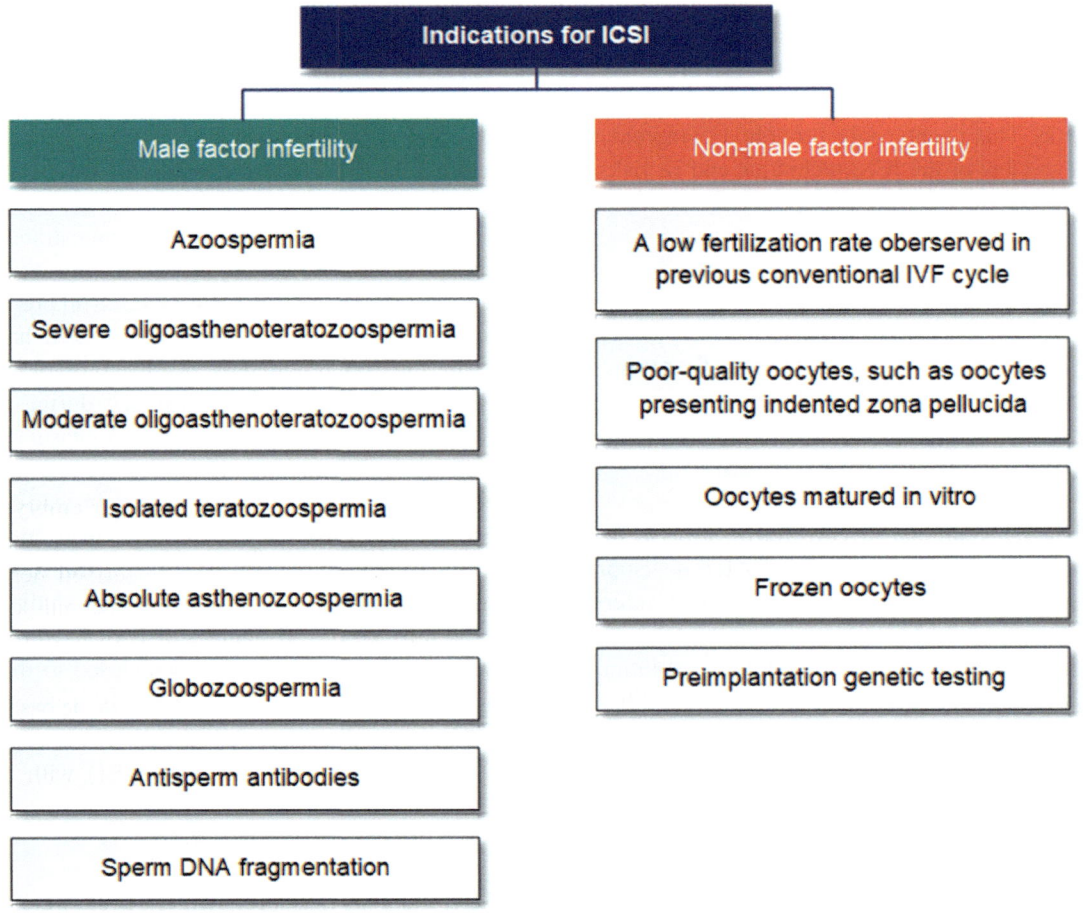

Fig. 10.1 Indications for ICSI

10.2 Equipment and Operating Pipettes for Micromanipulation

The micromanipulation station is the basic equipment for ICSI, and consists of an inverted microscope equipped with a modulated contrast system (to give a more three-dimensional effect to non-stained living specimens), motor modules containing X-, Y-, and Z-module (the pipette can be moved in all three spatial axes due to the layout of the modules), left and right pipette holders, hydraulic/pneumatic microinjectors, left and right control panels (including joysticks) and a heating stage (Fig. 10.2), which may vary among different brands of operating systems, however the basic structure is similar.

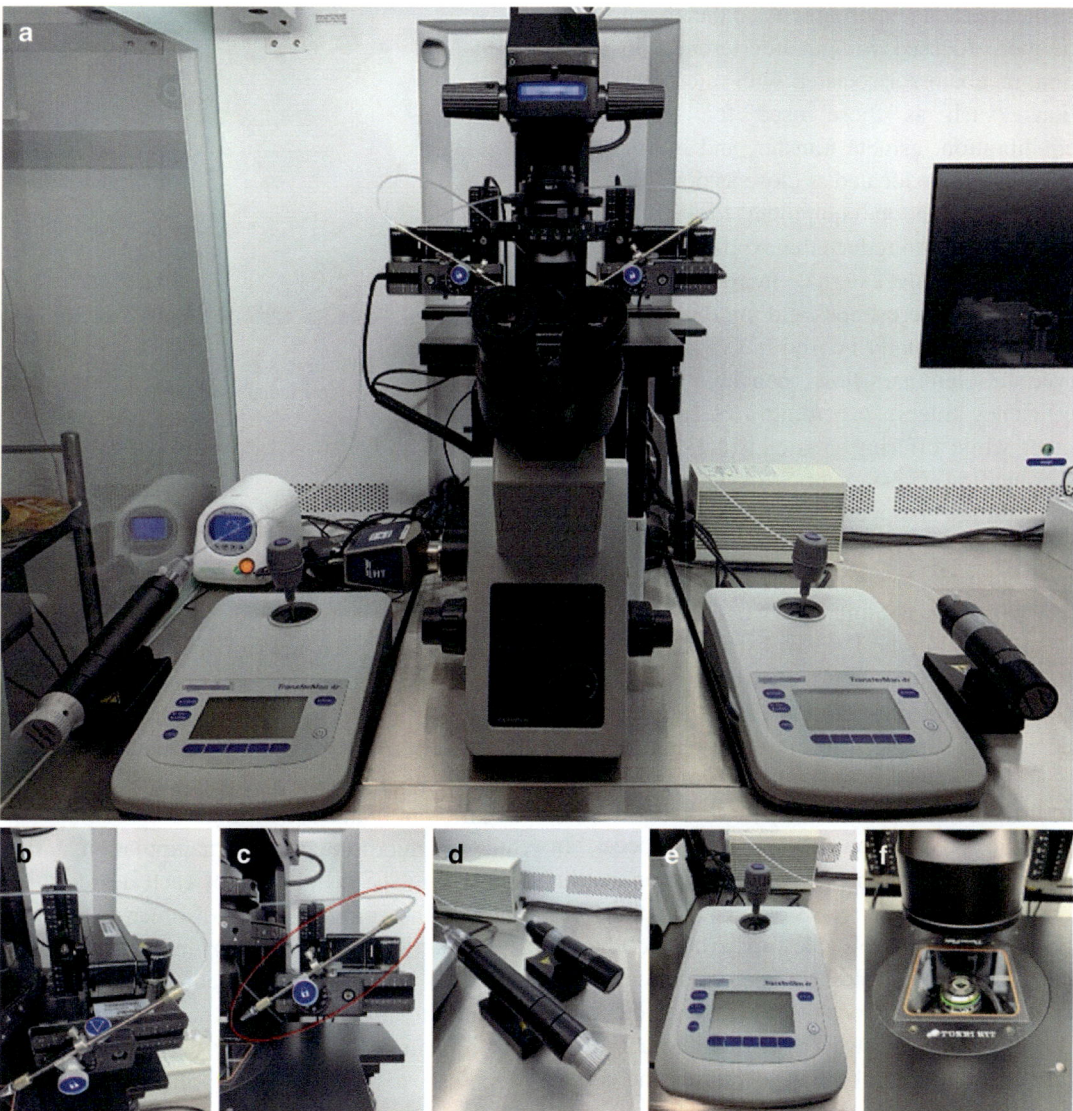

Fig. 10.2 Micromanipulation station. (**a**) The overall view of the micromanipulation station; (**b**) the motor modules containing X-, Y-, and Z-modules; (**c**) the pipette holder (red circle); (**d**) the hydraulic (left)/pneumatic (right) microinjector; (**e**) the control panel (including a joystick); (**f**) the thermostatic heating stage

10.2.1 The Installation of Micromanipulation Equipment and Precautions

Micromanipulation equipment should be installed in a relatively independent, quiet area in the laboratory with fewer personnel movements, away from doorways and transfer windows. Moreover, efforts should be made to avoid the operating field and the operator directly facing the high-efficiency filter air outlet to safeguard a stable operating environment, so the operator can be more focused without interference. In addition, incubators associated with micromanipulations (such as those used for temperature equilibration, gamete transfer, and in vitro culture) should be located as close as possible to the micromanipulation equipment to facilitate the workflow and to reduce the exposure of gametes or embryos to the external environment.

Inverted microscopes and micromanipulation stations are usually housed in IVF workstations (vertical laminar flow benches with high-efficiency filters), providing a cleaner environment while offering greater isolation from the surrounding environment. Workstations designed for ICSI are equipped with vibration dampening mechanisms to reduce vibrations caused by other manipulations or laboratory personnel activities. The vibration damping device should be independent within the IVF workstation (Fig. 10.3). It is worth noting that the inverted microscope should be placed on the vibration damping device and separated from other system components (such as microinjectors and control panels) to effectively avoid the impact of external and operational vibrations on the ICSI process. In addition, because the micromanipulation station has many power cords coiled in the rear (Fig. 10.4), if these cables are arranged chaotically, or if the cables generate significant tension, the independence of the vibration damping device will be destroyed, and the situation of "the clean bench vibration → pulling the cables → pulling the vibration damping device" may arise, which will significantly undermine the vibration-proof effect.

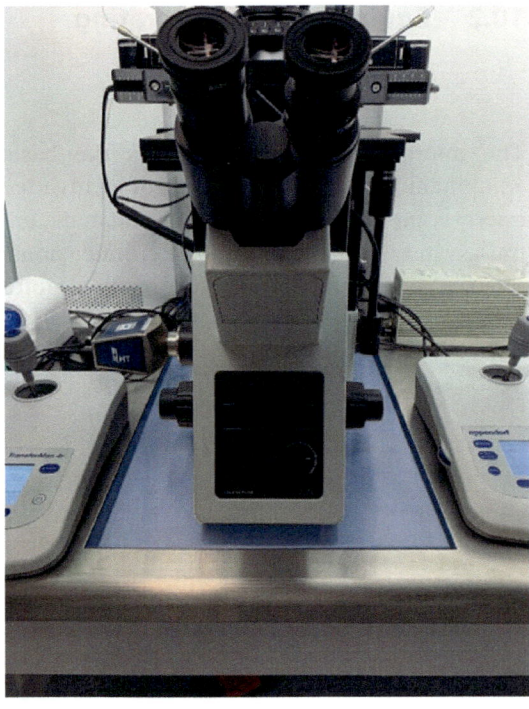

Fig. 10.3 The light blue area is a mechanical vibration damping device (stage) independent of other workbench parts

Before purchasing a micromanipulation station, it is important to ensure that it is compatible with your existing or pre-purchased inverted microscope. Micromanipulation station manufacturers normally provide adapters for major brands of inverted microscopes on the market. Proper installation and commissioning of each device within the system are crucial. Otherwise, it will directly affect the subsequent use. The installation process will involve multiple devices of different brands, such as the IVF workstation, inverted microscope, micromanipulation station, and laser. The installation of each device might involve the commissioning of other devices, for example: (a) After installing the inverted microscope, it is necessary to re-adjust the horizontal vibration damping stage of the IVF workstation; (b) after installing the laser device, it might be necessary to re-calibrate the optical system of the microscope; (c) the adjustment and setting of the microscope imaging output may also require the presence of the respective brand engineers of the

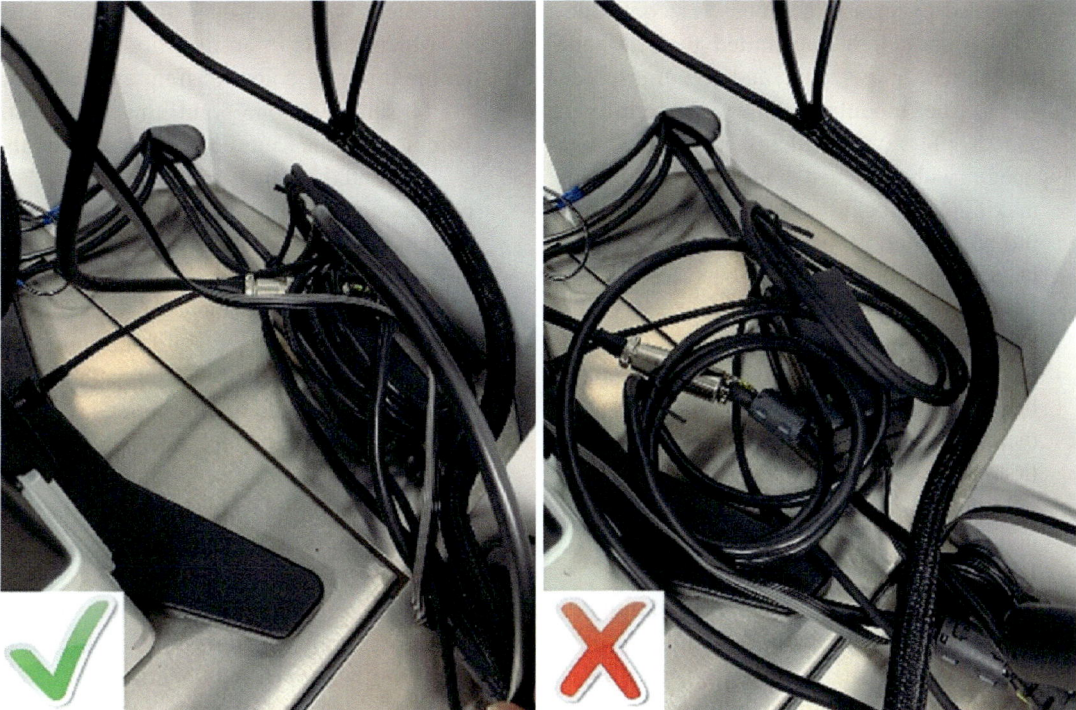

Fig. 10.4 The correct placement of the power cords at the rear of the microscope

workstation, laser, and other equipment simultaneously to complete the work in cooperation. Therefore, it is important to arrange the installation process reasonably and coordinate the engineers of each brand. Furthermore, when the engineers from the manufacturers make the initial installation, the personnel responsible for the micromanipulation should preferably be present so that they can better understand the basic structure and main components of the system, which will facilitate the subsequent daily use and maintenance. In addition, new equipment should be placed in a room away from the culture room for some time before installation to prevent it from generating excessive volatile organic compounds. In particular, new IVF workstations should be turned on and kept running for at least one month before formal use, but with attention to dust and contamination prevention.

Some brands of IVF workstations have different specifications for the height of the bench top from the floor, which should be chosen well according to the specific requirements of the laboratory personnel. It is also a very good setup to equip a comfortable and stable seat with good lumbar support and easy height adjustment based on full consideration of the ergonomics of the micromanipulation process. In short, ICSI and other micromanipulations are highly intensive and time-consuming, in which case the comfort of the personnel performing them will affect the quality of the manipulation.

10.2.2 Construction and Working Principle of the Microscope

IVF laboratory personnel should be proficient in the basic operating skills of the microscope and understand the operating principles of the relevant adapters in the optical path. Each microscope should come with a simple operation manual that can be readily accessed and a prepared standard operating procedure for the use of the equipment.

1. Hoffman modulation contrast (HMC): The HMC is an important optical system for inverted microscopes. It generates optical gradients through a special modulator with a slit

designed to form three zones for controlling the amount of light transmitted: the dark zone, the narrow gray zone, and the transparent zone. The modulated image has different shades of gray, producing a 3-dimensional image with brighter and darker domains, making the oocyte or embryo appear more 3-dimensional. Depending on the objective used, it can be matched to the corresponding modulator by rotating the concentrator dial to achieve the best visual effect. Based on the principle of HMC, various brands of microscope manufacturers have also introduced complementary technologies, such as Olympus' relief contrast, Nikon's advanced modulation phase contrast, and Leica's integrated Hoffman modulation contrast.

2. Eyepieces and objectives: Binocular eyepieces with 10× or 15× magnification and objectives with 4×, 10×, 20×, and 40× magnification are usually employed, and objectives with other magnifications can also be selected according to the work requirements. Attaching the objective lens in ascending order is a user-friendly practice so that turning the finger wheel clockwise/counterclockwise will stepwise increase/decrease the magnification. It is important to ensure that the objectives are fully installed into the objective plate, as the user cannot get the optimal magnification if they are not in place. The mounted eyepieces and objectives should be thoroughly cleaned—minor dirt (e.g., dust, fingerprints) can cause defects or blurring of the optical system. IVF laboratory personnel should briefly understand the different types of objectives and their specification parameters. Normally the objectives used for micromanipulation must cover a long working distance because there is a layer of glass/metal heating plate between the objective lens and the bottom of the culture dish, and the dish bottom also has a certain thickness. A planar achromatic objective should also be selected to correct for chromatic and spherical aberrations.

   (a) Chromatic aberration: Different wavelengths of light have different refractive indices when passing through a lens, which results in an inability to converge the different colors of light emitted from the sample at one point, thus generating color "streaks" at the border between the light and dark areas of the image.

   (b) Spherical aberration: It is an optical effect that arises when light strikes a lens, as the light passing through the edge is refracted to a greater extent than the light passing through the center part of the lens. The result of spherical aberration is that when a point is imaged, it will appear as a light patch with a brighter center and a gradually blurred rim.

   For example, our center is equipped with a semi-apochromatic objective for relief contrast observation (Fig. 10.5), which provides excellent plan images across high transmission visible light to the near-infrared spectrum. It offers a long working distance for relief contrast observation, facilitating the observation of gametes and embryos in culture dishes.

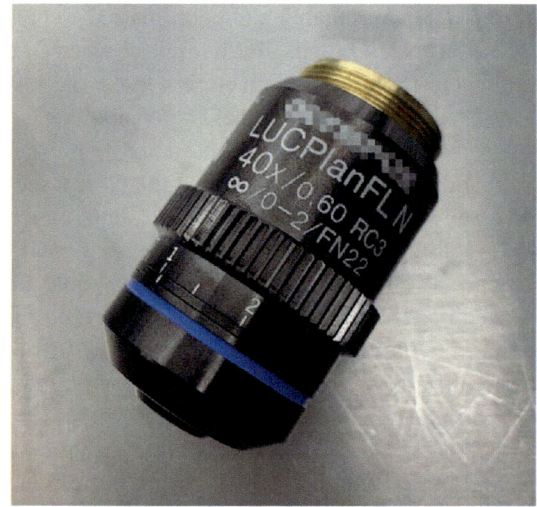

Fig. 10.5 A semi-apochromatic objective lens. Explanation of lens markings: L, long working distance (3–4.2 mm); *FL* Fluorite objective (i.e., semi-apochromatic objective); 40×, magnification; 0.60, aperture size; *RC* relief contrast; ∞ infinite distance, *0–2* correctable dish bottom thickness range (mm), *FN22* field number (mm)

10.2.3 Thermostatic Heating Plate

1. Types of heating plates: Heating plates can be divided into glass and metal. A glass heating plate is fully transparent and heats integrally, while a metal heating plate is non-transparent, with a round hole in the middle to let light through. However, regardless of which type of heating plate is applied to heat the culture dish, since the central area of the bottom of the culture dish is not in direct contact with the heating plate, the actual temperature of this part is lower than the surrounding area of the bottom of the dish. To mitigate this effect, some manufacturers have set up an airflow heating device below the heating plate to ensure uniform heating of the bottom of the culture dish (Fig. 10.6).

2. Heating plate setting: The accuracy range of the heating plate temperature should be ±0.1 °C. Because gametes and embryos are immersed in microdroplets, the temperature setting should be based on the actual temperature of the buffer microdroplets in the micromanipulation dish rather than the surface temperature of the heating plate [13]. The temperature of microdroplets during micromanipulation can be influenced by factors including the vertical laminar flow from the IVF workstation, the type and size of the heating plate, the size and material of the culture dish, the ambient temperature and

humidity, and the volume of the microdroplets and the volume of tissue culture oil used for covering the microdroplets [14]. Therefore, the heating plate is usually set at a temperature higher than 37.0 °C to compensate for the heat loss caused by the objective factors mentioned above. Strict and precise temperature control is necessary to secure a stable oocyte spindle during ICSI, allowing for better fertilization and pregnancy outcomes [15]. When a prepared micromanipulation dish is taken out from the incubator and placed on the heating plate, the temperature of the microdroplets will, in normal cases, drop significantly at first and then gradually get higher. The recommended temperature for the microdroplets is between 36.8 °C and 37.0 °C. Furthermore, since there is no definitive optimal temperature for in vitro manipulations, a slightly lower temperature may be safer than an overly high temperature [13]. A thermocouple may be utilized to measure the temperature of the microdroplets, and the heating plate controller can be calibrated according to the actual temperature measured (Fig. 10.7). The heating plate's temperature should be re-calibrated if a different brand (the contact surface of a different brand dish bottom with the heating plate is slightly different) or a different material dish is used (regular ICSI dishes are made of plastic, while some dishes for spindle observation are made of glass).

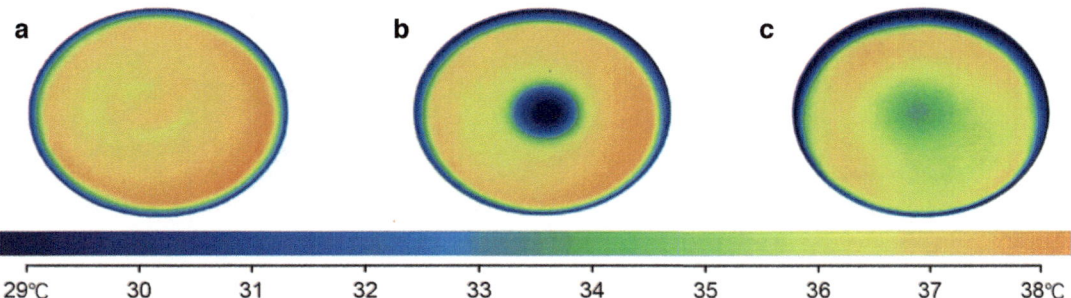

Fig. 10.6 Thermal imaging at the bottom of a culture dish on different types of heating plates. (**a**) A heated metal plate with an airflow heating device; (**b**) a heated metal plate without an airflow heating device; (**c**) a heated glass plate without an airflow heating device

10.2.4 Operation System

1. Operation system: This system provides a full range of operational control through mechanical, hydraulic (usually oil-filled), and electric means, and it is advisable for IVF laboratory

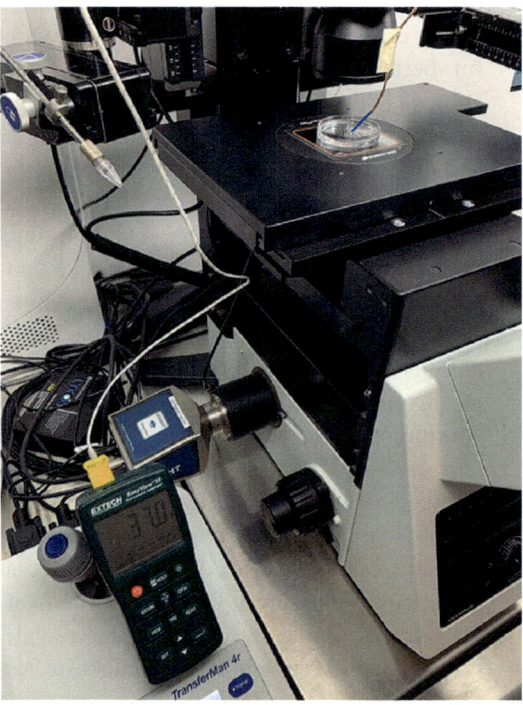

Fig. 10.7 Detecting droplet temperature using a thermocouple

personnel to have a good understanding of how each component of the system is linked. The user controls the X–Y–Z axis module via a joystick, enabling precise control and positioning of the micromanipulation pipettes. There are two common joystick types— upstanding and suspended (Fig. 10.8). Both types can be switched between coarse- and fine-tuning control based on operative needs to attain different movement speeds. Coarse control allows for bigger and faster movements and is mainly used for lifting, lowering, and positioning the pipette, while fine-tuning control is for delicate movements required during micromanipulations. Operation systems of different brands vary considerably in practice, but they all have excellent control capabilities, allowing users to be skilled in their application after systematic training. It may take an adjustment period for the user to change from one brand/type to another. However, for an embryologist who is skilled in microscopic manipulation, this process is nonetheless relatively simple. The latest generation of operating systems is equipped with a position memory function, which allows for quick positioning and thus shortens the operation time.

2. Precautions for use: (a) When the focus and start position of the manipulation pipette are set, there should be sufficient movement space

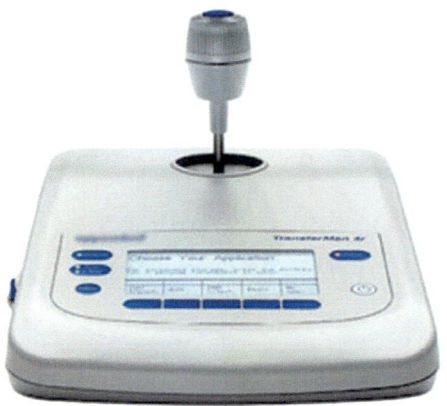

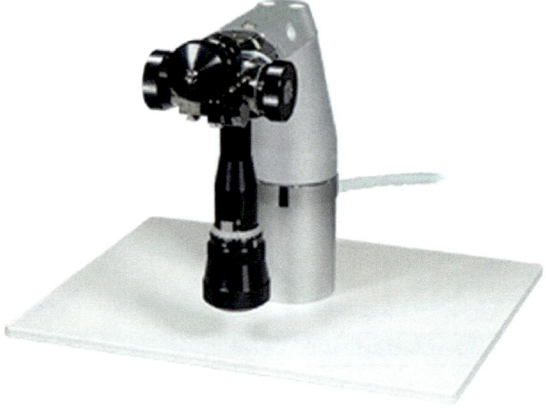

Fig. 10.8 Joysticks: the upstanding type (left) and the suspended type (right). (The left image kindly supplied by Eppendorf AG, Germany. www.eppendorf.com. The right image kindly supplied by NARISHIGE Group, Japan. www.narishige.co.jp)

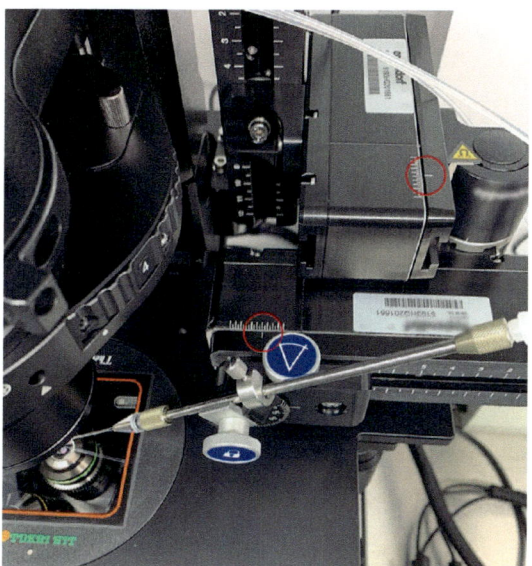

Fig. 10.9 *X*- and *Y*-axes module. Note: When the focus and start position of the manipulation pipette are set, the positioning mark should be located near the mid-point of the movement range scale as possible (red circle)

for the *X*- and *Y*-axes module to move back and forth (Fig. 10.9), thus allowing a greater range of movement for the manipulation pipette. (b) If the equipment is operated constantly in a range very close to its dimensional limits for a long period, the increased pressure it is subjected to will cause wear and tear. If a module reaches its defined range limits during operation, the gametes/embryos should be immediately returned to the incubator, and the equipment should be re-adjusted. (c) The equipment should be maintained clean. Dust settling into mechanical joints may interfere with the movement and cause equipment deterioration. (d) Regular maintenance and greasing of each mechanical part of the equipment should be carried out, as otherwise, the joints will be worn out. Abnormal or erratic movement may indicate a problem with the circuit board. In such cases, the equipment should promptly be returned to the manufacturer for repair. (e) When more than one person uses the equipment, the relevant settings of the operating system should be checked before starting work, in case the previous operator has made changes. (f) One must be

systematically trained and become sufficiently familiar with the micromanipulations before he/she is allowed to operate on the patient's oocytes or embryos.

10.2.5 Microinjector and Pipette Holder

1. Microinjector: According to the different filling materials, microinjectors can be divided into oil-hydraulic and pneumatic. The pipeline of an oil-hydraulic microinjector uses tissue culture oil as the conduction medium for pressure control. In contrast, the pipeline of a pneumatic injector uses air as the conduction medium. Usually, oil-hydraulic microinjectors are used for sperm immobilization, suction, and intracytoplasmic injection because of their more stable and precise control. When first installed, a new oil-hydraulic microinjector can be filled with tissue culture oil from the upper inlet valve (Fig. 10.10), and care must be taken to avoid air bubbles.

2. Pipette holder: Its function is to hold the micromanipulation pipette connected to the microinjector through a hose. Normally the holding pipette is mounted on the left pipette holder; the injection pipette is mounted on the

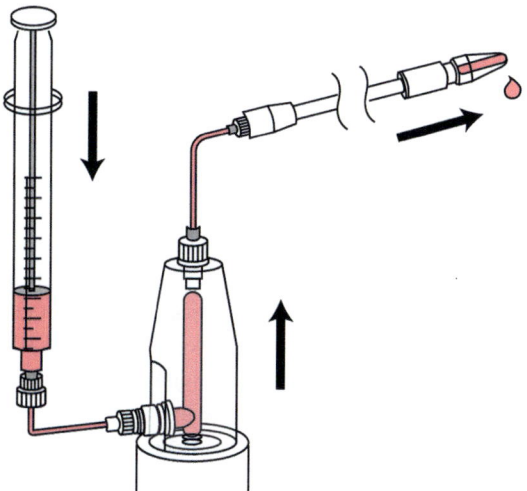

Fig. 10.10 Filling the oil-hydraulic microinjector via the oil inlet valve with a special syringe. (Image kindly supplied by Eppendorf AG, Germany. www.eppendorf.com)

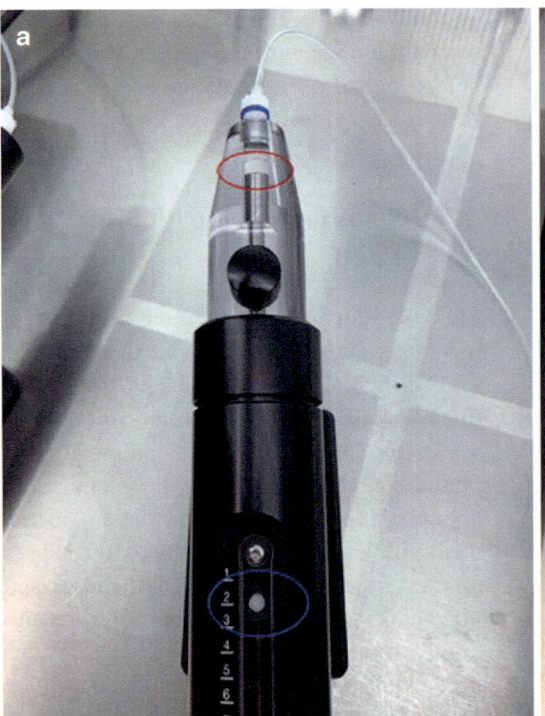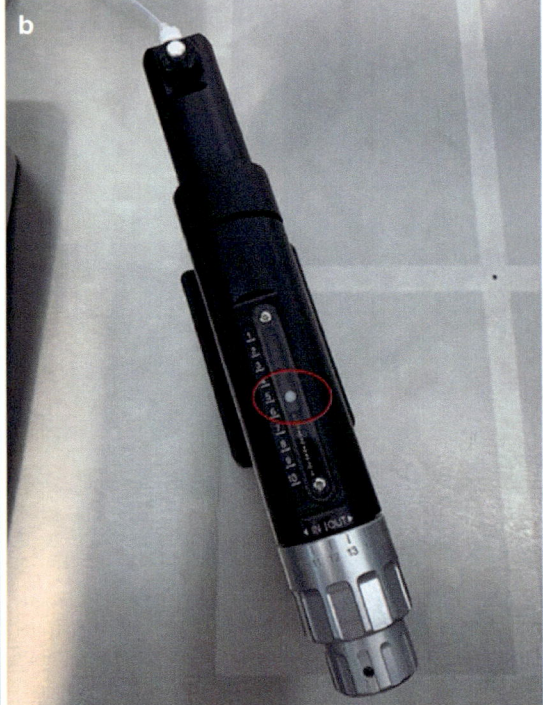

Fig. 10.11 Filling enough oil in front of the microinjector piston. (**a**) The oil section in front of the piston of the hydraulic microinjector of <0.5 cm (red circle) or the positioning scale of <2 (blue circle) indicates the need for an oil refill. (**b**) Keep the positioning scale of the pneumatic microinjector in the middle (red circle)

right pipette holder. The placement of the respective microinjectors depends on personal habits, and they can be placed on either side of the microscope or the same side.

3. Caution: (a) Before each operation, ensure enough oil is in front of the microinjector piston. When the piston is less than 0.5 cm from the front end, or the piston positioning scale reads <2, the microinjector needs to be refilled with oil (Fig. 10.11a). For pneumatic microinjectors, always position the piston so that the position reading remains in the middle of the scale range (Fig. 10.11b). (b) Tissue culture oil can also be aspirated through the front end of the pipette holder. However, it should be well sterilized to avoid contamination. It is important to prevent excessive or big air bubbles from being generated during the filling process, as this will increase the pressure in the microinjector and interfere with the operation. (c) Avoid forming a bent angle at the connection between the microinjector or pipette holder and the tubing (Fig. 10.12) and keep the tubing in a loose state.

10.2.6 Micromanipulation Pipettes and Their Installation

1. Micromanipulation pipettes: In IVF laboratory, commonly used micromanipulation pipettes include holding pipette, injection pipette, and biopsy pipette. Different specifications of manipulation pipettes (different angles, different inner diameters) are available from various brand manufacturers, and the choice of specifications depends on the type of operation and personal habits. Microinjection pipettes are used to capture, immobilize and inject sperm, and their tips can be classified as spiked or un-spiked (Fig. 10.13). An injection pipette with a spike and an internal diameter of 3–5 μm may reduce the incidence of oocyte degeneration.

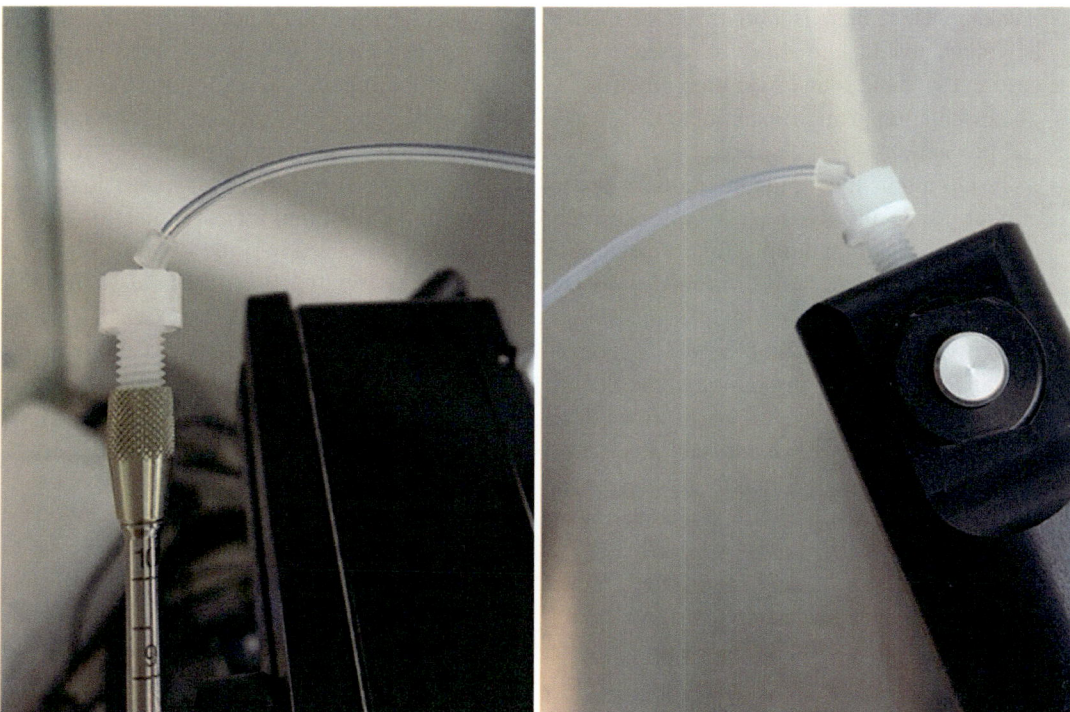

Fig. 10.12 The connections all have formed an obvious bent angle

Fig. 10.13 ICSI pipette without a spike (left); ICSI pipette with a spike (right)

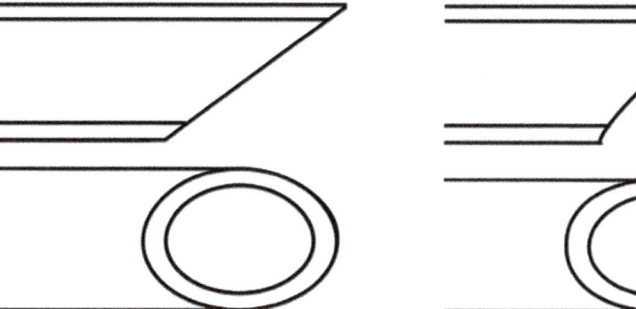

A sharp and finer pipette can minimize mechanical damage to the cell membrane during puncture, reduce the amount of aspirated cytoplasm during oolemma rupture, and the amount of polyvinylpyrrolidone (PVP) injected into the cytoplasm with the sperm [16]. It is also recommended that the laboratory keep spare pipettes of different inner diameters—for example, a slightly thicker pipette for testicular sperm retrieval to avoid blockage by tissue debris. Holding pipettes are used for holding oocytes or embryos. They all have flat tips with an inner diameter of 15–30 μm, while the outer diameter of different brands varies widely from 75 to 180 μm. All micromanipulation pipettes are made of glass and are very delicate and fragile. Extra care is required when removing them from their packaging. Before installation, each pipette should be carefully checked for breakage, especially whether the rear end is mutilated (the edge of the mutilated end is sharp and can easily damage the gasket inside the grip head of pipette holder). After installation, the tip of micromanipulation pipettes should be checked under the microscope for any breakage. Once there is a breakage, no matter how tiny, the pipette must be discarded to ensure a safe and sound operation process.

2. The installation of micromanipulation pipettes and precautions

Installing the micromanipulation pipette is critical, especially the injection pipette controlled by the oil-hydraulic microinjector. If the injection pipette is not installed properly or if a large number of air bubbles are generated, it will seriously compromise the operation and even make it impossible to work.

The installation process is as follows: Use one hand to hold the loose metal knurled screw on the pipette holder and the other hand to rotate the coarse adjustment screw of the microinjector clockwise to discharge all air bubbles left in the grip head. Then eject a little oil to prevent air bubbles from being generated when inserting the pipette (Fig. 10.14). Use one hand to hold the metal knurled screw when loading the pipette to avoid re-generating air bubbles. Then, slowly insert the injection pipette from the grip head opening. There will be a slight resistance when the pipette passes through the internal ring-shaped rubber gasket. Do not exert too much force at this point but keep a steady pressure to insert vertically until it reaches the stop, indicating that the injection pipette has been inserted into the bottom. When the injection pipette is successfully inserted, tighten the grip head clockwise. Finally, rotate the fine-tuning screw of the microinjector to stabilize the oil/air interface in the pipette at a position about 1 cm from the shoulder where the pipette starts getting thinner (this position allows for easier handling, see Fig. 10.15).

Precautions:

(a) If the pipette encounters high resistance during insertion, it may be due to an internal blockage in the pipette holder. Do not force insertion then, but first disassemble the pipette holder and check if any broken fragment is left inside.

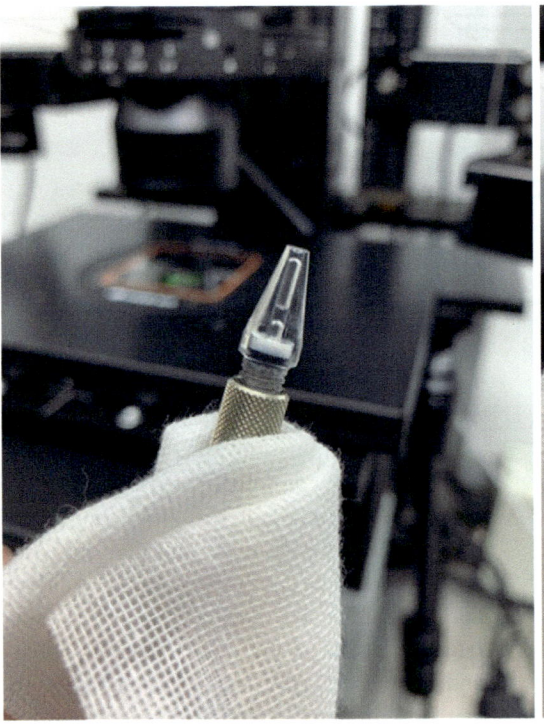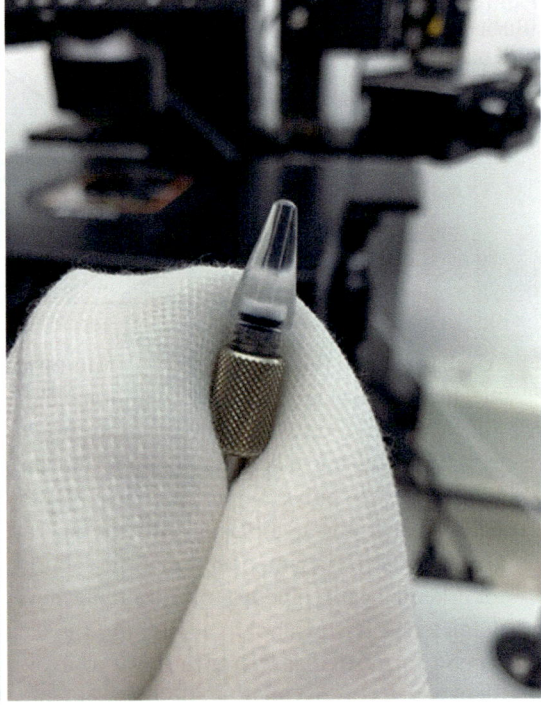

Fig. 10.14 Air bubbles remaining in the grip head (left); the air bubbles have been completely evacuated, and the oil surface is slightly emerging (right)

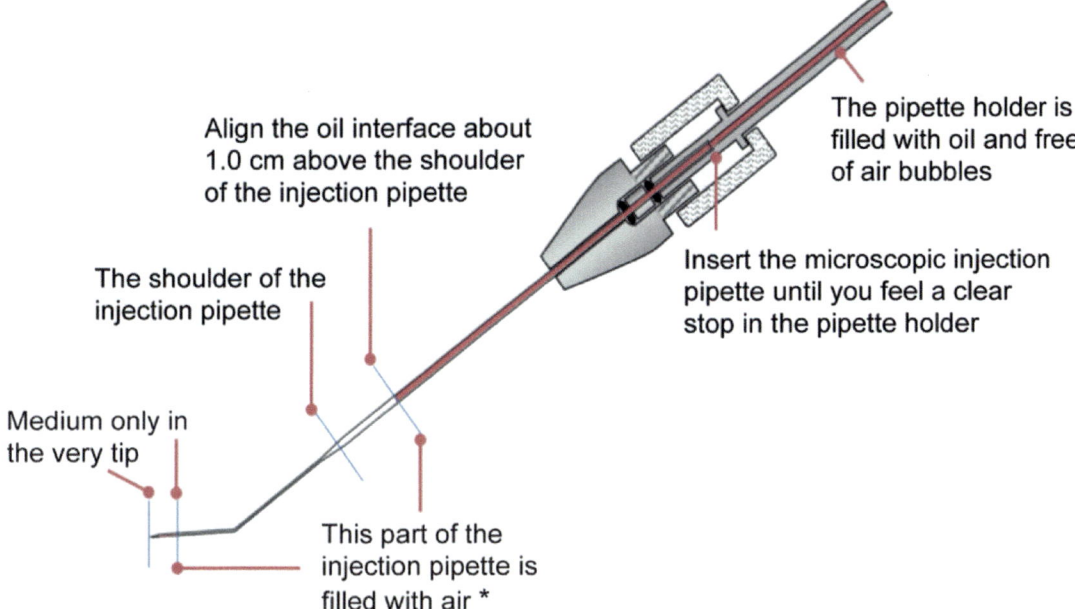

Align the oil interface about 1.0 cm above the shoulder of the injection pipette

The pipette holder is filled with oil and free of air bubbles

The shoulder of the injection pipette

Insert the microscopic injection pipette until you feel a clear stop in the pipette holder

Medium only in the very tip

This part of the injection pipette is filled with air *

Fig. 10.15 Schematic diagram of the overall structure after inserting the injection pipette into the pipette holder. Note: *A small oil volume inevitably exists between the air and the medium. As the ICSI operation dish is covered by an oil layer, which will be sucked by the injection pipette when it falls into the bottom of the dish. (Image kindly supplied by Eppendorf AG, Germany. www.eppendorf.com)

(b) If the pipette breaks during installation, the path inside the pipette holder must be thoroughly cleaned to ensure that no glass shards are left behind. One may use the special metal wire that comes with it to unclog and, at the same time, flush and clean with the oil inside the microinjector.

(c) If the pipette is not working right, especially if the sperm inside the injection pipette cannot be controlled steadily, the first thing to check is whether the pipette is in place or the grip head is tightened. If this problem continues, it could be that the gasket inside the grip head is worn out or broken and needs to be replaced.

3. Positioning: Slowly bring the installed micromanipulation pipettes down approaching the center of the stage and focus them under a low magnification objective (4× or 10×), such that the holding pipette and the injection pipette are positioned in a straight line. Before storing the positioning, raise both pipettes a little bit out of focus to avoid damage caused by their tips directly touching the bottom of the dish when they are automatically brought back down to the stored position later using the automatic repositioning function (Fig. 10.16).

4. Commissioning: The angle of the front end of the injection pipettes is mostly 30 °C or 35 °C, and the angle between the front end of the injection pipette and the bottom of the culture dish can be adjusted using the angle adjuster near the pipette holder. The front end of the injection pipette is not perfectly parallel to the bottom of the dish and is usually adjusted to a smaller angle to facilitate sperm immobilization (Fig. 10.17). Of course, the smaller this angle, the less damage will be done to the oocyte during puncture and the smoother the operation. The requirement for the angle between the holding pipette and the bottom of the dish is not so rigorous, and it can be adjusted until the front end of the holding pipette is horizontal to the bottom of the dish. Although the micromanipulation pipettes of major brands are generally of high quality, the angles between batches inevitably vary

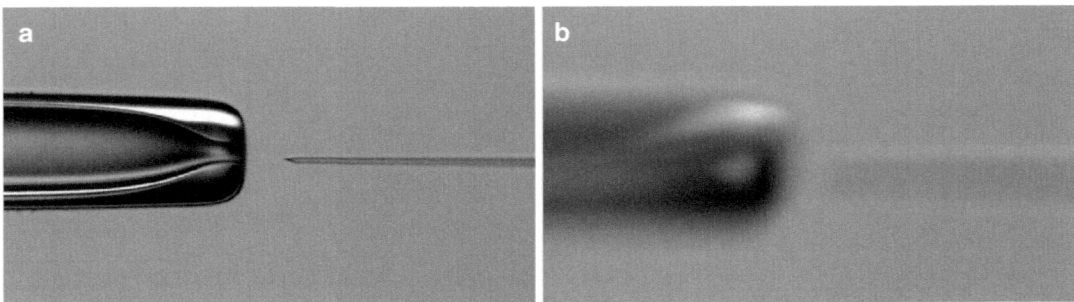

Fig. 10.16 Positioning. (**a**) The holding pipette and injection pipette are focused and in a straight line under the microscope; (**b**) store the positioning of the holding pipette and injection pipette after raising them just slightly

Fig. 10.17 The injection pipette taper is at a small angle to the bottom of the dish to facilitate sperm immobilization

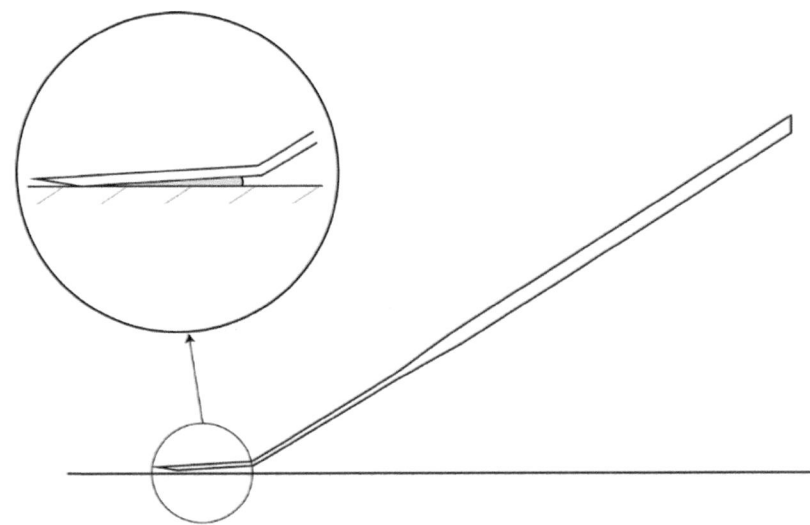

slightly. An angle adjuster has been introduced in China in recent years, allowing visual adjustment of the angle between the pipette taper and the bottom of the dish (Fig. 10.18). The pipette taper can be visually observed under the microscope or on the computer screen to see whether it is horizontal, which is quite convenient and practical.

10.2.7 Laser

A laser is a routine accessory for micromanipulations, usually integrated on an inverted microscope objective. It is mainly used for

assisting hatching, a biopsy of polar bodies and embryos, artificial shrinkage before blastocyst cryopreservation, sperm immobilization, assisting in ICSI, and identification of viable sperm [17]. According to the international laser safety standard (International Electrotechnical Commission, IEC 60825-1), only Class I laser products can be used for clinical micromanipulations. In assisted reproduction, common-brand laser devices usually utilize non-contact semiconductor lasers (Indium Gallium Arsenic Phosphorus, InGaAsP) with a wavelength of 1.48 μm or 1.46 μm (near-infrared). Such lasers do not cause DNA denaturation or contamination

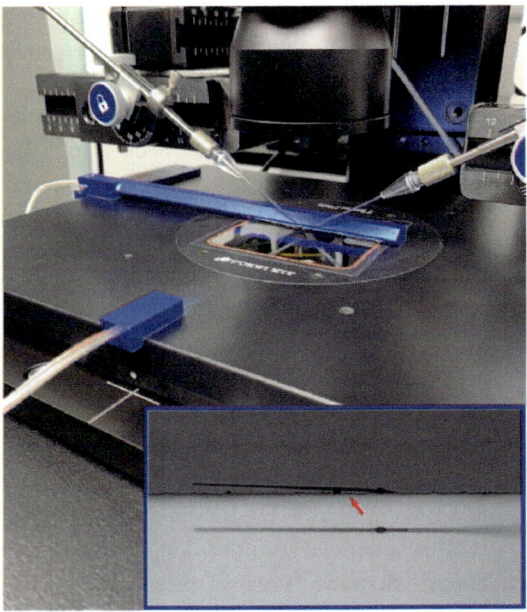

Fig. 10.18 Micromanipulation pipette angle adjuster. Note: The dark gray part in the blue box at the bottom right is the horizontal view; the light gray part is the under-microscope view; the red arrow points to the angle between the taper of the injection pipette and the horizontal plane (namely dish bottom)

(non-contact) in gametes or embryos, require no special equipment or additional steps and can be used with ordinary culture dishes [18]. The excitation energy of the laser should be strictly controlled, with different pulse durations chosen depending on which manipulation is being performed—the longer the pulse duration, the higher the energy, meaning more intense burning on the gametes or embryos. Early laser equipment emitted mostly fixed laser, requiring manually moving the microscope stage for positioning. With the continuous progress of this technology, major brands have launched mobile lasers. These laser devices can be preset on the computer for the number of strikes, strike position, and path (Fig. 10.19) according to the needs of the manipulation and then automatically triggered, making them convenient and efficient.

It is recommended to test the laser before using it to ensure accurate target location and proper intensity of pulse excitation. The laser may deviate with long-term use and must be recalibrated periodically.

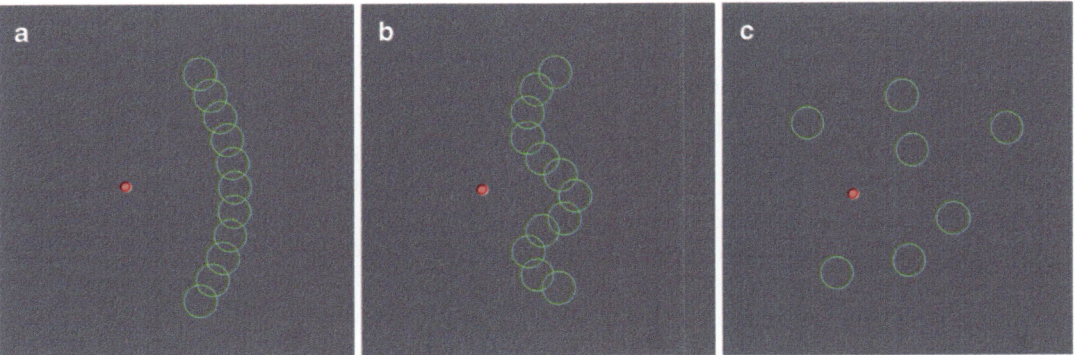

Fig. 10.19 Excitation trajectory of the mobile laser system (green circles). (**a**) striking arc trajectory; (**b**) custom trajectory; (**c**) and scatter points

## 10.3	Preparation of Culture Media and Culture Dishes for Micromanipulation

### 10.3.1	ICSI Media

Culture media containing 4-(2-hydroxyethyl)-1-piperazineethanesulfonic acid (HEPES) or 3-(N-morpholino)-propanesulfonic acid (MOPS) buffer system are recommended. Such media can maintain a stable physiological pH in the atmosphere for a certain time without depending on CO_2 for regulation. Conversely, media buffered with bicarbonate are not recommended for micromanipulation. The pH of such media rises dramatically during prolonged in vitro manipulation, thus affecting sperm viability, oocyte maturation, spindle polymerization, and embryo metabolism and development [19, 20]. Moreover, even when using media buffered with HEPES/MOPS, it is still recommended to keep the duration of the micromanipulation within 10 min for the following reasons: (a) The pH of the HEPES/MOPS buffer system increases when the temperature drops [20], and although there is a heating plate during the manipulation, it is still not possible to maintain a stable temperature continuously; (b) changes in external temperature can also cause damage to the oocyte spindle, which in turn compromises fertilization and embryo development [21]; (c) prolonged exposure of gametes to HEPES or MOPS can lead to oocyte degeneration, reduced fertilization rate, and impaired blastocyst formation. The number of oocytes injected in each dish in one go can be determined based on the operator's skill level. The optimal number of oocytes for a single-time operation can be determined by monitoring key performance indicators (KPIs) such as fertilization rate, high-quality embryo rate, blastocyst formation rate, and implantation rate.

### 10.3.2	PVP and Hyaluronan (HA)

1. Because of its high viscosity, PVP can significantly reduce sperm motility, and is therefore commonly used for sperm immobilization and capturing. Commercial PVP solutions with a content ranging from 7% to 10% can be used directly or after dilution with buffers. Our center routinely dilutes PVP by two times before use. However, it has been found that residual PVP can cause delayed calcium oscillation in oocytes and damage to sperm membrane, acrosome, and nucleus, thereby compromising fertilization and even the development of embryos [22]. Therefore, it is important to minimize the amount of oocyte cytoplasm drawn back into the injection pipette and PVP injection during the manipulation and shorten the time sperm are exposed to PVP. It has also been suggested that using micromanipulation media instead of PVP for ICSI is beneficial for improving clinical pregnancy outcomes. However, due to the low viscosity of micromanipulation media, strong manipulation control ability of the operator is required for sperm capturing, sperm immobilization, and oocyte injection.

2. HA features the same physical property as PVP (high viscosity) but also has physiological properties that PVP does not have. HA is the main component of the extracellular matrix of the cumulus oophorus and is a natural and easily degradable mucopolysaccharide. Only mature spermatozoa have HA binding sites on their plasma membrane, and the oocytes can metabolize HA. HA is a "physiological selector" for mature and intact sperm and can replace PVP for ICSI [23]. Current research evidence suggests that HA-ICSI is not significantly more effective than conventional PVP-ICSI in improving clinical pregnancy rate and live birth rate but may reduce the rate of miscarriage [24].

### 10.3.3	Preparation of Micromanipulation Dishes

ICSI dishes should be selected from those with internal coatings free of embryotoxicity. ICSI dishes usually contain PVP/HA microdroplets for sperm capturing and immobilization, and HEPES/MOPS-buffered medium microdroplets

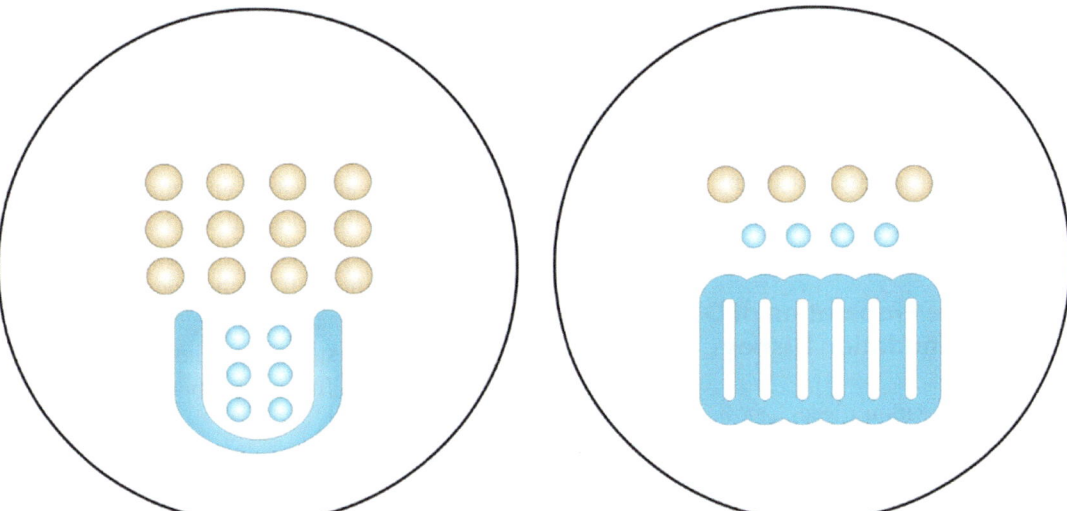

Fig. 10.20 Conventional ICSI dish. Note: HEPES/MOPS-buffered medium microdroplets (5 μL) are in yellow, and all blue ones are PVP microdroplets. The sperm is added to the U-shaped PVP droplet, and the preferentially selected sperm is transferred into the round PVP microdroplets before immobilization

Fig. 10.21 Special ICSI dish for the sperm from a patient with severe oligospermia or surgical sperm retrieval. Note: HEPES/MOPS-buffered medium microdroplets (5 μL) are in yellow, and all blue ones are PVP microdroplets. The sperm is added into the fence-shaped PVP droplet, and the preferentially selected sperm is transferred into round PVP microdroplets before immobilization

for oocyte injection, rinsing micromanipulation pipettes. Micromanipulation dishes should be placed in advance in a 37 °C non-ventilated incubator for equilibration (for at least 1 h). The specific layout of the microdroplets in the micromanipulation dish depends on personal habits (Fig. 10.20 is for reference only). The basic principles regarding dish preparation are as follows: (a) All microdroplets should be clustered in the center part of the dish as much as possible to avoid the restricted movement caused by the manipulation pipette touching the side wall of the dish. (b) Due to the small volume of microdroplets, tissue culture oil (about 4 mL) should be used to cover the microdroplets in time during the preparation process to prevent the change of osmolality, and air bubbles should be avoided when adding oil. (c) The microdroplets should have a certain distance between each other (especially those of different medium types) to avoid mixing. (d) For sperm samples containing many tissue fragments and cells, such as those from patients with severe oligospermia or surgical sperm retrieval, the dish needs to be prepared with a special droplet, such as a snake-, line-, or

fence-shaped droplet. (Fig. 10.21 for reference only), so that more specimens can be added to facilitate the search for motile sperm, which usually swim to the edge of the droplet.

10.3.4 Hyaluronidase

Oocytes obtained from the follicular fluid are surrounded by cumulus and corona cells, so hyaluronidase must digest the hyaluronan between the cumulus and corona cells to loosen them off before performing ICSI. It has been demonstrated that high concentrations of hyaluronidase (approximately 760 IU/mL) may cause degeneration and parthenogenic activation of the oocyte. Thus, the concentration of hyaluronidase currently used in various laboratories is usually 80 IU/mL [25]. Some studies diluted hyaluronidase concentrations to 39 IU/mL and 10 IU/mL, showing no significant effect on fertilization, embryonic development, or pregnancy outcomes [25]. It has even been suggested that a ten-fold dilution of hyaluronidase (8 IU/mL) could be cost-effective while achieving better outcomes [26]. The most reasonable and safe practice should be to minimize the concentration of hyaluronidase while securing the time and effect of degranulation. Our center usually uses twice diluted hyaluronidase (40 IU/mL) for the digestion of cumulus and corona cells.

10.3.5 The Preparation of Oocyte Denudation Dishes

Oocyte denudation dishes can be prepared with 60 mm diameter dishes with the upper half of the dish set up with hyaluronidase microdroplets and the lower half with HEPES/MOPS-buffered medium microdroplets. All microdroplets should be covered with tissue culture oil (about 6–7 mL) (Fig. 10.22). Moreover, the dishes should be placed in advance in an unventilated 37 °C incubator for equilibration (for at least 1 h). The volume of every hyaluronidase microdroplet should be as large as possible (100 μL) to facilitate the digestion and the pipetting of the cumulus-oocyte complex using a Pasteur pipette.

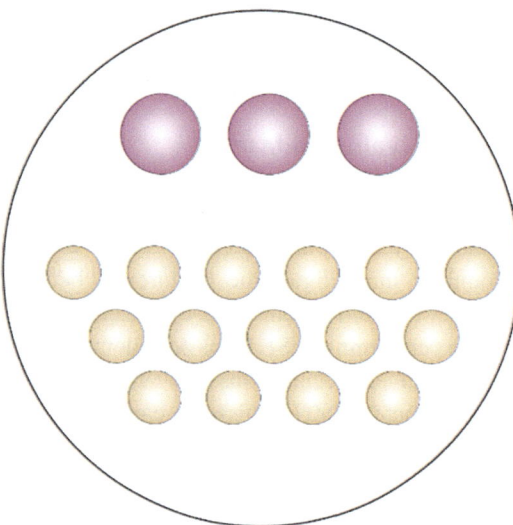

Fig. 10.22 Oocyte denudation dish. Note: Hyaluronidase microdroplets (100 μL/droplet) are in pink; HEPES/MOPS-buffered medium microdroplets (50 μL/droplet) are in yellow

10.4 Semen Preparation and Sperm Selection

Different preparation protocols should be chosen for semen specimens of different quality and origin. A proper and reasonable preparation protocol facilitates the selection and capture of sperm during the subsequent ICSI process. Moreover, it is more beneficial for subsequent fertilization, embryo development, and pregnancy outcomes if sperm that are structurally intact, mature, and have a low DNA fragmentation rate can be identified and screened.

10.4.1 Preparation of Semen Specimens

1. For semen specimens with normal parameters or mild oligospermia, density gradient centrifugation with the swim-up method is recommended to select the sperm with higher viability, better morphology, and more intact DNA [27]. The protocol currently used in our center is as follows:

   (a) Centrifuge ($300 \times g$, 15 min) the semen with 40% density gradient medium +80% density gradient medium (1.5 mL each).

   (b) Remove the supernatant as much as possible. The pellet is washed twice ($200 \times g$, 5 min) in a 2 mL sperm washing medium.

   (c) Discard the supernatant and place the suspended pellet in the bottom of the 1 mL sperm washing medium in the tube to perform the swim-up method.

   (d) The following two points should be noted during processing. Firstly, it is recommended that sperm specimens be placed in an incubator at 35–36 °C or room temperature (with care to avoid light and direct cold air flow) rather than 37 °C. Secondly, sperm specimens for ICSI are usually placed in a sperm washing medium containing HEPES instead of a fertilization medium because ICSI does not require sperm acquisition in vitro.

However, the sperm placed in the fertilization medium for a long time may have accelerated aging.

2. For specimens from patients with severe oligospermia, direct centrifugation (300 × g, 15 min) combined with the swim-up method is recommended in order to obtain a higher recovery of motile sperm.

3. For specimens from patients with cryptozoospermia (sperm visible only in the centrifuged sediment), it is recommended that the pellet be suspended with a small amount of sperm washing medium after direct centrifugation (1000 × g, 20 min). Then the suspended pellet is added directly to a specially prepared ICSI dish for sperm capture when ICSI is performed (Fig. 10.21), or the sperm capture microdroplet is prepared directly using the suspended pellet.

4. For patients requiring surgical sperm retrieval, the sperm can be surgically retrieved prior to the ovulation cycle, and the retrieved sperm can be cryopreserved before use. This measure ensures the availability of sperm on the day of oocyte retrieval and avoids the need for both spouses to undergo surgery (and anesthesia) on the same day. After thawing, the processing method is determined by the number of motile sperm. If a thawed specimen does not have sufficient sperm or no sperm at all, some or all of the oocytes can be cryopreserved. If the patient has signed informed consent, donor sperm can be prepared in advance for use on the day of oocyte retrieval.

5. Sperm obtained from the epididymis or testes are usually less motile or even very inactive, but they are often viable. Artificial sperm activation can be performed using theophylline activators (commonly known as "sperm Viagra"), which have been shown to be effective in increasing sperm motility (especially in frozen-thawed testicular sperm) and improving treatment outcomes [28].

6. For patients who have difficulty with sperm retrieval or cannot come for sperm retrieval on the day of oocytes retrieval, the semen can be obtained and frozen in advance.

7. If the sperm quality is poorer than expected or the number of motile sperm is insufficient, a second sperm retrieval might be suggested. In some patients, the sperm parameters may improve at the second retrieval [29].

10.4.2 Sperm Selection

Sperm selection in ICSI is still based on the morphology and motility of the sperm [30], with the criteria being: straight and fast movement; oval head without vacuoles; no residual cytoplasm in the neck (no more than 1/2 the size of the head), and an intact tail. Compared to conventional IVF, it is more important to screen for sperm capable of activating the oocyte and forming the male pronucleus during ICSI, which is why more and more advanced sperm selection techniques are being applied. These techniques preferentially select sperm based on surface charge, apoptosis, head birefringence, ability to bind hyaluronan, and morphology under ultra-high magnification microscopy (6000×), but there is no reliable evidence that these techniques are more beneficial for clinical outcomes [24].

10.5 Procedures, Techniques, and Precautions for ICSI

The complete ICSI process includes oocyte denudation, sperm selection, capture and immobilization; oocyte puncture and oolemma rupture; and injection of sperm into the oocyte. Each step of this procedure is critical and has profound effects on the subsequent manipulations, the development of the embryo, and ultimately the treatment outcomes.

10.5.1 Oocyte Denudation

This step facilitates the assessment of oocyte maturity and morphology and the subsequent injection. A method combining chemical digestion and mechanical stripping is utilized to remove the granulosa cells around the oocyte as quickly as possible. It is recommended to limit the time for this step to 1–3 min, so it is inadvisable to denude too many oocytes at one time.

The procedure of oocyte denudation is as follows: (a) Use a glass Pasteur pipette to remove most granulosa cells in a hyaluronidase-containing medium. Try to limit the operation time of this step to 30 s and not longer than 1 min. (b) Transfer the oocytes to HEPES/MOPS-buffered medium microdroplets for washing (1 to 2 drops), and then perform further mechanical stripping. It is recommended to use commercial oocyte denudation pipettes with decreasing inner diameters for mechanical denudation. Oocyte denudation is done by first gentle and repeated pipetting with a 170 μm or 165 μm diameter denudation pipette, followed by further pipetting with a thinner (140 μm or 145 μm diameter) pipette until the oocyte is clearly visible. During the pipetting process, always use a fresh HEPES/MOPS-buffered medium microdroplets to wash away the stripped granulosa cells and the trace amount of residual hyaluronidase. (c) The final step is to observe the maturity of the oocyte and transfer it to a culture medium that has been equilibrated with CO_2 overnight for further incubation, pending the execution of ICSI. It is worth noting that because the opening diameter of the oocyte denudation pipette is slightly smaller than the overall diameter of the oocyte with granulosa cells, overly vigorous pipetting is likely to cause extrusion rupture of the zona pellucida that leads to oocyte degeneration, and may also cause damage to the oolemma or cytoskeleton, thus making the cytoplasm more prone to outflow after injection and, again, leads to oocyte degeneration [31]. Furthermore, the shear stress from vigorous pipetting can also cause potential damage to the oocyte/embryo [32].

In summary, oocyte denudation should be performed with pipettes of appropriate diameters; vigorous pipetting should be avoided; the enzyme concentration should be reduced; the exposure time should be shortened to minimize the adverse effects of physicochemical stresses on the oocytes [33].

On the other hand, there is currently no consensus on how "clean" the oocyte should be denuded. It has been reported that incomplete removal of granulosa cells may improve Day-2 or Day-3 embryo quality and blastocyst formation. However, it may also increase oocyte degeneration after ICSI. The authors suggested that this is due to residual granulosa cells hindering the optimal position of needle entry or more invasive needle entry due to unstable fixation of the oocyte by the holding pipette [34, 35]. How thoroughly the granulosa cells are removed also depends on the maturity of the oocyte—the more mature the oocyte, the easier the granulosa cells can be stripped. This is because, during the growth and maturation of the oocyte, the granulosa cells become attached to and interact with the oocyte through axon-like structures extending through the zona pellucida. These connections diminish progressively during the maturation of the oocyte [36, 37], making the removal of granulosa cells easier. Therefore, for oocyte denudation, it is sufficient as long as there is no interference with the observation of the first polar body and the implementation of ICSI (Fig. 10.23) while avoiding damage to the cell membrane or even to the oocyte. However, for oocytes from PGT patients, granulosa cells should still be removed as much

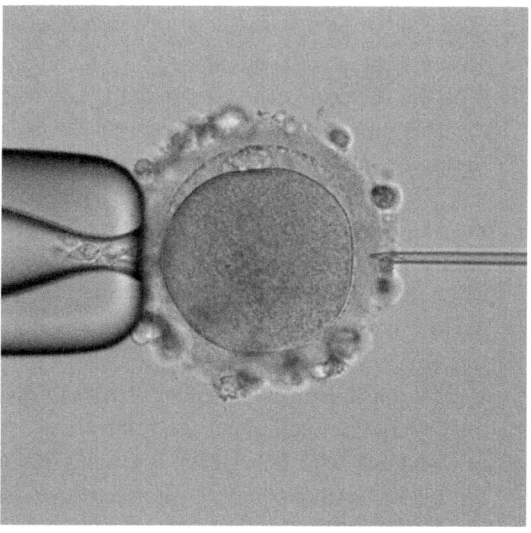

Fig. 10.23 An oocyte with incomplete denudation

as possible to avoid maternal contamination [38]. When using a time-lapse imaging system, one should also try to remove most granulosa cells to avoid interfering with focus of lens.

10.5.2 Sperm Immobilization and Capture

1. Sperm addition: First, add sperm to the PVP microdroplets. For sperm with good density and viability, adding only about 1 μL of the specimen is sufficient. Adding too many specimens will dilute PVP and lose its viscosity, and the high concentration of sperm will make the next step of preferential selection and capturing more difficult. For sperm with very poor motility or those that lose motility quickly after being added to PVP, they can be added to the HEPES/MOPS-buffered medium microdroplets to perform sperm capture and sperm immobilization.

2. Drop the injection pipette: After adding sperm to the microdroplet, place the micromanipulation dish in the center of the heating plate, focus on the edge of the microdroplet under a low magnification microscope (4× or 10×), and bring the injection pipette down into the sperm-free PVP microdroplet. During the

descent of the injection pipette, first, a small portion of the tissue culture oil and then PVP will be aspirated due to the siphon phenomenon, thus forming a PVP-oil interface. It is recommended to always keep this interface within the microscopic visual range during the manipulation (Fig. 10.24).

3. Sperm immobilization: After the injection pipette is focused and the PVP-oil interface is balanced and stabilized, move it into the PVP microdroplet containing sperm. Use the fine-tuning mode of the joystick to raise the injection pipette just a little bit, select sperm and then quickly drop the injection pipette to press the sperm tail. It is important to control the downward pressure at this point. The best pressure is to keep the injection pipette taper in focus while suppressing the sperm. Too little downward pressure will not suppress the sperm, while too much will cause the injection pipette taper to cock. Following pressing the sperm tail, quickly withdrawn the injection pipette until the tail forms an obvious bend, which means a successful immobilization. Keep the injection pipette taper in focus during withdrawal, i.e., do not move the injection pipette in Z-axis. Sperm immobilization is not just about stopping sperm movement but mainly intends to damage the sperm mem-

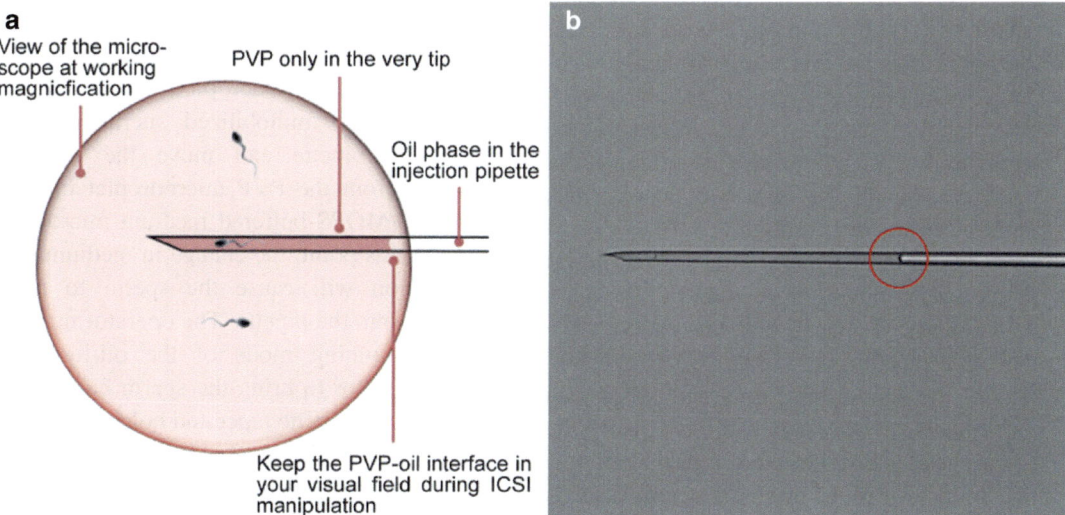

Fig. 10.24 (**a**) In view of the microscope, keep the PVP-oil interface at the taper of the injection pipette; (**b**) the interface between PVP and oil is indicated by a red circle

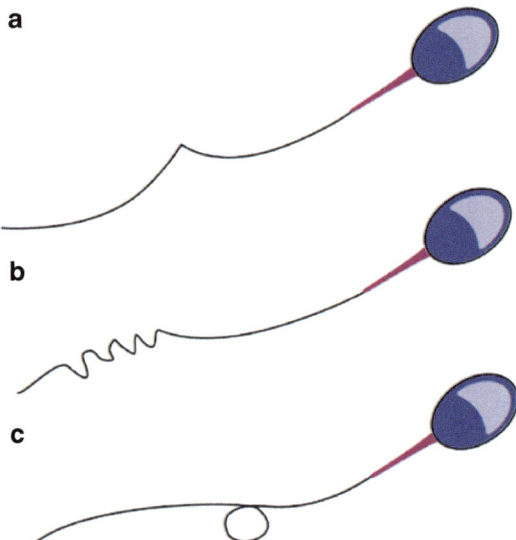

Fig. 10.25 Aggressive immobilization: the sperm has a permanently kinked (**a**), convoluted (**b**) or looped (**c**) tail

brane. In order to damage the membrane sufficiently, some operators would press or grind the sperm tail several times. However, it has been indicated that compared to multiple aggressive immobilization maneuvers, a single sperm immobilization does not reduce the fertilization rate but rather results in a higher high-quality embryo rate on day 3 [39]. On the other hand, for immature sperm (e.g., fresh or frozen-thawed epididymal sperm), the prevailing view advocates adequate aggressive sperm immobilization such that the sperm has a permanently kinked, convoluted or looped tail (Fig. 10.25). These morphological changes can increase the permeability of the sperm membrane and facilitate the release of active factors, thus improving the fertilization rate [40].

4. Precautions during sperm immobilization: (a) If the sperm cannot be pressed by the injection pipette, it means that the taper of the injection pipette is "too parallel" to the bottom of the dish or even upturned, which can be adjusted by the angle adjuster. (b) If the sperm head is disconnected from the tail during immobilization, or if the sperm neck is accidentally touched, another sperm should

be selected. This is because sperm centrosomes are located in the neck. Damage to the centrosomes will compromise the outcome of fertilization and embryo development [41]. (c) The sperm tend to swim toward the edge of the droplet. When the injection pipette tip is placed at the interface between the droplet and the tissue culture oil (Fig. 10.26), it can intercept the sperm to stop their movement, and the sperm may even swim into the injection pipette on their own. This approach is suitable for semen specimens containing large amounts of debris (e.g., testicular tissue), as the injection pipette is prone to get partially or completely blocked when searching for and aspirating sperm in such specimens. (d) When handling semen specimens from patients with very severe oligospermia, to avoid potential damage caused by prolonged exposure of sperm to PVP, the sperm found can be placed in a HEPES/MOPS-buffered medium microdroplets without sperm immobilization first. After enough sperm are captured, they can then be transferred into the PVP microdroplet for sperm immobilization just before injection to ensure their viability.

10.5.3 ICSI Operation Procedure

1. Transfer the denuded mature oocyte into the HEPES/MOPS-buffered medium microdroplets. It is recommended to put only one oocyte per microdroplet.
2. Aspirate the immobilized sperm into the injection pipette and move the injection pipette from the PVP microdroplet into the HEPES/MOPS-buffered medium microdroplet. At this point, the change in medium concentration will cause the sperm to move inward into the pipette. The operator may use the fine-tuning mode of the oil-hydraulic microinjector to bring the sperm back to the front of the pipette taper and hold it steady.
3. First, adjust the microscope to focus the oolemma, followed by rotating the oocyte with the injection pipette so that the first polar body is at the 6 o'clock or 12 o'clock position.

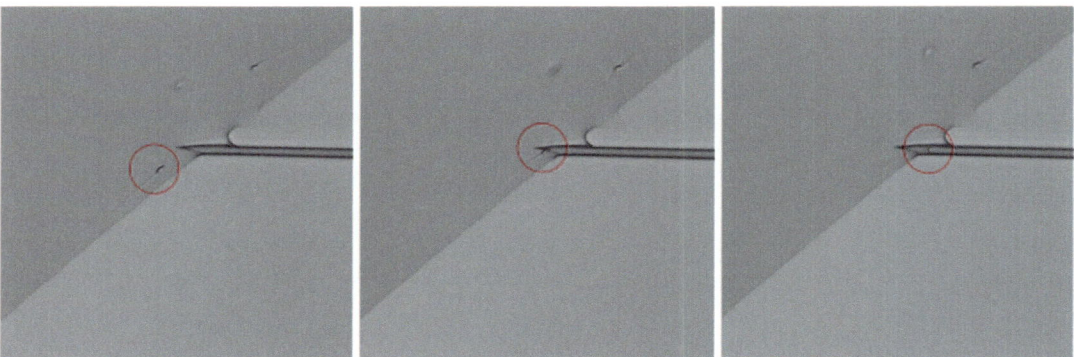

Fig. 10.26 When the injection pipette tip is placed at the interface between PVP (dark gray) and oil (light gray), the sperm with good motility (red circle) may automatically swim into the pipette

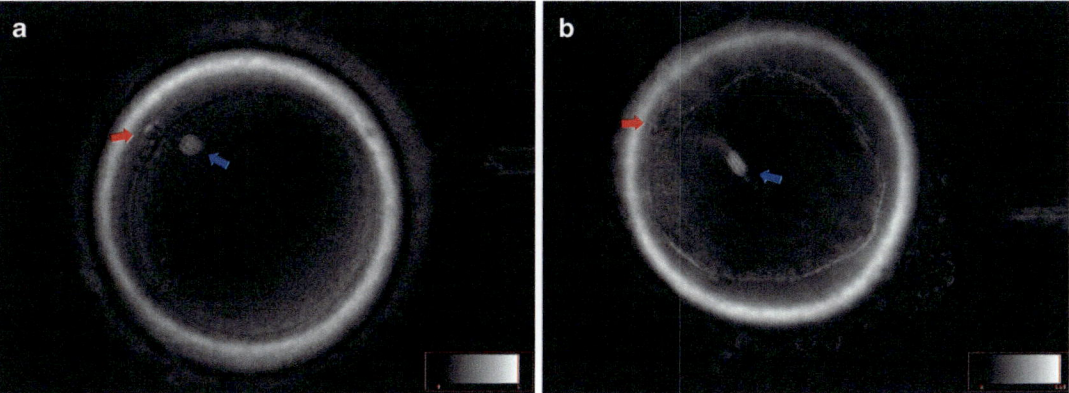

Fig. 10.27 (**a**) Spindle near the first polar body; (**b**) spindle deviating from the first polar body. Blue arrows point to the spindle, and red arrows point to the first polar body

Then hold the oocyte in place by suction with the holding pipette at the 9 o'clock position, followed by puncturing it with the injection pipette from the 3 o'clock spot. It is generally accepted that the spindle is close to the first polar body (Fig. 10.27a) and that puncturing from the 3 o'clock position can minimize the probability of spindle damage. During meiosis, the spindle is responsible for the normal arrangement and segregation of chromosomes. Any damage to the spindle may cause rearrangement of chromosomes in the cytoplasm, ultimately leading to aneuploidy. Not all oocytes have a spindle close to the first polar body [42–44] (Fig. 10.27b), and it is speculated that the denudation process may cause the shift of the polar body [45]. However, 74% of oocytes have spindles shifted within 45 degrees [43], which means that the spindle is, in most cases, still close to the first polar body. In addition, oocytes with better developmental potential tend to have their spindle close to the first polar body. These oocytes would have a relatively low chance of having their spindle damaged when punctured [44], as described above. Therefore, the current ICSI procedure still takes the 3 o'clock position as the puncture site.

4. Adjust the position of the oocyte and the injection pipette, so the oolemma and the pipette tip are focused in the same plane under the microscope. The oolemma can be gently pressed with the injection pipette before injection to ensure puncture from the equatorial plane of the oocyte. Push the sperm to the injection pipette tip and then puncture along

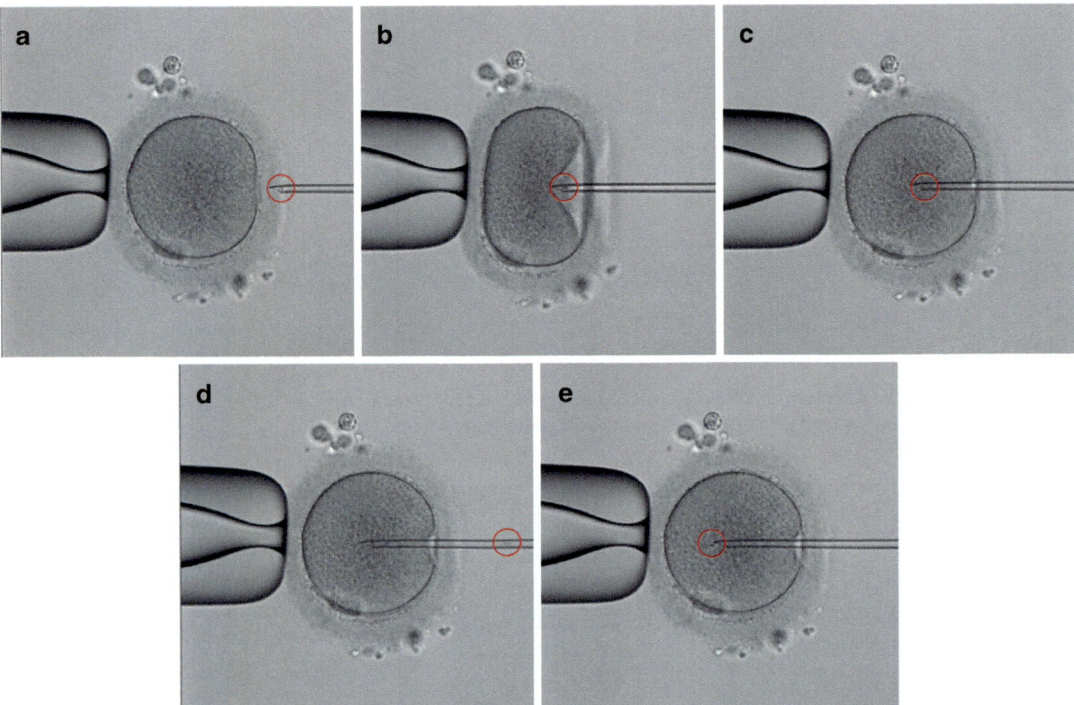

Fig. 10.28 ICSI injection procedure. (**a**) After the sperm is moved to the tip of the injection pipette, the pipette tip is gently placed against the zona pellucida; (**b**) the pressure of the pipette slightly deforms the oocyte (which has not yet broken through the zona pellucida); (**c**) the zona pellucida is successfully broken through, the oolemma is rebounded, and aspiration of cytoplasm starts to occur; (**d**) the membrane has been successfully ruptured with rapid aspiration of cytoplasm; (**e**) slow injection of sperm into the cytoplasm (red circle shows the position of the sperm)

the centerline of the oocyte, as deviation from the centerline greatly increases the likelihood of damage to the oocyte. The injection pipette first breaks through the zona pellucida, with relatively high resistance in this process. It is important to control the force to avoid excessive pressure on the cytosolic membrane from a sudden breakthrough. Usually, after a successful breakage of the zona pellucida, the injection pipette has already entered one-third or deeper into the oocyte. For oocytes with a more elastic cell membrane, the cell membrane will form a funnel shape by the pressure of the injection pipette. The cell membrane will start to regain its original position when the pipette reaches 1/2 or 2/3 into the oocyte, at which point transient reflux of sperm and cytoplasm can be observed, which proves that the membrane has been success-fully ruptured. Once the membrane is broken, the suction should be stopped, and the sperm should be slowly injected into the cytoplasm. It is important to minimize the amount of cytoplasm drawn back into the pipette at this time, as too much cytoplasm being aspirated from the oocyte can disrupt the ultrastructure of the oocyte and compromise the formation of the blastocyst (Fig. 10.28).

5. After the sperm is injected into the cytoplasm, withdraw the injection pipette, and release the oocyte from the holding pipette. Immediately after all injections of a batch of oocytes are completed, they are transferred into an overnight equilibrated cleavage culture medium for further culture. It is recommended to have no more than ten oocytes in a single ICSI manipulation or to limit the total manipulation time to less than 10 min.

10.5.4 Timing of Oocyte Denudation and ICSI

The timing of oocyte denudation after oocyte retrieval and ICSI have not been established. The general opinion is that granulosa cells contribute to the further maturation of the cytoplasm, so proper incubation before ICSI is beneficial. However, the range of "optimal incubation time" obtained from different studies varies widely (1–12 h) [16]. A recent study confirmed a progressive trend toward poor clinical outcomes due to oocyte aging as the time between oocyte retrieval and ICSI increases [46]. Therefore, the timing of these two procedures needs to be determined on a lab-specific basis and in conjunction with KPIs. In our center, oocyte denudation is usually performed 39–40 h after human chorionic gonadotrophin (hCG) administration, and ICSI is commonly performed after 30 min of incubation upon oocyte denudation. Also, the following two factors need to be considered:

1. Oocyte count: If there are many mature oocytes, a longer injection time may be required to have a longer time interval between the first and the last oocyte injected.
2. Sperm preparation: In the case of very severe oligospermia or surgically obtained sperm, it may take a long time to capture the sperm, so an earlier sperm capture may be required to avoid missing the optimal injection time.

10.5.5 Precautions and Tips for ICSI Manipulation

1. When injected into the cytoplasm, the sperm may slip or dive as it leaves the tip of the injection pipette. Sometimes, even with a successful oolemma rupture, the sperm will move slowly outward along the insertion channel following the withdrawal of pipette. This phenomenon is usually because the sperm did not really make it through the ruptured oolemma into the cytoplasm but was injected into the "folds" of the retracted oolemma, which may affect the fertilization outcome.

2. It has been suggested that the direction of the sperm head and tail within injection pipette during ICSI injection does not affect oocyte survival, fertilization, embryo development, or implantation potential. A head-first aspiration (the tail pointing forward as the sperm is aspirated into the injection pipette) facilitates aspiration of the sperm, shortens the injection time, and permits the sperm to enter the oocyte more adequately, which may facilitate fertilization [47]. In contrast, a head pointing forward facilitates placing the sperm at the very tip of the injection pipette to avoid injecting too much PVP. Given that the ICSI manipulation technique is already very well established and sperm aspiration and injection are no problem for experienced embryologists, "head forward" is still recommended as the primary way for ICSI injections.

3. Aspiration of multiple sperm at a time can shorten the time of ICSI manipulation provided that the distance between sperm is kept sufficient, but some risks are still involved. In the case of an oocyte with a tough membrane, when the membrane is ruptured, the rapid aspiration of cytoplasm may force two sperms to come closer together due to the significant pressure. This nearness makes it difficult to separate the two sperm, resulting in injecting multiple sperm in one shot, which is why aspirating one sperm at a time is the safest way to perform the ICSI injection.

4. If the sperm "sticks" to the tip of the pipette after injection and is carried out of oolemma when the injection pipette is withdrawn, reinjection can be done after the other oocytes in the dish have been injected. When reinjecting, change the injected site by rotating the oocyte so that the polar body is in a different position. If the sperm always sticks to the injection pipette, it should be replaced promptly with a new injection pipette. This is usually more likely to happen when semen is prepared by direct centrifugation and sedimentation without a swim-up procedure, such as in the case of very severe oligozoospermia or testicular puncture for sperm retrieval. At this point, an adequate number of sperm may be captured in

one go, and a new injection pipette may be taken to perform the injection.

5. In the case of an oocyte that is difficult to rupture, the operator may slowly spit the oolemma that was aspirated into the injection pipette back out, withdraw the injection pipette, and then perform a second injection parallel to the first insertion channel and rupture the oolemma by aspiration, as the "stretched" oolemma is usually easier to rupture.

6. In some patients, the oolemma is less elastic and is usually ruptured after the zona pellucida is breached, which results in a significantly higher rate of oocyte degeneration after ICSI [48]. Therefore, it is important to apply gentle pressure when puncturing the zona pellucida to reduce the pressure of the pipette tip on the membrane after the zona pellucida is breached. It has been suggested that using a laser to drill a 5–7 μm channel in the zona pellucida to reduce the pressure on the oolemma during puncture may help reduce the oocyte degeneration rate in such cases [49]. Another study also confirmed that laser-ICSI could improve the Day 2 high-quality embryo rate, the Day 5 hatching rate, and clinical pregnancy rate while significantly reducing the degeneration rate [50]. However, an RCT study in 2006 yielded quite different results, with no statistically significant difference between laser-ICSI and conventional ICSI in terms of all indicators, and laser-ICSI did not improve the outcome of oocytes with high membrane fragility [51].

7. Some researchers have also performed ICSI (piezo-ICSI) using a piezoelectric membrane breaker, characterized by rapid membrane breakage without sucking the cytoplasm and no compression of the oocyte during the puncture process that could cause degeneration. Thus, it can significantly reduce the oocyte degeneration rate (especially in oocytes with fragile membranes) and increase the fertilization rate, high-quality embryo rate, blastocyst formation rate, and live birth rate [52, 53]. A recent study has shown that piezo-ICSI is more suitable for patients of advanced age (>35 years old) and can improve the fertiliza-

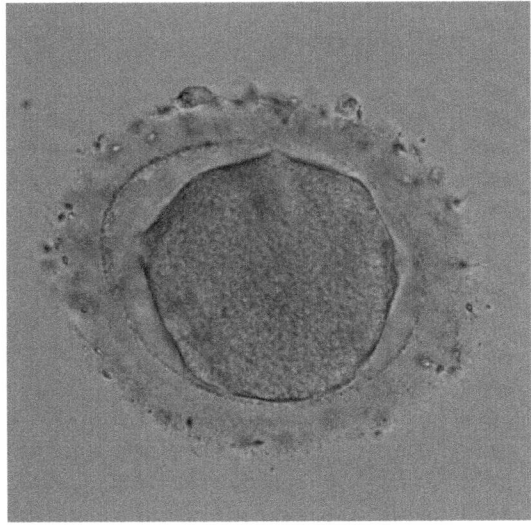

Fig. 10.29 Elevated osmolality of microdroplets, resulting in the crumpled and deformed oolemma

tion rate and the Day 5/Day 6 blastocyst formation rate [54]. However, this technique is not commonly applied worldwide.

8. If all or some of the oocytes are found to have some degree of cell membrane crumpling and deformation (Fig. 10.29), it may be due to elevated osmolality of the manipulation medium, which can be caused by: too low relative humidity in the room, too small manipulation medium microdroplets, too slow preparation of the dish, and tissue culture oil not completely covering the microdroplets.

10.5.6 Fertilization Results Observation

According to the *Istanbul Consensus* [55], the oocyte should be observed 16–18 h after ICSI for fertilization. The presence of double pronuclei (2PN) and two polar bodies are considered normal fertilization. The morphological score of the pronucleus is also an important indicator of embryo potential [56], including the location and size of the pronucleus and the number, size, and arrangement of nucleolar precursor bodies within the pronucleus. In addition to 2PN, the following abnormalities may also occur:

1. Monopronuclear (1PN): i.e., only one pronucleus is seen. The mechanism of 1PN may be [57]: (a) The male pronucleus and female pronucleus developed asynchronously, or the two became fused, a condition that should theoretically lead to the formation of a diploid embryo; (b) oocyte parthenogenesis activation, which results in an abnormal embryo. The *2017 Vienna Consensus* recommends that the incidence of ICSI-1PN should be less than 3% [58], and an ICSI-1PN rate higher than this may indicate problems with culture conditions or gamete manipulation. It has been suggested that the incidence of ICSI-1PN may be associated with a prolonged time between hCG administration and ICSI, presumably due to parthenogenesis activation following in vitro oocyte aging [59]. Although there is a high incidence of abnormal embryos developed from ICSI-1PN [57], a certain fraction of normal embryos was found by PGT after blastocyst culture, and normal live births were obtained [60, 61].

2. Multipronuclear (≥3PN): i.e., three or more pronuclei are observed, with 3PN being the most common. The mechanism of multipronuclei is as follows [62]: (a) Nonextrusion of the second polar body will result in digynic triploidy. (b) Although the second polar body is released, the maternal chromosomes split to form two aneuploid pronuclei. (c) The second polar body was released carrying some of the chromosomes, and the remaining chromosomes formed an aneuploid pronucleus. 3PN embryos derived from either conventional IVF or ICSI cannot be implanted [33].

3. Nonpronuclear (0PN): The absence of the pronucleus is mostly due to fertilization failure. In rare cases, the pronucleus disappears too early, or its formation is delayed, thus staggering its presence from the time of observation. The most important cause of fertilization failure is the failure of oocyte activation. Other causes include the failure of sperm chromatin decondensation, premature condensation of sperm chromatin, defects in the spindle or sperm aster, and injection failure due to manipulation. It has been reported that 1% to 3% of ICSI cycles are followed by the non-fertilization of the oocytes. Before proceeding to the next cycle, the mouse oocyte activation test can be utilized to determine whether the fertilization failure is due to sperm or oocyte [63]. For some patients who have failed oocyte activation owing to sperm, artificial oocyte activation can be performed to improve treatment outcomes [64]. However, there is still no effective treatment for fertilization failure due to oocyte spindle abnormalities caused by certain gene mutations (e.g., TUBB8) [65].

4. Degeneration: Some oocytes degenerate already during the injection process, while in some other cases, degeneration is detected when observing fertilization after ICSI. The *2017 Vienna Consensus recommends* that the oocyte degeneration rate for ICSI cycles should be less than 10%. The main cause of oocyte degeneration is the quality of the oocytes involved. Although ICSI manipulation requires extensive experience, there is no evidence that degeneration is correlated with the manipulation [16]. Oocyte degeneration may be reduced by applying recombinant hyaluronidase, selecting sharper and finer inner diameter injection pipettes, and applying laser-ICSI or piezo-ICSI technique [16].

10.6 Training in Microscopic Manipulation

In 2005, the American Society for Reproductive Medicine mandated that novice ICSI operators complete intracytoplasmic sperm injection of 20 unfertilized oocytes and 50 oocytes from actual patients under the supervision of a senior embryologist [66]. Moreover, they can perform the procedure independently only after achieving a fertilization rate ≥50% and an oocyte degeneration rate <15%. With the continuous advancement and sophistication of assisted reproduction technology, the KPIs related to ICSI are also on the rise, with the *2017 Vienna Consensus* recommending that the competency and benchmark levels for ICSI fertilization and oocyte degeneration rates should be ≥65% and <10% [58], respectively. Novice operators can initially practice ICSI using unfertilized or immature oocytes, or they can culture immature oocytes in vitro before practicing. However, all training involving gametes or embryos requires informed consent from the patients.

References

1. Gordon JW, Grunfeld L, Garrisi GJ, et al. Fertilization of human oocytes by sperm from infertile males after zona pellucida drilling. Fertil Steril. 1988;50(1):68–73.
2. Cohen J, Malter H, Fehilly C, et al. Implantation of embryos after partial opening of oocyte zona pellucida to facilitate sperm penetration. Lancet. 1988;2(8603):162.
3. Lanzendorf SE, Maloney MK, Veeck LL, et al. A preclinical evaluation of pronuclear formation by microinjection of human spermatozoa into human oocytes. Fertil Steril. 1988;49(5):835–42.
4. Palermo G, Joris H, Devroey P, et al. Pregnancies after intracytoplasmic injection of single spermatozoon into an oocyte. Lancet. 1992;340(8810):17–8.
5. Practice Committees of the American Society for Reproductive Medicine, Society for Assisted Reproductive Technology. Intracytoplasmic sperm injection (ICSI) for non-male factor infertility: a committee opinion. Fertil Steril. 2012;98(6):1395–9.
6. Li M, Ma SY, Yang HJ, et al. Pregnancy with oocytes characterized by narrow perivitelline space and heterogeneous zona pellucida: is intracytoplasmic sperm injection necessary? J Assist Reprod Genet. 2014;31(3):285–94.
7. Tannus S, Son WY, Gilman A, et al. The role of intracytoplasmic sperm injection in non-male factor infertility in advanced maternal age. Hum Reprod. 2017;32(1):119–24.
8. Guo N, Hua X, Li YF, et al. Role of ICSI in non-male factor cycles as the number of oocytes retrieved decreases from four to one. Curr Med Sci. 2018;38(1):131–6.
9. Liu H, Zhao H, Yu G, et al. Conventional in vitro fertilization (IVF) or intracytoplasmic sperm injection (ICSI): which is preferred for advanced age patients with five or fewer oocytes retrieved? Arch Gynecol Obstet. 2018;297(5):1301–6.
10. Drakopoulos P, Garcia-Velasco J, Bosch E, et al. ICSI does not offer any benefit over conventional IVF across different ovarian response categories in non-male factor infertility: a European multicenter analysis. J Assist Reprod Genet. 2019;36(10):2067–76.
11. Catford SR, McLachlan RI, O'Bryan MK, et al. Long-term follow-up of intra-cytoplasmic sperm injection-conceived offspring compared with in vitro fertilization-conceived offspring: a systematic review of health outcomes beyond the neonatal period. Andrology. 2017;5(4):610–21.
12. Esteves SC, Roque M, Bedoschi G, et al. Intracytoplasmic sperm injection for male infertility and consequences for offspring. Nat Rev Urol. 2018;15(9):535–62.
13. Cairo 2018 Consensus Group. 'There is only one thing that is truly important in an IVF laboratory: everything' Cairo Consensus Guidelines on IVF Culture Conditions. Reprod Biomed Online. 2020;40(1):33–60.
14. Butler JM, Johnson JE, Boone WR, et al. The heat is on: room temperature affects laboratory equipment-an observational study. J Assist Reprod Genet. 2013;30(10):1389–93.
15. Wang WH, Meng L, Hackett RJ, et al. Rigorous thermal control during intracytoplasmic sperm injection stabilizes the meiotic spindle and improves fertilization and pregnancy rates. Fertil Steril. 2002;77(6):1274–7.
16. Rubino P, Viganò P, Luddi A, et al. The ICSI procedure from past to future: a systematic review of the more controversial aspects. Hum Reprod Update. 2016;22(2):194–227.
17. Davidson LM, Liu Y, Griffiths T, et al. Laser technology in the ART laboratory: a narrative review. Reprod Biomed Online. 2019;38(5):725–39.
18. Ebner T, Moser M, Tews G, et al. Possible applications of a non-contact 1.48 microm wavelength diode laser in assisted reproduction technologies. Hum Reprod Update. 2005;11(4):425–35.
19. Swearman H, Koustas G, Knight E, et al. pH: the silent variable significantly impacting meiotic spindle assembly in mouse oocytes. Reprod Biomed Online. 2018;37(3):279–90.
20. Will MA, Clark NA, Swain JE, et al. Biological pH buffers in IVF: help or hindrance to success. J Assist Reprod Genet. 2011;28(8):711–24.
21. Wale PL, Gardner DK. The effects of chemical and physical factors on mammalian embryo culture and their importance for the practice of assisted human reproduction. Hum Reprod Update. 2016;22(1):02–22.
22. Simopoulou M, Gkoles L, Bakas P, et al. Improving ICSI: a review from the spermatozoon perspective. Syst Biol Reprod Med. 2016;62(6):359–71.
23. Parmegiani L, Cognigni GE, Bernardi S, et al. Comparison of two ready-to-use systems designed for sperm-hyaluronic acid binding selection before intracytoplasmic sperm injection: PICSI vs. Sperm Slow: a prospective, randomized trial. Fertil Steril. 2012;98(3):632–7.
24. Lepine S, McDowell S, Searle LM, et al. Advanced sperm selection techniques for assisted reproduction. Cochrane Database Syst Rev. 2019;7(7):CD010461.
25. Van de Velde H, Nagy ZP, Joris H, et al. Effects of different hyaluronidase concentrations and mechanical procedures for cumulus cell removal on the outcome

of intracytoplasmic sperm injection. Hum Reprod. 1997;12(10):2246–50.

26. Moura BR, Gurgel MC, Machado SP, et al. Low concentration of hyaluronidase for oocyte denudation can improve fertilization rates and embryo quality. JBRA Assist Reprod. 2017;21(1):27–30.

27. Xue X, Wang WS, Shi JZ, et al. Efficacy of swim-up versus density gradient centrifugation in improving sperm deformity rate and DNA fragmentation index in semen samples from teratozoospermic patients. J Assist Reprod Genet. 2014;31(9):1161–6.

28. Sandi-Monroy NL, Musanovic S, Zhu D, et al. Use of dimethylxanthine theophylline (SpermMobil®) does not affect clinical, obstetric or perinatal outcomes. Arch Gynecol Obstet. 2019;300(5):1435–43.

29. Shen ZQ, Shi B, Wang TR, et al. Characterization of the sperm proteome and reproductive outcomes with in vitro, fertilization after a reduction in male ejaculatory abstinence period. Mol Cell Proteomics. 2019;18(Suppl 1):S109–17.

30. Karimi N, Mohseni Kouchesfahani H, Nasr-Esfahani MH, et al. DGC/zeta as a new strategy to improve clinical outcome in male factor infertility patients following intracytoplasmic sperm injection: a randomized, single-blind, clinical trial. Cell J. 2020;22(1):55–9.

31. Nagy ZP, Liu J, Joris H, et al. The influence of the site of sperm deposition and mode of oolemma breakage at intracytoplasmic sperm injection on fertilization and embryo development rates. Hum Reprod. 1995;10(12):3171–7.

32. Xie Y, Wang F, Puscheck EE, et al. Pipetting causes shear stress and elevation of phosphorylated stress-activated protein kinase/jun kinase in preimplantation embryos. Mol Reprod Dev. 2007;74(10):1287–94.

33. Gianaroli L, Plachot M, van Kooij R, et al. Revised guidelines for good practice in IVF laboratories (2015). Hum Reprod. 2016;31(4):685–6.

34. Ebner T, Yaman C, Moser M, et al. A prospective study on oocyte survival rate after ICSI: influence of injection technique and morphological features. J Assist Reprod Genet. 2001;18(12):623–8.

35. Ebner T, Moser M, Sommergruber M, et al. Incomplete denudation of oocytes prior to ICSI enhances embryo quality and blastocyst development. Hum Reprod. 2006;21(11):2972–7.

36. Coticchio G, Dal Canto M, Mignini Renzini M, et al. Oocyte maturation: gamete-somatic cells interactions, meiotic resumption, cytoskeletal dynamics and cytoplasmic reorganization. Hum Reprod Update. 2015;21(4):427–54.

37. El-Hayek S, Yang Q, Abbassi L, et al. Mammalian oocytes locally remodel follicular architecture to provide the foundation for germline-soma communication. Curr Biol. 2018;28(7):1124–1131.e3.

38. Harton GL, Magli MC, Lundin K, et al. ESHRE PGD Consortium/Embryology Special Interest Group-best practice guidelines for polar body and embryo biopsy for preimplantation genetic diagnosis/screening (PGD/PGS). Hum Reprod. 2011;26(1):41–6.

39. Velaers A, Paternot G, Debrock S, et al. Triple touch sperm immobilization vs. single touch sperm immobilization in ICSI-a randomised trial. Reprod Biol Endocrinol. 2012;10:65–5.

40. Palermo GD, Schlegel PN, Colombero LT, et al. Aggressive sperm immobilization prior to intracytoplasmic sperm injection with immature spermatozoa improves fertilization and pregnancy rates. Hum Reprod. 1996;11(5):1023–9.

41. Schatten H, Sun QY. The role of centrosomes in mammalian fertilization and its significance for ICSI. Mol Hum Reprod. 2009;15(9):531–8.

42. Hardarson T, Lundin K, Hamberger L. The position of the metaphase II spindle cannot be predicted by the location of the first polar body in the human oocyte. Hum Reprod. 2000;15(6):1372–6.

43. Rienzi L, Ubaldi F, Martinez F, et al. Relationship between meiotic spindle location with regard to the polar body position and oocyte developmental potential after ICSI. Hum Reprod. 2003;18(6):1289–93.

44. Mahfoudh AM, Moon JH, Henderson S, et al. Relationship between pre-ICSI meiotic spindle angle, ovarian reserve, gonadotropin stimulation, and pregnancy outcomes. J Assist Reprod Genet. 2017;34(5):609–15.

45. Rienzi L, Ubaldi F, Iacobelli M, et al. Meiotic spindle visualization in living human oocytes. Reprod Biomed Online. 2005;10(2):192–8.

46. Pujol A, García D, Obradors A, et al. Is there a relation between the time to ICSI and the reproductive outcomes? Hum Reprod. 2018;33(5):797–806.

47. Woodward BJ, Campbell KH, Ramsewak SS, et al. A comparison of headfirst and tailfirst microinjection of sperm at intracytoplasmic sperm injection. Fertil Steril. 2008;89(3):711–4.

48. Palermo GD, Alikani M, Bertoli M, et al. Oolemma characteristics in relation to survival and fertilization patterns of oocytes treated by intracytoplasmic sperm injection. Hum Reprod. 1996;11(1):172–6.

49. Nagy ZP, Oliveira SA, Abdelmassih V, et al. Novel use of laser to assist ICSI for patients with fragile oocytes: a case report. Reprod Biomed Online. 2002;4(1):27–31.

50. Moser M, Ebner T, Sommergruber M, et al. Laser-assisted zona pellucida thinning prior to routine ICSI. Hum Reprod. 2004;19(3):573–8.

51. Richter KS, Davis A, Carter J, et al. No advantage of laser-assisted over conventional intracytoplasmic sperm injection: a randomized controlled trial [NCT00114725]. J Exp Clin Assist Reprod. 2006;3:5.

52. Takeuchi S, Minoura H, Shibahara T, et al. Comparison of piezo-assisted micromanipulation with conventional micromanipulation for intracytoplasmic sperm injection into human oocytes. Gynecol Obstet Investig. 2001;52(3):158–62.

53. Hiraoka K, Kitamura S. Clinical efficiency of Piezo-ICSI using micropipettes with a wall thickness of 0.625 μm. J Assist Reprod Genet. 2015;32(12):1827–33.

54. Furuhashi K, Saeki Y, Enatsu N, et al. Piezo-assisted ICSI improves fertilization and blastocyst devel-

opment rates compared with conventional ICSI in women aged more than 35 years. Reprod Med Biol. 2019;18(4):357–61.

55. Alpha Scientists in Reproductive Medicine and ESHRE Special Interest Group of Embryology. Istanbul consensus workshop on embryo assessment: proceedings of an expert meeting. Reprod Biomed Online. 2011;22(6):632–46.

56. Papale L, Fiorentino A, Montag M, et al. The zygote. Hum Reprod. 2012;27(Suppl 1):22–49.

57. Mateo S, Parriego M, Boada M, et al. In vitro development and chromosome constitution of embryos derived from monopronucleated zygotes after intracytoplasmic sperm injection. Fertil Steril. 2013;99(3):897–902.e1.

58. ESHRE Special Interest Group of Embryology and Alpha Scientists in Reproductive Medicine. The Vienna consensus: report of an expert meeting on the development of ART laboratory performance indicators. Reprod Biomed Online. 2017;35(5):494–510.

59. Fabozzi G, Rega E, Starita MF, et al. The influence of clinical and laboratory factors on the formation of monopronucleated zygotes after intracytoplasmic sperm injection (ICSI). Zygote. 2019;27(2):64–8.

60. Bradley CK, Traversa MV, Hobson N, et al. Clinical use of monopronucleated zygotes following blastocyst culture and preimplantation genetic screening, includ-

ing verification of biparental chromosome inheritance. Reprod Biomed Online. 2017;34(6):567–74.

61. Mateo S, Vidal F, Parriego M, et al. Could monopronucleated ICSI zygotes be considered for transfer? Analysis through time-lapse monitoring and PGS. J Assist Reprod Genet. 2017;34(7):905–11.

62. Rosenbusch BE. Selective microsurgical removal of a pronucleus from tripronuclear human oocytes to restore diploidy: disregarded but valuable? Fertil Steril. 2009;92(3):897–903.

63. Bonte D, Ferrer-Buitrago M, Dhaenens L, et al. Assisted oocyte activation significantly increases fertilization and pregnancy outcome in patients with low and total failed fertilization after intracytoplasmic sperm injection: a 17-year retrospective study. Fertil Steril. 2019;112(2):266–74.

64. Murugesu S, Saso S, Jones BP, et al. Does the use of calcium ionophore during artificial oocyte activation demonstrate an effect on pregnancy rate? A meta-analysis. Fertil Steril. 2017;108(3):468–482.e3.

65. Chen B, Li B, Li D, et al. Novel mutations and structural deletions in TUBB8: expanding mutational and phenotypic spectrum of patients with arrest in oocyte maturation, fertilization or early embryonic development. Hum Reprod. 2017;32(2):457–64.

66. Keck C, Fischer R, Baukloh V, et al. Staff management in the in vitro fertilization laboratory. Fertil Steril. 2005;84(6):1786–8.

Trophectoderm Biopsy

11.1 Overview of the Development of Embryo Biopsy

In 1990, Handyside et al. reported a successful pregnancy utilizing preimplantation genetic diagnosis (PGD) technology for embryo sex selection in IVF for the first time [1]. Nowadays, the technology has been used in IVF centers worldwide. The term PGD has been replaced by preimplantation genetic testing (PGT) in 2017 [2]. PGT refers to a test performed to analyze the DNA from oocytes (polar bodies) or embryos (cleavage stage or blastocyst) for HLA-typing or for determining genetic abnormalities. These include PGT for aneuploidies (PGT-A); PGT for monogenic/single gene defects (PGT-M); and PGT for chromosomal structural rearrangements (PGT-SR). With the continuous development of molecular biology techniques, some tests can be performed using non-invasive or minimally invasive methods to obtain genetic material [3, 4]. However, the accuracy of the test results based on such sampling methods is still controversial [5]. For this reason, genetic material is still predominantly retrieved by invasive means, i.e., biopsy. The biopsy consists of two micro-manipulation steps: zona pellucida (ZP) opening and cell removal. PGT biopsies are usually performed in three different ways: (a) polar body biopsy: the first and second polar bodies are biopsied at the oocyte or zygote stage; (b) cleavage stage biopsy: one or two blastomeres are taken for biopsy at the cleavage stage; and (c) blastocyst biopsy: 5 to 10 trophectoderm (TE) cells are taken for biopsy at the blastocyst stage. Biopsy of polar bodies is mainly used for diagnosing maternal genetic mutations and specific laws and regulations prohibit embryo biopsy in some regions. Before 2010, approximately 90% of PGD biopsies were performed on cleavage stage embryos [6]. However, a prospective cohort study found that the number of blastomeres biopsied at the cleavage stage would affect blastocyst formation and pregnancy outcomes [7]. Another randomized paired study also showed that biopsy of even only one blastomere of a cleavage embryo would significantly reduce its implantation potential. In contrast, biopsies of blastocysts had no measurable impact on implantation rate [8]. Therefore, following the improvement of controlled ovarian stimulation and blastocyst vitrification technology, blastomere biopsy has been gradually replaced by trophectoderm biopsy in the last decade [9, 10].

11.2 Trophectoderm Biopsy

11.2.1 Advantages and Controversies of Trophectoderm Biopsy

The following advantages of TE biopsy are observed: (a) The number of cells that can be obtained is higher, thereby improving the

D. Li, Y. Gao, *Quality Management in the Assisted Reproduction Laboratory*,
https://doi.org/10.1007/978-981-99-6659-2_11

amplification efficiency and diagnostic accuracy and reducing the incidence of test failure [11]. (b) Lesser embryonic damage: despite acquiring more cells, a quite small proportion of the whole embryo was obtained. Furthermore, the TE cells will develop into the placenta and not be involved in fetal development [8]. (c) Blastocyst stage embryos have undergone embryonic genome activation and are therefore more tolerant to invasive micromanipulations than cleavage stage embryos. (d) Frozen-thawed blastocyst transfer has achieved a satisfactory pregnancy rate [12, 13].

While blastocyst biopsy has significant advantages, it is still associated with two major controversies: (a) The diagnosis of mosaic embryos might "miscategorize" some embryos that have the potential to develop into a fetus [14]. Chromosome mosaicism is typically defined as the presence, in a single sample, of two or more cell lines with different chromosome sets, which has been observed commonly in a minority of embryos at all preimplantation development stages [15]. Whether TE cells can exactly reflect the chromosome of the whole embryo remains unclear, since not all cells of a mosaic embryo share identical chromosomal complements. Furthermore, some mosaic blastocysts may be able to self-correct and thus have the potential to develop normally [16]. Therefore, when both euploidy and mosaic embryos are available, euploidy embryos should be undoubtedly preferred for transfer; when only mosaic embryos are present, the risk should be carefully assessed based on the type and level of chromosomal mosaicism. Prenatal diagnosis of the fetus and placenta is highly recommended, with amniocentesis currently considered most representative of fetal tissues [17]. (b) Some patients have to give up due to the absence of blastocyst formation. However, the blastocyst formation rate has satisfactorily increased with continuous improvement and refinement of IVF laboratory culture techniques. Moreover, this issue should also be considered dialectically: fewer blastocysts are formed due to natural elimination; however, they have more developmental potential and reduced the financial burden on patients while avoiding "unnecessary" embryo testing.

11.2.2 Choosing the Blastocyst Biopsy Method

The trophectoderm biopsy consists of two main steps: assisted hatching (AH) and TE-cell removal. The 1.48 μm (or 1.46 μm) non-contact diode laser is generally used for AH and TE-cell removal due to greater safety and easier handling [18]. According to the different AH timing, TE biopsy is mainly divided into three methods. (a) Day 3/4 hatching-based method (Fig. 11.1c-i, ii): A ZP opening is made via AH on the cleavage stage embryo on day 3 or 4, and biopsy is performed after TE cells are hatched on day 5 or 6 [19]. (b) Day 5–6 hatching-based method (Fig. 11.1c-iii): A ZP opening of the expanding blastocyst is made via AH in the morning of day 5 or 6. The blastocyst is further incubated for 2–4 h, followed by a biopsy after some TE cells have been hatched [20]. (c) Day 5–7 sequential ZP opening and TE-cell removal (Fig. 11.1a): This method involves consecutive manipulation of the fully expanded stage blastocyst (stage 4–6) on day 5 or 6, with TE-cell aspiration and removal immediately after the ZP opening [21].

The third method is more recommended here, because it does not involve AH on day-3 or day-4 embryos, which can keep the embryo undisturbed in culture up to the expanded blastocyst stage. In addition, the biopsy by the third method can be performed at any time if a stage 4–6 blastocyst is formed. The first method requires opening the ZP during the cleavage stage, which may disrupt the internal environment for cell growth and thus affect blastocyst formation. Also, when using the first method, the location of the inner cell mass (ICM) within the blastocyst cannot be predicted. Sometimes the ICM may hatch through the ZP opening when they are close, making the biopsy more difficult to perform and increasing the risk of laser burns on the ICM [22, 23]. In addition, the blastocyst may not be able to expand sufficiently due to the disruption of the integrity of the ZP [24], thus affecting the accuracy of the blastocyst assessment according to the Gardner blastocyst scoring system. Although the second method also does not interfere too much with the embryonic growth process, the time and number of cells hatched after AH varies among different quality embryos, putting embryologists in a restricted

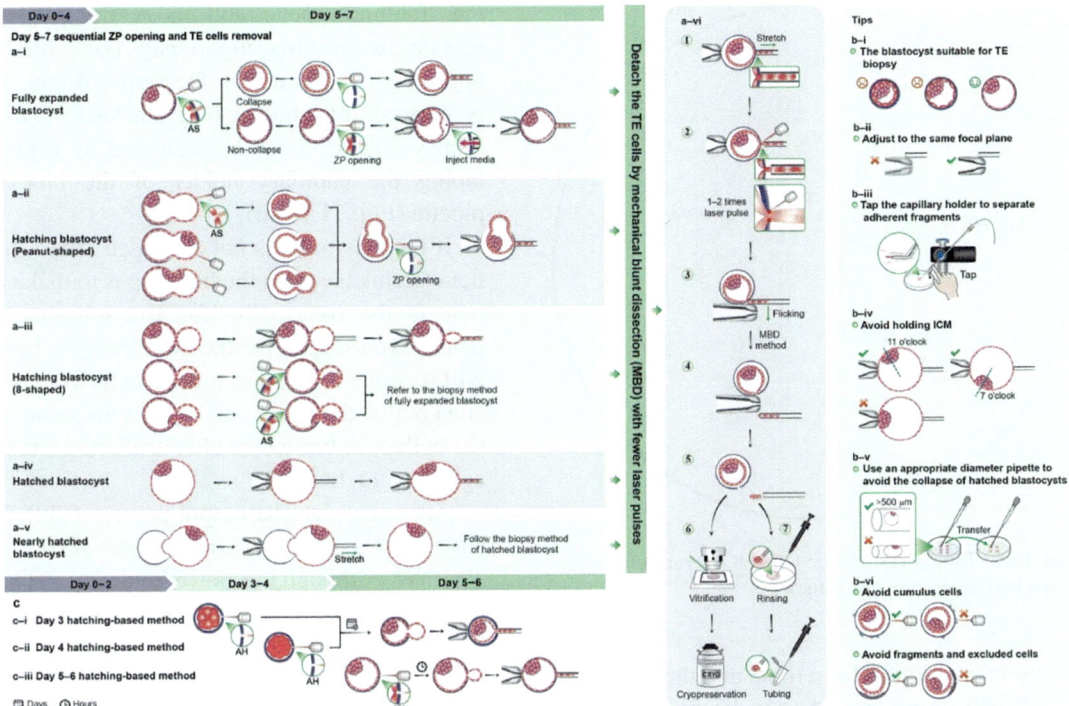

Fig. 11.1 Steps and tips for the trophectoderm biopsy. The techniques for trophectoderm (TE) biopsy are demonstrated for fully expanded blastocysts (a–i), peanut-shaped hatching blastocysts (a–ii), 8-shaped hatching blastocysts (a–iii), hatched blastocysts (a–iv), and nearly hatched blastocysts (a–v) utilizing the Day 5–7 sequential zona pellucida (ZP) opening and trophectoderm cell removal method. (a–vi) The steps of the mechanical blunt dissection (MBD) method and the transfer of biopsy specimens. (b–i) The blastocysts suitable for TE biopsy. (b–ii) During mechanical blunt dissection, the biopsy and holding pipette should

be adjusted to the same focal plane. (b–iii) Tap the capillary holder to separate adherent fragments. (b–iv) Both the biopsy pipette and the holding pipette should be kept away from the inner cell mass (ICM). (b–v) Transfer hatched blastocysts using a pipette of an appropriate diameter to prevent collapse. (b– vi) The biopsy procedure should avoid aspirating cumulus cells, excluded cells and fragments that remain under the ZP. The techniques for TE biopsy are demonstrated using the Day 3 (c–i), Day 4 (c–ii), and Day 5–6 (c–iii) hatching-based methods. AS, artificial shrinkage; AH, assisted hatching

position to perform biopsies. In addition, this method may result in an "8"-shaped hatched blastocyst. It is controversial whether the "8"-shaped hatching affects embryo implantation and increases the occurrence of monozygotic twin [25, 26].

11.2.3 Procedure of Trophectoderm Biopsy

At our center, trophectoderm biopsy is performed using the third method described above (Day 5–7 sequential ZP opening and TE-cell removal). Only blastocysts that have reached full expansion or beyond are subjected to biopsy, i.e., stage 4, 5, or 6 blastocysts (Fig. 11.1b-i). Here, we summarize a set of effective approaches to the trophecto-

derm biopsy for different characteristics of blastocysts by "mechanical blunt dissection (MBD)" (Fig. 11.1) [27].

1. Main equipment, consumables, and the preparation of biopsy dishes: (a) Equipment: laser (1.46 μm); inverted microscope equipped with a micro-manipulation system. (b) Consumables: biopsy pipettes with flat opening, 27 μm outer diameter (21 μm inner diameter) or 20 μm outer diameter (16 μm inner diameter); oocyte denudation pipettes with 140 μm inner diameter (for transferring biopsy specimens); biopsy dishes (same as ICSI dishes). (c) Preparation of biopsy dishes: HEPES microdroplets are prepared and numbered for trophectoderm biopsy manipulation (Fig. 11.2). Usually, a maximum of six blasto-

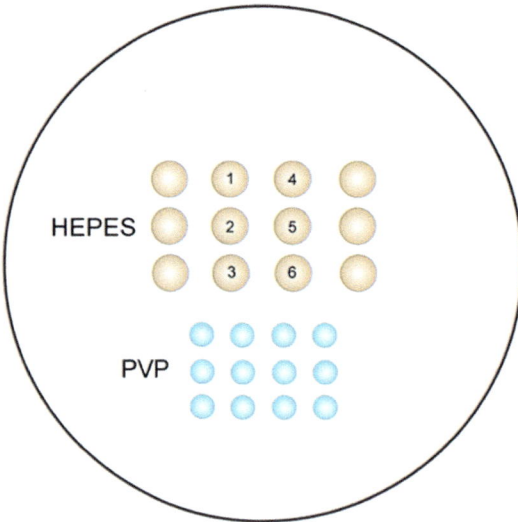

Fig. 11.2 Biopsy dish. Note: HEPES microdroplets (yellow); PVP microdroplets (blue)

cysts are biopsied at a time, and the rest of the HEPES microdroplets can be used to clean the pipette. The PVP microdroplets are used for wetting the manipulation pipette and rinsing the biopsy pipette. After each biopsy, the manipulation pipette should be fully cleaned in the PVP microdroplets

2. Biopsy of fully expended (stage-4) blastocysts: For fully expended blastocysts (Fig. 11.1a-i, vi), artificial shrinkage should first be performed using a 400–500 µs pulsed laser (approx. 5–7 µm aperture). Generally, the blastocyst will collapse after artificial shrinkage. The blastocyst is positioned by the holding pipette, and then a narrow channel in the zona pellucida is made using a 200–250 µs pulsed laser (approx. 3–5 µm aperture), away from the trophectoderm cells and ICM. Next, the biopsy pipette is carefully pressed against the opening. 5–10 cells are aspirated into the biopsy pipette by applying gentle suction. The biopsy pipette is moved away from the blastocyst to stretch the selected fragment and expose the junctions between cells. After two to three times of 200–250 µs pulsed laser, aiming at cell junctions or weak spots, the holding pipette is maneuvered to the rim of the biopsy pipette. Then, the biopsy and holding pipette are adjusted to the same focal plane under a microscope (Fig. 11.1b-ii). Fix

the holding pipette and move the biopsy pipette downwards vigorously (i.e., MBD approach). Subsequently, the biopsy fragment is released. If the biopsy fragment sticks to the biopsy pipette, it can be separated by gently taping the capillary holder of the biopsy pipette (Fig. 11.1b-iii).

If the blastocyst is not collapsed after artificial shrinkage, then the first step is to make a hole in the zona pellucida. The subsequent gentle expulsion of the medium from the hole will separate the trophectoderm cells from the zona pellucida. The next biopsy is the same as the collapsed blastocyst after artificial shrinkage (Fig. 11.1a-i, vi).

Attention: (a) The output power of different laser brands varies from 110 to 400 mW. Although this power intensity can be adjusted, it is typically set to 100% output. The size of the ZP ablation aperture produced by a single laser strike is modified by adjusting the pulse duration. The longer the pulse duration, the larger the aperture. As the maximum (100%) output power varies among different laser brands, the ZP ablation aperture size may be different even when using the same pulse duration. Therefore, the laser pulse duration should be adjusted based on the actual ablation aperture produced by the laser used in the laboratory. (b) For easier MBD, the angle should be set between the tip of manipulation pipettes (holding pipette and biopsy pipette) and the bench surface of 0°, i.e., they are parallel (details in Chap. 10). This is different from the ICSI pipette, which is usually set at a small angle to the horizontal surface for adequate sperm immobilization.

3. Biopsy of stage-5 blastocyst.

(a) "Peanut"-shaped hatching (Fig. 11.1a-ii, vi): Because of the large ZP opening in "peanut"-shaped hatching cases, there is a risk of drawing the blastocyst out of the opening completely, if the biopsy is performed from the herniated TE cells. It increases the difficulty of biopsy if the ICM cells are herniated, and tends to damage the ICM. Our approach can prevent the blastocyst from completely hatching out of the zona pellucida. First, the laser pulse is aimed at the herniation of the trophectoderm cells from the zona pellucida to make it collapse. Meanwhile, the cells remaining in ZP will be separated from ZP. Then, the holding pipette is positioned perpendicularly to the axis of the herniation of the trophectoderm. After reducing the trophectoderm herniation, the steps of the trophectoderm biopsy are the same as the fully expanded blastocyst.

(b) "8"-shaped hatching (Fig. 11.1a-iii, vi): This type of blastocyst biopsy is relatively simple. The embryo is secured by the holding pipette at the opposite side of the herniation of the trophectoderm cells, and an appropriate amount of TE cells needs to be directly aspirated and biopsied using a laser combined with MBD. Suppose the inner cell mass of the "8"-shaped blastocyst has hatched out. In that case, artificial shrinkage with a laser pulse, aiming at a trophectoderm cell junction located inside the ZP, should be performed first. Then, the blastocoel inside the ZP will collapse. The biopsy method afterward can be performed following the biopsy method of the fully expanded blastocyst.

4. Biopsy of stage-6 blastocyst: MBD works best for a fully hatched blastocyst (Fig. 11.1a-iv, vi). The embryo is secured by the holding pipette. The trophectoderm opposite to the inner cell mass is brought into the fine biopsy pipette, and the subsequent steps of the trophectoderm biopsy are the same as the fully expanded blastocyst. Notably, biopsy pipettes (outer diameter 20 μm) can effectively control the target number of trophectoderm cells, making the biopsy of fully hatched blastocysts easier. During the biopsy, both the biopsy pipette and the holding pipette should be away from the ICM (Fig. 11.1b-iv) to avoid damage to the ICM. In addition, since blastocysts are no longer protected by ZP, it is important to avoid excessive suction exerted by the holding pipette. Also, the aspiration of TE cells should be gentle and steady. In addition, a larger diameter (>500 μm) pipette should be used to transfer the embryo before biopsy to

avoid the blastocoel collapsed (Fig. 11.1b-v). Because the collapse of the blastocyst prior to biopsy can lead to poor recognition of ICM, and the thicker cell layer will increase the difficulty of MBD.

5. For nearly hatched blastocysts (Fig. 11.1av), i.e., when only a small portion of TE cells remain in the ZP, the blastocyst should be pulled out of the ZP, and the subsequent biopsy is referenced to that of a stage-6 blastocyst.

6. Transfer of biopsy specimens: (a) Biopsy specimens should be transferred to an IVF workstation with laminar airflow, and the operator should wear gloves. (b) The polymerase chain reaction (PCR) tube should be marked with the "medical record number, names of the couple, and embryo number," where the medical record number combined with the embryo number can ensure the identification of each embryo. Then, the prepared PCR tubes should be placed in a box with ice for later use. (c) Aspirate the tissue culture oil covering the biopsy dish (this step can be selected based on SOPs of the IVF laboratory) to reduce the oil residue in the transfer pipette, but take care to prevent the microdroplets containing biopsy specimens from being conjoined with each other. (d) Prepare four 20-μL HEPES microdroplets, used for rinsing biopsy specimens, on the lid of a 60 mm culture dish and conjoin the last three microdroplets (Fig. 11.3). (e) Use a 140 μm oocyte denudation pipette for biopsy specimen transfer, and the optimal volume of culture medium carried with the biopsy specimen should be determined according to the requirements of the amplification kit. First, aspirate a volume of the rinse medium, and then the biopsy specimen from the biopsy dish. A small amount of rinse medium can be expelled toward the biopsy specimen to flush it up before aspirating the biopsy specimen. This action facilitates an easier biopsy specimen aspiration in case the biopsy specimen adheres to the bottom of the culture dishes. (f) The aspirated biopsy specimen is first released into a separate rinse microdroplet. Then the residual medium and oil in the oocyte denudation pipette are evacuated. The biopsy specimen is

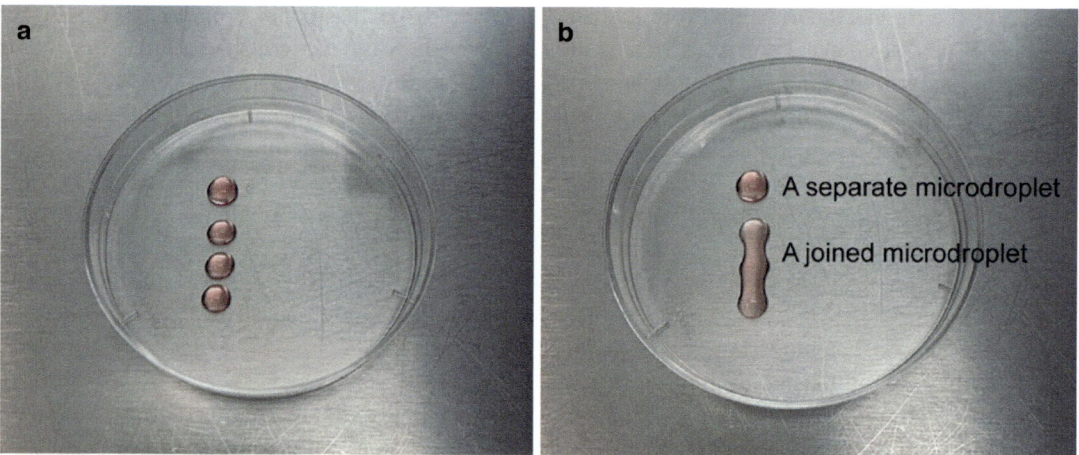

Fig. 11.3 The medium microdroplets used for rinsing biopsy specimen

re-aspirated, transferred into the above-described joined rinse microdroplets, and thoroughly rinsed from top to bottom. (g) Finally, the biopsy specimen is aspirated and placed to the tip of the oocyte denudation pipette, and transferred into the PCR tube while taking care not to touch the bottom of the tube. Each biopsy specimen should be transferred using a new oocyte denudation pipette. (h) After transferring all specimens, the PCR tubes are centrifuged for a few seconds, sealed, and stored in a − 20 °C refrigerator until testing.

7. Cryopreservation, thawing, and embryo transfer: The blastocysts should be vitrified within 30 min after the biopsy to avoid re-expansion. After thawing, stage-4 blastocysts should be subjected to assisted hatching before embryo transfer (the cryopreservation and thawing procedure is described in detail in Chap. 9).

11.3 Quality Management of Trophectoderm Biopsy

11.3.1 The Number of Biopsied Trophectoderm Cells

Zhang et al. found that the number of biopsied trophectoderm cells does not affect the survival rate of frozen-thawed blastocysts [28].

Meanwhile, the diagnostic efficiency improves with an increased number of biopsied cells. When more than six cells were obtained for biopsy, the incidence of diagnostic failure is <0.7%. However, for blastocysts with grade B or C TE cells, the implantation rate decreases as the number of biopsied cells increases. They, therefore, recommend that one to five cells be biopsied for such blastocysts. The study by Guzman et al. concluded that even for high-quality blastocysts, pregnancy outcome is impaired when more than six cells are retrieved for biopsy [29]. The ESHRE PGT Consortium and SIG-Embryology Biopsy Working Group in 2020 recommends that: it is appropriate to biopsy 5–10 TE cells for genetic testing (according to the stage of development and number of cells constituting the blastocyst) [30]. Fewer than five cells may impact on amplification profiles (noise) and mosaic detection levels [15]. The impact of removal of more than 10 TE cells on embryo development remains an area of further investigation.

11.3.2 Key Points for Biopsy Operation

1. Adequate and high-quality blastocysts are the prerequisite for blastocyst biopsy. Therefore, a separate incubator is recommended for

patients undergoing PGT, aiming to keep the culture environment stable.

2. Only one embryo can be placed in each microdroplet for biopsy. It is optimal to change the biopsy pipette for each blastocyst. Alternatively, thoroughly rinsing the biopsy pipette is acceptable. After each biopsy, the biopsy and holding pipettes should be fully rinsed in a clean PVP microdroplet. The oil inside the biopsy pipette can be pushed to the very tip and even slightly expelled (Fig. 11.4) to ensure no cellular residue remains in the pipette. The safety of repeatedly using a biopsy pipette should be verified in the laboratory to avoid cross-contamination. A new biopsy pipette should be used after a biopsy of

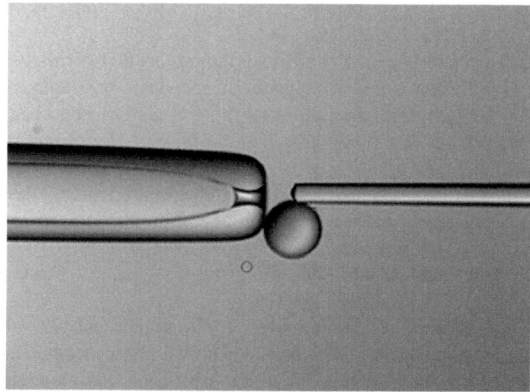

Fig. 11.4 Cleaning of the biopsy pipette

many blastocysts or many lysed cells in the biopsy pipette.

3. Aspiration of cumulus cells and excluded cells and fragments remaining under the ZP should be avoided during a biopsy (Fig. 11.1b-vi). Some studies have found that the remaining cells are usually abnormal and can lead to misdiagnosis or an increased chance of being diagnosed as mosaicism [31].

4. The integrity of biopsy cells should be preserved as best as possible. It is recommended to retain photographs of biopsy specimens so that in case of amplification failure or low-quality test results, it can be retrospectively observed whether this is due to a low-quality biopsy specimen (Fig. 11.5).

5. The process of transferring biopsy specimens and cryopreservation should be strictly double-checked.

6. The blastocysts should be frozen within 30 min after the biopsy to avoid re-expansion.

7. The benchmark value of successful biopsy rate should be ≥95% [32]. The mosaicism detection rate varies from center to center (2% to 40%). If the mosaicism detection rate is consistently high, clinical treatment, laboratory operations, and patient-related factors should be analyzed, and the underlying causes should be identified [15].

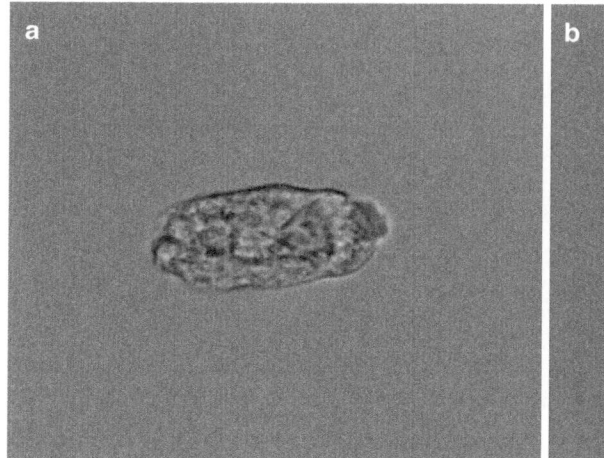
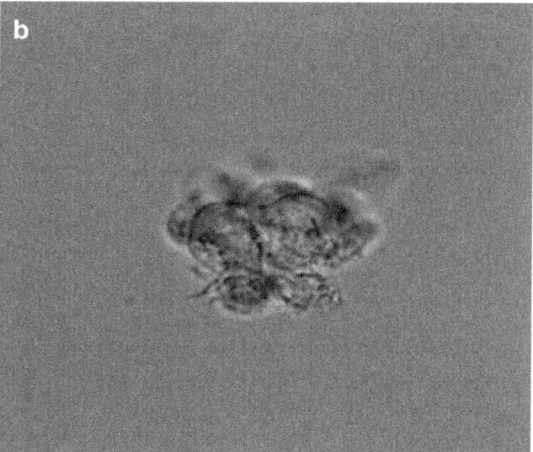

Fig. 11.5 (**a**) The intact cells from TE biopsy and (**b**) the lysed cells

References

1. Handyside AH, Kontogianni EH, Hardy K, et al. Pregnancies from biopsied human preimplantation embryos sexed by Y-specific DNA amplification. Nature. 1990;344(6268):768–70.
2. Zegers-Hochschild F, Adamson GD, Dyer S, et al. The international glossary on infertility and fertility care, 2017. Fertil Steril. 2017;108(3):393–406.
3. Xu J, Fang R, Chen L, et al. Noninvasive chromosome screening of human embryos by genome sequencing of embryo culture medium for in vitro fertilization. Proc Natl Acad Sci U S A. 2016;113(42):11907–12.
4. Jiao J, Shi B, Sagnelli M, et al. Minimally invasive preimplantation genetic testing using blastocyst culture medium. Hum Reprod. 2019;34(7):1369–79.
5. Leaver M, Wells D. Non-invasive preimplantation genetic testing (niPGT): the next revolution in reproductive genetics? Hum Reprod Update. 2020;26(1):16–42.
6. Harton GL, Magli MC, Lundin K, et al. ESHRE PGD Consortium/Embryology Special Interest Group—best practice guidelines for polar body and embryo biopsy for preimplantation genetic diagnosis/screening (PGD/PGS). Hum Reprod. 2011;26(1):41–6.
7. De Vos A, Staessen C, De Rycke M, et al. Impact of cleavage-stage embryo biopsy in view of PGD on human blastocyst implantation: a prospective cohort of single embryo transfers. Hum Reprod. 2009;24(12):2988–96.
8. Scott RT Jr, Upham KM, Forman EJ, et al. Cleavage-stage biopsy significantly impairs human embryonic implantation potential while blastocyst biopsy does not: a randomized and paired clinical trial. Fertil Steril. 2013;100(3):624–30.
9. Scott KL, Hong KH, Scott RT Jr. Selecting the optimal time to perform biopsy for preimplantation genetic testing. Fertil Steril. 2013;100(3):608–14.
10. Schoolcraft WB, Treff NR, Stevens JM, et al. Live birth outcome with trophectoderm biopsy, blastocyst vitrification and single-nucleotide polymorphism microarray-based comprehensive chromosome screening in infertile patients. Fertil Steril. 2011;96(3):638–40.
11. Gardner DK, Weissman A, Howles CM, et al. Textbook of assisted reproductive techniques. 4th ed. Boca Raton: CRC Press; 2012.
12. Glujovsky D, Farquhar C, Quinteiro Retamar AM, et al. Cleavage stage versus blastocyst stage embryo transfer in assisted reproductive technology. Cochrane Database Syst Rev. 2016;6:CD002118.
13. Wei D, Liu JY, Sun Y, et al. Frozen versus fresh single blastocyst transfer in ovulatory women: a multicentre, randomised controlled trial. Lancet. 2019;393(10178):1310–8.
14. Vera-Rodriguez M, Rubio C. Assessing the true incidence of mosaicism in preimplantation embryos. Fertil Steril. 2017;107(5):1107–12.
15. Cram DS, Leigh D, Handyside A, et al. PGDIS position statement on the transfer of mosaic embryos 2019. Reprod Biomed Online. 2019;39(Suppl 1):e1–4.
16. Popovic M, Dhaenens L, Boel A, et al. Chromosomal mosaicism in human blastocysts: the ultimate diagnostic dilemma. Hum Reprod Update. 2020;26(3):313–34.
17. Gleicher N, Albertini DF, Barad DH, et al. The 2019 PGDIS position statement on transfer of mosaic embryos within a context of new information on PGT-A. Reprod Biol Endocrinol. 2020;18(1):57.
18. Davidson LM, Liu Y, Griffiths T, et al. Laser technology in the ART laboratory: a narrative review. Reprod Biomed Online. 2019;38(5):725–39.
19. McArthur SJ, Leigh D, Marshall JT, et al. Pregnancies and live births after trophectoderm biopsy and preimplantation genetic testing of human blastocysts. Fertil Steril. 2005;84(6):1628–36.
20. Kokkali G, Traeger-Synodinos J, Vrettou C, et al. Blastocyst biopsy versus cleavage stage biopsy and blastocyst transfer for preimplantation genetic diagnosis of beta-thalassaemia: a pilot study. Hum Reprod. 2007;22(5):1443–9.
21. Capalbo A, Rienzi L, Cimadomo D, et al. Correlation between standard blastocyst morphology, euploidy and implantation: an observational study in two centers involving 956 screened blastocysts. Hum Reprod. 2014;29(6):1173–81.
22. Zhao H, Tao W, Li M, et al. Comparison of two protocols of blastocyst biopsy submitted to preimplantation genetic testing for aneuploidies: a randomized controlled trial. Arch Gynecol Obstet. 2019;299(5):1487–93.
23. Capalbo A, Romanelli V, Cimadomo D, et al. Implementing PGD/PGD-A in IVF clinics: considerations for the best laboratory approach and management. J Assist Reprod Genet. 2016;33(10):1279–86.
24. Maggiulli R, Giancani A, Cimadomo D, et al. Human blastocyst biopsy and vitrification. J Vis Exp. 2019;26(149):e59625.
25. Yan Z, Liang H, Deng L, et al. Eight-shaped hatching increases the risk of inner cell mass splitting in extended mouse embryo culture. PLoS One. 2015;10(12):e0145172.
26. Gu YF, Zhou QW, Zhang SP, et al. Inner cell mass incarceration in 8-shaped blastocysts does not increase monozygotic twinning in preimplantation genetic diagnosis and screening patients. PLoS One. 2018;13(1):e0190776.
27. Yang D, Feng D, Gao Y, et al. An effective method for trophectoderm biopsy using mechanical blunt dissection: a step-by-step demonstration. Fertil Steril. 2020;114(2):438–9.
28. Zhang S, Luo K, Cheng D, et al. The number of biopsied trophectoderm cells is likely to affect the implantation potential of blastocysts with poor trophectoderm quality. Fertil Steril. 2016;105(5):1222–7.
29. Guzman L, Nuñez D, López R, et al. The number of biopsied trophectoderm cells may affect pregnancy outcomes. J Assist Reprod Genet. 2019;36(1):145–51.

30. ESHRE PGT Consortium and SIG-Embryology Biopsy Working Group, Kokkali G, Coticchio G, et al. ESHRE PGT Consortium and SIG Embryology good practice recommendations for polar body and embryo biopsy for PGT. Hum Reprod Open. 2020;2020(3):hoaa020.

31. Lagalla C, Tarozzi N, Sciajno R, et al. Embryos with morphokinetic abnormalities may develop into euploid blastocysts. Reprod Biomed Online. 2017;34(2):137–46.

32. ESHRE Special Interest Group of Embryology and Alpha Scientists in Reproductive Medicine. The Vienna consensus: report of an expert meeting on the development of ART laboratory performance indicators. Reprod Biomed Online. 2017;35(5):494–510.

Embryo Transfer

12

The success of assisted reproductive technology depends on maximizing the efficiency of each step. Embryo transfer (ET) is considered the final and critical step in the laborious process of in vitro fertilization treatment. The embryo transfer aims to place embryos accurately in the uterine cavity without trauma to the endometrium to allow for healthy embryonic development. Any problems in this step will ruin the accumulated efforts of the laboratory and significantly reduce pregnancy rates. A smooth embryo transfer depends on many factors, such as the embryologist's experience, reagents, types and pieces of equipment, and the degree of difficulty encountered during uterine cavity entry. Nowadays, the most accepted and extended ET method for cleavage-stage embryos and blastocysts is to transfer the embryos to the uterine cavity through the cervical canal, i.e., transcervical ET. This chapter focuses on laboratory practices; only after standardizing an ET protocol will it be possible to maximize IVF success. While each laboratory has its ET regimen, herein, we provide a set of standard operating procedures and quality management schemes based on international consensus and evidence-based medicine.

12.1 Preparations for Embryo Transfer

12.1.1 Embryo Transfer Training for Embryologists

Embryo transfer is an operator-dependent technique. A proficient embryologist is crucial to a smooth embryo transfer. How long does it take a trainee to master this technique? Firstly, a trainee must master basic knowledge, standard operating procedures, and principles. A discarded biological material, for example, a developmentally arrested embryo, is suitable for catheter loading training. Secondly, 50–60 embryo transfers supervised by a senior embryologist constitute essential requirements for a trainee to achieve competency. A competent embryologist should be able to troubleshoot any problems, such as embryo retention, re-loading of embryos, and managing complex transfers. When a beginner starts clinical practice, much attention should be paid to his/her ET outcomes, such as embryo implantation and clinical pregnancy rates. An embryologist is authorized to perform ETs without supervision if the outcomes reach the average laboratory rates. The training process should be well documented.

12.1.2 Preparation of Reagents and Pieces of Equipment

12.1.2.1 Embryo Transfer Catheter

Various catheters are commercially available for human ET, and these generally fall into two categories: soft and stiff, according to the softness and hardness of the inner catheter [1]. Soft catheters are the first choice for today's embryo transfer. The routine use of transabdominal ultrasound scan guidance during ET enhances the functionality of a soft embryo transfer catheter, and there is sufficient evidence that using a soft embryo transfer catheter significantly improves pregnancy rates [1]. Soft catheters adapt more easily to the contour of the endometrial cavity, thus causing less trauma or endometrial disruption. However, soft catheters are disadvantaged by more difficult insertions and passages. In cases of technically challenging ETs, such as encountering cervical stenosis or acute cervical-uterine angles, a malleable stylet helps a soft catheter to negotiate the cervical canal. Transfer catheters available on the market have a variety of specifications and designs, including tip structure, flexibility, presence of a separate outer sheath, location of the distal port (end- or sideloading), degree of stiffness, thickness, length, diameter, and echogenic visibility.

12.1.2.2 Embryo Transfer Dish Preparation

Blastocyst media with 20% standard protein supplementation can be used for ET. Some assisted conception units select a culture medium corresponding to the embryo stage for ET. This medium is prepared by filling the central well with 0.5–1 mL of blastocyst media and 4 mL into the outer ring of the dish. The ET dishes are pre-equilibrated in an incubator at 37 °C overnight. The number of ETs scheduled for that day is checked, and 2–3 additional ET dishes are prepared as a precaution in case of unanticipated events.

12.1.2.3 Syringe Type

Using a disposable 1 mL syringe to connect with the transfer catheter for ET is appropriate. The resistance of a syringe can be assessed by pumping and depressing the plunger in advance, ensuring smooth embryo discharge. A suitable syringe selected for ET should have a moderate resistance when depressing the plunger.

12.1.2.4 Trial Embryo Transfer

A trial transfer could be done during the first appointment, before the cycle begins, at the time of oocyte retrieval, immediately before the actual ET procedure, or as part of the actual ET procedure (known as an afterload ET method). Usually, ET is performed without anesthesia. A trial embryo transfer is routinely performed to gain a better understanding of the patient's anatomy, including the length and direction of the cervical canal and endometrial cavity, as well as the degree of difficulty in entering the uterine cavity, thereby facilitating selecting a suitable transfer catheter and reducing the incidence of challenging transfers that could adversely impact clinical outcomes.

12.2 Procedures for Embryo Transfer

Direct single-step and afterload double-step ET methods are widely used in clinics. Regarding the direct single-step method, embryos are preloaded within the catheter while negotiating the cervical canal. In the afterload double-step method, while the guide catheter negotiates the cervical canal, embryos are being loaded within the transfer catheter, which is then introduced into the uterine cavity through a guide catheter. The direct method is more suitable for a straightforward transfer, especially in a patient with an axial uterus and a straight, short cervical canal. However, an afterload method is better at dealing with a complex uterine cavity and cervical canal. Setti found that an afterload method significantly reduced the difficult transfer rate, likely to impair pregnancy rates by causing uterine contractions capable of displacing the embryo or inducing unwanted endometrial damage [2]. Furthermore, the afterload method may reduce the time of embryo exposure to potentially unsafe conditions.

12.2.1 The Procedure for ET

Here, we provide an afterload double-step procedure for ET.

1. Warm the embryo catheter by placing it on the heated workbench.
2. Connect a 1 mL syringe to a sterile transfer catheter, always ensuring its sterility.
3. Once the patient is in the operating room, double-check the patient's identity and confirm the transfer embryo number and grade/quality with the patient.
4. Wait for the clinician to prepare access to the uterus.
5. Once the guide catheter has been placed in a satisfactory position, give the embryologist clear instructions authorizing embryo loading.
6. Move the culture dish containing the patient's embryos selected for ET from the incubator and double-check the identification on the dishes for ET. Transfer the patient's embryos to an ET dish containing ET media pre-equilibrated a day earlier.
7. Wash the warmed catheter with the culture medium in the ET dish's external ring.
8. Load the embryos into the catheter following the laboratory procedure, and then bring the embryos into the operating room.
9. Insert the transfer catheter into the guide catheter already placed in the cervix.
10. Push the transfer catheter into the uterus until the catheter tip is visualized in the upper or middle area of the uterine cavity, more than 1 cm from the fundus via ultrasound [1].
11. Press the syringe plunger to expel the embryos into the uterine cavity.
12. Maintain pressure on the plunger to avoid a "plunger effect," and slowly withdraw both inner and guide catheters simultaneously from the uterus.
13. After ET, double-check under the stereomicroscope that no embryos are retained in the catheter by flushing it with media in the transfer dish.
14. If no embryos are retained, give the clinician an "OK" signal; otherwise, request the practitioners to repeat the embryo transfer.
15. Clean the workbench.
16. Document the ET procedure on the embryology worksheet, including the patient's name, the number of embryos transferred, the embryos' grade/quality, the date and time of performing the ET, the embryologist and witness' names, and the number of attempts at entering the uterus. Also, record the use of a malleable stylet or tenaculum and whether blood or mucus remained in the catheter. Any difficulties in passing the guide catheter through the cervical canal into the uterine cavity should be documented.

12.2.2 Embryo Transfer Catheter Loading Techniques

Embryo loading refers to embryos aspirated from a culture medium into a transfer catheter by an embryologist. There are two widely used catheter loading techniques: air-fluid and fluid-only methods (Fig. 12.1). In the air-fluid method, after washing the catheter and ensuring that the catheter is filled with culture medium, 10 µL of air is aspirated, followed by 15–20 µL of the culture medium containing embryos, and another 10 µL of air at the catheter tip. In the fluid-only method,

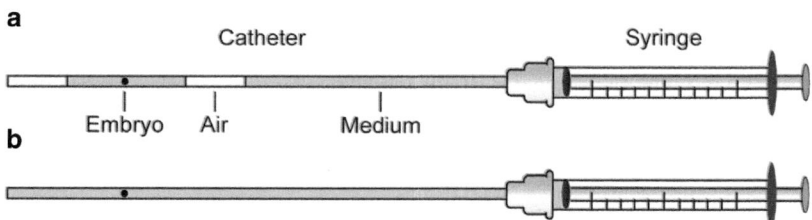

Fig. 12.1 Catheter loading techniques. (**a**) air-fluid; (**b**) fluid-only methods

after washing and filling the catheter with culture medium, the 20–25 μL medium containing embryos is aspirated without being bracketed by air columns.

There is insufficient evidence to suggest that one method is superior to the other based on existing evidence [3]. Advocates of the air-fluid method suggest that using air columns between the embryo-containing medium may help protect embryos from the cervical mucus and accidental discharge before reaching the ideal location for embryo placement within the uterine cavity. More importantly, the presence of air columns inside the transfer catheter is beneficial for ultrasound visualization during the ET, thereby precisely identifying the embryo catheter tip and allowing appropriate distancing from the uterine fundus. Conversely, advocates of the fluid-only method emphasize that air is not generally found in the uterus under physiologic conditions; even a tiny amount of air in the uterus is considered a non-physiological factor that may change the pH of the expelled medium, resulting in an adverse effect on embryo implantation.

12.3 Quality Management of Embryo Transfer

12.3.1 Should Embryos Be Loaded from a Center-Well Dish or Culture Microdroplets Under the Oil?

A center-well dish is commonly used dish for ET. Some specialists suggest drawing the embryos directly into the ET catheter from culture microdroplets under the oil, considering the benefits of growth factors secreted by embryos and remaining in the microdroplets. However, using microdroplets to load embryos does not increase cycle outcomes [4]. In addition, the oil, which theoretically could be detrimental to embryo implantation, remains on the catheter tip.

12.3.2 Should the Transfer Catheter Be Withdrawn Immediately or Delayed After ET?

Once the embryo is injected into the uterine cavity, the clinician can immediately withdraw the transfer catheter or delay withdrawal for a few seconds (30–60 s). No differences in terms of pregnancy rates were found between the two methods mentioned above [5, 6]. Sroga et al. reported that, in the patients who underwent ET with both methods in subsequent cycles, the delayed withdrawal method had a significantly higher pregnancy rate than the immediate withdrawal method [5]. The findings suggest that in patients who experience a failed ET with the immediate withdrawal method, the delayed method may improve pregnancy outcomes in the next ET cycle.

12.3.3 The Time Interval Between Loading and Discharging the Embryos

The longer the time interval between loading and discharging the embryos, the lower the pregnancy and implantation rates, especially for poor-quality embryos [7]. This phenomenon may be attributed to environmental stress, for instance, temperature reduction, osmotic pressure increase, and pH increase, which are caused by exposure to the medium outside the incubator. Thus, a recommended time interval is 60 s or less. Once the interval exceeds 120 s, the pregnancy rate decreases significantly [8].

12.3.4 The Volume of Transfer Media

A recommended volume of media injected into the uterine cavity with embryos during ET is 20 to 40 μL; a volume less than 10 μL may negatively affect implantation rates [9].

12.3.5 Does Hyaluronic Acid Improve Embryo Implantation?

Hyaluronic acid is a naturally occurring molecule added as a specific adherence compound to embryo transfer media. A meta-analysis suggests that adding functional (0.5 mg/mL) hyaluronic acid to the transfer medium probably increases the number of live births and slightly decreases the miscarriage rate [10].

12.3.6 Embryo Expulsion Speed

A slow embryo expulsion speed is recommended for ET, as a slow speed can reduce the driving force on the embryo, preventing injury to it [11].

12.3.7 Embryo Retention

After embryo transfer, checking for retained embryos within catheters is critical ET procedures. Once embryos are retained, an immediate re-transfer is required. The retained embryos should be transferred to a new ET dish, and a new catheter should be used to re-transfer the embryos. It is recommended that the clinician leave the outer sheath in place until the embryologist checks for retained embryos. If the outer sheath has been pulled out, return the retained embryos to the incubator while waiting for the guide catheter's transcervical passage.

Embryo retention incidence is higher in fresh transfer cycles than in frozen transfer cycles [12]. The mechanism of embryo retention is associated with mucus on or in transfer catheters in fresh transfer cycles [12]. This may be attributed to the increased secretion of cervical mucus caused by high estrogen levels in fresh cycles and highlights the importance of removing cervical mucus in fresh ET cycles [13]. Besides uterine smooth muscles' spontaneous and rhythmic contraction and relaxation waves, the transcervical passage of the transfer catheter or the application of a tenaculum may stimulate the uterine contractions. The pressure changes caused by uterine contractions can alter the flow and direction of the transfer fluid containing embryos. Under certain conditions, the transfer fluid can flow backward in the catheter, leading to embryo retention in catheters or expulsion of embryos toward the cervical canal. It is advised to gently transfer embryos with soft catheters to avoid excessive cervix stimulation and achieve maximal relaxation of the uterus. Other treatments to decrease the frequency of uterine contractions during ET include acupuncture [14], transcutaneous electrical acupoint stimulation [15], or an oxytocin inhibitor [16]. In addition, it is recommended to maintain pressure on the plunger of a syringe until the complete withdrawal of the catheter from the uterus to avoid the embryo's re-aspiration.

Whether embryo retention impairs pregnancy outcomes is inconclusive. Some studies report that retained embryos in the transfer catheter and immediate re-transfer do not affect pregnancy rates. However, a retrospective study found that retained embryos have lower implantation, clinical pregnancy, and live-birth rates and increase the risk of ectopic pregnancy [12].

12.3.8 Does Contamination of the Catheter with Mucus or Blood After Catheter Removal Affect ET Success?

Once it is withdrawn, mucus on the embryo transfer catheter does not impair clinical pregnancy or live-birth rates [1]. There is fair evidence that cleaning cervical mucus during embryo transfer improves clinical pregnancy and live-birth rates [1]. Cervical mucus should be gently removed before ET to avoid the potential risk of cervical mucus blocking the catheter's opening and causing embryo retention.

Many studies have analyzed the influence of different locations and amounts of blood contamination on pregnancy outcomes and yielded conflicting results. Some cohort studies demonstrated that the pregnancy rate is not affected by catheter contamination with blood [17, 18], while others demonstrated the opposite finding [19, 20].

Blood on the ET catheter may come from cervical or uterine bleeding. Traumatic catheter passage through the cervical canal or endometrial cavity may cause tissue damage and bleeding. The blood may circulate in the endometrial cavity and get deposited with the embryos, disrupting the embryo's implantation environment. An emphasis on atraumatic transfer techniques, specifically using soft catheters and gentle manipulation under ultrasound guidance during ET, should contribute to improved pregnancy outcomes.

References

1. Practice Committee of the American Society for Reproductive Medicine. Performing the embryo transfer: a guideline. Fertil Steril. 2017;107(4):882–96.
2. Levi Setti PE, Cirillo F, Morenghi E, et al. One step further: randomised single-centre trial comparing the direct and afterload techniques of embryo transfer. Hum Reprod. 2021;36(9):2484–92.
3. Christianson MS, Zhao Y, Shoham G, et al. Embryo catheter loading and embryo culture techniques: results of a worldwide web-based survey. J Assist Reprod Genet. 2014;31(8):1029–36.
4. Halvaei I, Khalili MA, Razi MH, et al. Impact of different embryo loading techniques on pregnancy rates in in vitro fertlization/embryo transfer cycles. J Hum Reprod Sci. 2013;6(1):65–9.
5. Sroga JM, Montville CP, Aubuchon M, et al. Effect of delayed versus immediate embryo transfer catheter removal on pregnancy outcomes during fresh cycles. Fertil Steril. 2010;93(6):2088–90.
6. Martínez F, Coroleu B, Parriego M, et al. Ultrasound-guided embryo transfer: immediate withdrawal of the catheter versus a 30 second wait. Hum Reprod. 2001;16(5):871–4.
7. Ciray HN, Tosun S, Hacifazlioglu O, et al. Prolonged duration of transfer does not affect outcome in cycles with good embryo quality. Fertil Steril. 2007;87(5):1218–21.
8. Matorras R, Mendoza R, Expósito A, et al. Influence of the time interval between embryo catheter loading and discharging on the success of IVF. Hum Reprod. 2004;19(9):2027–30.
9. Ebner T, Yaman C, Moser M, et al. The ineffective loading process of the embryo transfer catheter alters implantation and pregnancy rates. Fertil Steril. 2001;76(3):630–2.
10. Heymann D, Vidal L, Or Y, et al. Hyaluronic acid in embryo transfer media for assisted reproductive technologies. Cochrane Database Syst Rev. 2020;9(9):CD007421.
11. Ding D, Shi W, Shi Y. Numerical simulation of embryo transfer: how the viscosity of transferred medium affects the transport of embryos. Theor Biol Med Model. 2018;15(1):20.
12. Xu J, Yin MN, Chen ZH, et al. Embryo retention significantly decreases clinical pregnancy rate and live birth rate: a matched retrospective cohort study. Fertil Steril. 2020;114(4):787–91.
13. Franasiak JM. Finding a retained embryo after attempted embryo transfer: how does it impact outcomes? Fertil Steril. 2020;114(4):745.
14. Manheimer E, van der Windt D, Cheng K, et al. The effects of acupuncture on rates of clinical pregnancy among women undergoing in vitro fertilization: a systematic review and meta-analysis. Hum Reprod Update. 2013;19(6):696–713.
15. Zhang R, Feng XJ, Guan Q, et al. Increase of success rate for women undergoing embryo transfer by transcutaneous electrical acupoint stimulation: a prospective randomized placebo-controlled study. Fertil Steril. 2011;96(4):912–6.
16. Moraloglu O, Tonguc E, Var T, et al. Treatment with oxytocin antagonists before embryo transfer may increase implantation rates after IVF. Reprod Biomed Online. 2010;21(3):338–43.
17. Moragianni VA, Cohen JD, Smith SE, et al. Effect of macroscopic or microscopic blood and mucus on the success rates of embryo transfers. Fertil Steril. 2010;93(2):570–3.
18. Silberstein T, Weitzen S, Frankfurter D, et al. Cannulation of a resistant internal os with the malleable outer sheath of a coaxial soft embryo transfer catheter does not affect in vitro fertilization-embryo transfer outcome. Fertil Steril. 2004;82(5):1402–6.
19. Alvero R, Hearns-Stokes RM, Catherino WH, et al. The presence of blood in the transfer catheter negatively influences outcome at embryo transfer. Hum Reprod. 2003;18(9):1848–52.
20. Goudas VT, Hammitt DG, Damario MA, et al. Blood on the embryo transfer catheter is associated with decreased rates of embryo implantation and clinical pregnancy with the use of in vitro fertilization-embryo transfer. Fertil Steril. 1998;70(5):878–82.

GPSR Compliance

The European Union's (EU) General Product Safety Regulation (GPSR)
is a set of rules that requires consumer products to be safe and our
obligations to ensure this.

If you have any concerns about our products, you can contact us on
ProductSafety@springernature.com

In case Publisher is established outside the EU, the EU authorized
representative is:

Springer Nature Customer Service Center GmbH
Europaplatz 3
69115 Heidelberg, Germany

Batch number: 10091943

Printed by Printforce, the Netherlands